ALSO BY ROBERT COOKE

Improving on Nature

Earthfire

DR. FOLKMAN'S WAR

DR. FOLKMAN'S WAR

Angiogenesis and the

Struggle to Defeat Cancer

ROBERT COOKE

Random House New York

RANDOM HOUSE and colophon are registered trademarks
of Random House, Inc.

Library of Congress Cataloging-in-Publication Data
Cooke, Robert
Dr. Folkman's War: Angiogenesis and the struggle to defeat
cancer/Robert Cooke.
p.   cm.
ISBN 0-375-50244-0
1. Neovascularization inhibitors—Therapeutic use.   2. Cancer—
Chemotherapy.   3. Folkman, M. Judah.   4. Cancer—Research.
I. Title.

RC271.N46 C66   2000
616.99'4061—dc21   00-34165

Random House website address: www.atrandom.com
Printed in the United States of America on acid-free paper
24689753
First Edition

To my wife, Sue C. Cooke,

who loves greatly,

cares deeply, and

makes all things possible

Foreword

C . E v e r e t t K o o p , M . D . , S c . D .

IN AN INSPIRED MOVE by a smart university, Harvard appointed Judah Folkman surgeon-in-chief of the Boston Children's Hospital despite his lack of specific training in the surgery of children—an established specialty with its own rigorous board of certification. Harvard chose Dr. Folkman for his potential, not his past performance in pediatric surgery.

I have no idea whether Harvard knew they were appointing a rare bird in surgery—the surgeon scientist. Harvard sent Judah Folkman to me at the Children's Hospital of Philadelphia for an abbreviated training period in pediatric surgery. I'm told it is the first time Harvard sent a full professor anywhere for training. The six-month period we were together was unusually stimulating. Surgeons get in the habit of doing things a certain way because "it works," but Judah never let me do anything without a reason that I could defend.

He had powers of observation that were unusual, and I enjoyed being around him and trying to show him more.

Two anecdotes illustrate the depth of Judah's powers of observation. Remember that Judah Folkman was a well-trained surgeon but had no experience handling the very delicate tissues of young children. At the end of the first week that we worked together, I was about to bring down the undescended testicles of a small baby, a wonderful teaching opportunity: I would do one side, explaining every step I took, and then coach Judah as he did the other side. I finished my side in a little longer than the seventeen minutes that it usually took because I was explaining as much as I thought was necessary. About an hour and a quarter after Judah started his side he was in trouble: The hernial sac was in fragments, real skill was going to be needed to repair the situation, and Judah was unbelievably frustrated. Together, we made things right and closed his side, about one hour and forty-five minutes after he had started. I did the best I could to reassure him, telling him that in one fell swoop he had learned the difference between delicate pediatric tissues and the tougher ones of adults and that the experience, although somewhat humiliating, would stand him in good stead.

The next morning I met him in the hallway when he arrived early to make rounds. He rushed up to me, all smiles, and said, "Fingernails! Fingernails!" I said, "What do you mean?" He replied, "Fingernails! You have fingernails and I don't. Your technique is largely dependent upon your ability to use your left thumbnail to steady things against your left forefinger, while you dissect the delicate tissues attached to the parts of spermatic cord you have mobilized." He was absolutely right, but I had never realized how important my nondominant hand's thumbnail was to my surgical prowess. I'm told that when Judah got back to Boston's Children's Hospital, he made his residents grow a thumbnail on their nondominant hand.

Later, after Judah had gone back to Boston and was settled into his new job, he invited me to give a lecture at the Boston City Hospital. I chose to talk about my experiences with the difficult surgery on malignant tumors in children, and to illustrate it with some dramatic slides. One of the slides showed a child lying in the operating room with his abdomen stitched closed after a procedure. On his abdomen and chest was the blood clot I had removed from the renal vein, the vein that goes from the kidney into the vena cava, the major vessel of the abdomen carrying blood back to the heart. The blood clot in question had extended about an inch and a half down the renal vein, taken a sharp left turn up the vena cava through the chest and then a left U-shaped turn into the right atrium, the upper chamber of the heart. The clot was composed of blood and tumor tissue. The purpose of including it in my lecture was simply to show that you can remove even such a huge clot containing tumor through an incision in the vena cava, get the child off the table alive, and, indeed, see him recover completely.

The next slide I showed was a microscopic one taken through the tip of the clot in the chamber of the heart. I said, "This is just to show you that this was a metastasis in the making because here you see, in the tip of the thrombus, Wilms' tumor [a malignant tumor of the kidney that occurs in children]." I had the slide on the screen for perhaps ten seconds when Judah yelled, "Stop, stop!" He then showed the audience that right in the tip of the clot all that distance from the kidney was a tumor trying to survive, and right in the center you could see a capillary. This was, of course, Judah's mind, off on its own where no one else had been, observing the angiogenesis factor, the then-mysterious force that called that blood vessel into the tumor so far from its parent in the kidney.

It wasn't long after Judah began his career in Boston that he discovered the importance of blood vessels in pathological processes and began the research that led him to the angiogenesis factor, the factor that stimulates the growth of blood vessels in usual and unusual places. Some seminal research projects take a relatively short time—such as Crick's and Watson's discovery of the double helix, which took about two years. Other projects, like Perutz's work on hemoglobin, can take a quarter of a century. That kind of research takes the stamina and the commitment of a long-distance runner—the ability to stay the course and persevere. That is and was the modus operandi of Judah Folkman, as he persisted over the years, learning more and more about angiogenesis and its antagonists.

The outstanding quality of Judah's research is that it has such broad applicability. So far, his research has found applications in twenty-six diseases as varied as cancer, diabetic retinopathy, macular degeneration, psoriasis, arthritis, and endometriosis. Ordinarily, researchers working in any of these fields do not communicate with each other. They do dig parallel trenches, as it were, and like train tracks they go in the same direction but never meet. The angiogenesis and antiangiogenesis factors research has impact across disciplines. Specialized researchers did not know that they were dealing with the same molecule. Judah connected the parallel trenches, and the resultant cross-fertilization has led to discoveries that are important to oncologists, ophthalmologists, gynecologists, dermatologists, and many others.

Dr. Folkman's discoveries did not meet with instant approval and acclaim; there were many doubters over the years. In the 1970s, laboratory scientists didn't believe any of it. Angiogenesis was not something to be taken seriously: Tumors didn't call in blood vessels, period. In the 1980s, the critics began to believe in the theory of angiogenesis, but not that specific molecules were involved. Then textbooks began to include angiogenesis and it was considered to be a well-established phenomenon; the critics' objections were hushed for good in 1989. In the 1990s, the criticisms came chiefly from the clinical side, and the pharmaceutical companies didn't want anything to do with angiogenesis. In the end, of course, Judah Folkman's beautiful idea has triumphed over the doubters. A few still persist, but their time will come.

Acknowledgments

———

IT IS HARDLY POSSIBLE to thank Dr. Judah Folkman enough for sparing his time, insight, humor, and depth of knowledge to make the preparation of this book possible. As Dr. C. Everett Koop said during one interview, anyone who spends much time with Judah Folkman comes away changed—for the better. That is true.

Deep appreciation must also be expressed for the dedication and skill of writer/editor Richard Firstman, who signed on in mid-book to help me fashion a loosely organized project into a coherent story that I think readers will enjoy. He was masterly at asking the right questions, getting me to fill in blanks, and putting flesh on bare bones that were rattling badly. Rick Firstman's ability to see the big, overall picture while I was mired in technical detail was especially valuable. Thanks, too, for his patience and for his ability to beat my stumbling words into decent shape.

There are, of course, many others who deserve thanks, and Paula Folkman ranks high among them for her patience, good humor, and steadfastness. Also, thanks to Judah Folkman's willing staff at Children's Hospital in Boston, especially office experts Polly Breen, Wendy Foss, and Emy Chen, who field so many calls with unfailing grace and empathy. Most of the others who deserve thanks are mentioned in the text, but I must express appreciation for Rakesh Jain, Pat D'Amore, and Susan Connors and others who were involved in various parts of the angiogenesis research program.

In addition, thanks must be expressed for the time and effort given to me by David Cheresh at the Scripps Research Institute; his patient Barry Riccio and Barry's wife, Kathryn Anthony; former American Cancer Society employee Leo Allard; the ACS media representative Joanne Schellenbach; Dr. Gerald Soff at Northwestern University Medical School in Chicago; David

Anderson at the California Institute of Technology; Dr. Richard Klausner, director of the National Cancer Institute; Don Gibbons and his staff at the Harvard Medical School News Office; Bess Andrews at Children's Hospital in Boston; and my two dedicated transcribers, Linda Goetzfried and Jean Fessenden. Special thanks, too, must go to Faith Hamlin, my agent at Sanford J. Greenburger Associates in New York, whose ability to nurse an author through the creation process was invaluable.

Thanks also to the able team at Random House who were central to getting this book published. They include president and publisher Ann Godoff, Mary Bahr, Amy Edelman, Sunshine Lucas, Kate Niedzwiecki, Carol Schneider, Tom Perry, Sally Marvin, Tracy Howell, Tracy Pattison, Linda Pennell, Martha Schwartz, Andy Carpenter, Richard Elman, and Barbara Bachman. Special thanks to senior editor Scott Moyers, whose enthusiasm and editorial skills improved the book immeasurably.

Gratitude is also due to my employer, Newsday Inc., and my editors there for helping me finagle enough time and energy to pursue this project. Because of their flexibility and understanding, it was possible to make several dozen trips to Boston and back for crucial interviews and important events, sometimes on short notice.

Saying thank you is hardly enough, though, for the care and support I continue to receive from good friends in and around Sudbury, Massachusetts, whose deep friendship will always be cherished. These beautiful people include Ted and Jan Carvalho, Floyd and Marge Stiles, Ed and Nancy Ross, Bob and Alice Vannerson, and in Vermont, Bill and Barbara McBride. Such friends are irreplaceable.

Contents

———

Foreword by C. Everett Koop / ix

Acknowledgments / xiii

PART ONE / 1

PART TWO / 107

PART THREE / 219

Index / 351

PART ONE

Chapter One

———

IT WAS A TANTALIZING idea that Judah Folkman had nurtured for nearly four decades—he had hatched it, worked it, published it, defended it, romanced it. He had withstood the ridicule of his peers. He had fought battles of medical and scientific politics. And he had endured, seemingly obsessed, never straying from the ideas in his head, the conviction in his heart, and the truth he saw in his laboratory. That was where the real battles were waged, where Folkman had been trying for nearly forty years to read and understand Nature's book, page by page. Now the time had come to see what it all amounted to. The answers were starting to trickle in from medical wards around the country, and there was little more for Folkman to do than wait, and hope.

At the core was a simple notion that had gradually matured in Folkman's mind ever since that day in 1961 when he was noodling in a navy lab in Bethesda, Maryland, a twenty-eight-year-old draftee trying to make cells grow under artificial conditions. That was when he'd first noticed a strange thing about tumors: They wouldn't grow unless they first recruited their own blood vessels. Over time he convinced himself that there had to be some way to block the growth of those blood vessels. To starve the tumor to death—and save the patient.

So Folkman had been trying to conquer cancer for nearly four decades when, in the waning days of the twentieth century, the first patients began to be infused with the natural drugs that had come from his long campaign. The new compounds had worked marvelously in mice—"We've never lost a mouse yet," Folkman liked to say—and now they were being given the first crucial tests in men and women. Three clinical trials were under way to test one of the potent substances, endostatin, that had been discovered in Folkman's laboratory. And as many as two hundred biotechnology companies, some large and others tiny, were exploring the once-ridiculed field that Folkman had years before named "angiogenesis," meaning the growth of the blood vessels de novo needed to support tumor growth.

In Boston, where Folkman had lived, studied, and worked since leaving Ohio behind in 1953, the volunteers trooped to the Dana-Farber Cancer Institute for their daily infusions of the possible wonder drug. The infusion center was on the ground floor, equipped with a collection of beds, some of which were fashioned after chairs, designed for patients who could take their medicine sitting up. Each would take his or her place, and the dose would then be thawed. Endostatin was a precious commodity that couldn't be wasted—the first one-kilogram batch was said to be worth seven million dollars—so it was never thawed before the patient actually arrived, in case the patient didn't show up. But they always did. These were people facing terminal cancer, desperate for the cure and very relieved to find that this drug, unlike the standard chemotherapy they had received, did not make them awfully sick. Of course, they hoped the treatments would also be different in a much more important way: Chemotherapy had not worked. That's why they were here. The infusion process, during which the drug was given through an IV line, lasted twenty minutes. Then the patients would leave, returning the same time the next day, Saturdays and Sundays included.

Would the new treatment live up to its billing, actually erase tumors without dangerous side effects? Would patients who had been given little or no chance of survival emerge unscathed, as if touched by magic? No one could tell—but everyone was watching. Although the first phase of the trials was only meant to test for signs of toxicity, those involved could not resist the natural impulse to peek beyond the government-enforced protocols, hoping for signs, even the barest hint, of efficacy. The doctors running the trials, gagged by their institutions, refused to utter a public word. But the rumors were flying. The doctors talked sub rosa, and so did the nurses and interns who were close to the trials. Word got around the biomedical grapevine that at Dana-Farber and both of the other experiment centers conducting the trials in Texas and Wisconsin some patients' tumors had stopped growing. One man, it was said, had experienced remarkable progress. As one insider put it, the mystery man's cancer, both the primary tumor and its dangerous metastases, had been "galloping." But since he began getting endostatin—in only small doses during the toxicity phase of the trial—his tumors had shrunk by half. One patient was just one patient, but it was an encouraging start.

But that start had been an end in itself. To reach the point where real patients were showing real progress against aggressive end-stage tumors was an amazing achievement for Folkman. He and the legion of researchers who had come through his lab had marched down countless blind alleys, encountered formidable roadblocks, and endured almost unending ridicule from colleagues, especially those who claimed to be experts about cancer. Folkman was, after all, *just a surgeon*, a biomechanical plumber not likely to know much about tumors other than how to take them out. The scorn had once been so incessant and so intense that Folkman had almost left Harvard over it.

Naturally, Folkman preferred to remember the people who *did* appreciate him. There was Heidi Patriquin, a Canadian radiologist who was struggling with all her might against breast cancer. It was an aggressive tumor that the best treatments had one by one failed to stop. In 1996, she attended a lecture at which Folkman showed a slide listing drugs then known to have some antiangiogenic properties, and on that list was only one that might be available for patients. It was thalidomide, the infamous drug that had caused thousands of birth defects when it had been used decades earlier by pregnant women, especially in Europe. A member of the Folkman laboratory, Dr. Robert D'Amato, had figured out that thalidomide acts as a mild inhibitor of blood vessel growth. And here Folkman was saying it might help against cancer if combined with standard chemotherapeutic drugs. Patriquin wasn't worried about birth defects—she was then past sixty—and decided to try thalidomide. Maybe the drug would stabilize her cancer long enough for an agent like endostatin to reach the clinic. And it did. Patriquin once told Folkman that if she could live long enough to get into one of those trials, she would consider her life complete. As a patient who had gone through surgery, radiation treatments, and many rounds of chemotherapy, Patriquin felt she represented a bridge between the old world and the new one being opened up by angiogenesis research. When the trials of endostatin did start, Patriquin was on the waiting list.

When Folkman began pursuing his ideas about angiogenesis in the early 1960s, most of the body's biochemistry was still a deep and enduring enigma, a closed box with mysterious and poorly understood things going on inside. Among the least understood, perhaps, was the circulatory system. To reach his goal, Folkman had made a career of learning whatever he could about blood vessels. He liked to say that he hoped to someday put himself out of business. The only way to do that, he imagined, was to persist in his work, no matter the odds. It was a fine line, he knew, between being persistent and being stubborn. And the difference, in the end, was in results: "If your idea succeeds everybody says you're persistent. If it doesn't succeed, you're stubborn."

Folkman allowed himself the luxury of thinking that persistence seemed to have finally paid off. He was at last approaching the summit of his work, the culmination of an arduous expedition of the imagination, the intellect, and the heart. He had been building toward this time throughout his entire life. And sometimes, when asked about his personal history, his mind would drift back to a defining moment, a consequential event from decades past that he could recall from memory like a carefully filed monograph. It was an image of his father, the rabbi, a man who had high hopes for his eldest child. Folkman could still see him leaning down in the sanctuary of the synagogue in Bexley, Ohio, on the morning of his confirmation, the whispered words still ringing in his ears. There was no way the young boy could predict how his own life would play out, but he was ready to live up to this, his father's private admonition: "Be a credit to your people."

Chapter Two

———

THINK. IN THE CHILDHOOD home of Moses Judah Folkman it was more than an admonition, it was a moral imperative. Each night, at Jerome and Bessie Folkman's dinner table, the moment would come when Rabbi Jerome Folkman would ask his wife and children: "Well, what did everyone learn today?" Inevitably, before Judah or his younger brother, David, or the youngest sibling, Joy, could finish offering up whichever piece of newfound knowledge they'd brought with them to the table, their father would launch into his own experiences—the day's visits, the questions he had heard and the answers he had given, the problems that had come up and his solutions. Sometimes, he would ask his eldest child what *he* might have said or done were he the rabbi, in a not-so-subtle attempt to plant a seed. One night when Judah was five, his father told of a visit that day from a couple grieving the loss of their newborn child. Why would God do this to us? they were desperate to know. "Judah," the rabbi asked, "what should I have said?" The answer is long lost in time, but the father's question never faded from the boy's memory. *Think.*

Jerome Folkman had descended from an extended clan of rabbis, a family line that originated in central Europe and sent a branch to the United States from a region near the Hungarian-Austrian border in the late 1800s. His father, Benjamin—Judah's grandfather—had grown up in Cleveland, the eleventh of twelve children, and had interrupted the rabbinical succession in pursuit of secular American aspirations. Simple bad luck changed the course of these ambitions: He and a brother both wanted to be doctors, but the family had only enough money to send one of them to school. The other would have to stay home and support their widowed mother. They flipped a coin; Benjamin lost and went into the ladies' coat and suit business. Not one to curse his lot, he pursued his trade energetically, so energetically that he became wildly rich, rich enough to afford a mansion with both upstairs and downstairs ballrooms. But the splendor was not to last. Judah's grandfather invested heavily in silk just as rayon came on the market and he felt he had to unload what was suddenly thought to be an all-but-obsolete material, selling his business for a ruinously low amount. He moved on to real estate and did well in that business, too, eventually owning several apartment buildings in Cleveland. Though he had only a high school education, Benjamin read extensively—he had a fine command of Latin and could quote from Cicero— and was regarded by his son, Jerome, as quite learned. Jerome chose to embrace that side of his father's talents when it came time for him to decide on his own life's work, eschewing business for the rabbinate.

Bessie Schomer's family arrived in the United States from Germany and settled in Cincinnati, where she met Jerome Folkman while he was a rabbinical student at Hebrew Union College. Bessie had attended the Shuster-Martin School of Drama and was acting in local theater productions when she and Jerome became engaged. Bessie had no formal academic degree but was thoroughly educated by attending classes with her husband-to-be, who was busy cramming six or seven years of school into four—taking undergraduate classes in the morning and pursuing rabbbinical studies later in the day. Bessie was tall and sweet-natured, not quite so eccentric or gregarious as Jerome. The young rabbi was tall and on the heavy side, and he had taken to wearing pince-nez glasses because he thought they made him look more mature as a rabbi.

Soon after Jerome and Bessie married in 1930, the young rabbi went looking for his first job. He wanted his own congregation instead of being an older rabbi's associate, so he applied for an opening at a small synagogue in Jackson, Michigan. Folkman and two other candidates were invited to Jackson to address the congregants, as a kind of command performance. Folkman composed a thoughtful and carefully researched speech that explored the tiny congregation's history. He spent a day honing it, repeating it over and over in his hotel room. The next day, scheduled as the second speaker, he arrived at the synagogue, ready to perform.

The first candidate strode to the front of the room and launched into his sermon, and Rabbi Folkman couldn't believe his ears: It was his own sermon, nearly word for word. His competitor had apparently overheard the speech through the hotel's thin walls. Folkman had to think quickly. He didn't have another speech and didn't have time to dream up something new. So when his turn came, he got up, faced the audience, and said: "In fifteen minutes you can't really judge any of the qualities of a rabbi. So I'll show you only one: that I have a really good memory. I will now give the exact same sermon my counterpart gave." It was a story that would be handed down from father to son like a moral heirloom, a lesson in mental agility and nerve—especially nerve. To be successful, one had to surmount all manner of unanticipated obstacles. And sometimes, one had to be fearless. Rabbi Folkman got the job.

The Folkmans' first child, Moses Judah, was born in Cleveland on February 24, 1933, shortly before they moved from Jackson to Grand Rapids, where Rabbi Folkman was hired to lead a larger congregation. With Fourth of July parades down back alleys and a healthy furniture industry (which eventually moved to Chicago), Grand Rapids was the kind of prosperous and close-knit midwestern town that might have inspired a *Saturday Evening Post* cover by Norman Rockwell—or a satirical story by Sinclair Lewis. Its Jewish population was a small percentage of the city's population of 200,000, but it was concentrated: Rabbi Folkman's new congregation consisted of some two hundred families.

The intellectual challenges posed by their parents became central to the Folkman children's lives from their earliest years. If their answer to "What did you learn today?" was "Nothing," the rabbi or his wife might respond, "The whole day? Do you think we should pay our taxes for that?" They were sure the children were blessed with intelligence and that to squander the gift was very nearly a sin—as was the failure to share their knowledge. "You have your intelligence by genetic accident," was their drumbeat, "so you should help people who aren't so fortunate." This admixture of confidence, altruism, intellectual curiosity, and a measure of mettle helped put Judah on his path.

From the beginning, encouraged by his mother, that path involved science. A bedtime story from Mom meant a children's biography of Newton, or a book called *The Microbe Hunters*, about Louis Pasteur. One of the first books Judah read himself was a biography of Madame Marie Curie.

Raising their children during the Depression, the Folkmans were always on the lookout for inexpensive educational opportunities. They took the children on tours of factories owned by members of the congregation. If they went to the doctor's office for vaccinations, they asked if he would let the children look through the microscope—and would he mind explaining what they were seeing? They took the children for walks in the woods and fields, or to visit museums, always discussing, always pushing. If the children asked questions, the Folkmans would urge them to explore further—an implicit life lesson that the world was theirs to explore. Among the three Judah needed the least encouragement. One of David's abiding memories of his brother as a child is of Judah on his hands and knees in the yard examining something in the grass with one of his most useful possessions, a magnifying glass.

In Grand Rapids, Judah had a chance to develop a sort of fearlessness different from the kind his father had summoned to get his first job. As a skinny, brainy, and somewhat awkward-looking Jewish kid, Judah presented a tempting target for anti-Semitic bullies. He was beaten up regularly while at Ottawa Hills Junior High School. Finally, he asked his father what he should do about it. Should he complain to the principal? Rabbi Folkman thought for a moment. "No," he said. "This won't end until you knock one of them down. These boys only respect strength." So the rabbi hired a special tutor: a member of the congregation who was a professional boxer. Next time out, Judah flattened one of his tormenters, and that was that. He'd learned the power of a little skill and a lot of nerve.

Rabbi Folkman wanted to impart something even more consequential to his children. Naturally, he wanted them to fully embrace Judaism—its meanings, duties, and traditions. But being tied so closely to the temple also meant that the rabbi's children were expected to act like *the rabbi's children.* They certainly had to be seen attending services each week, and they always had to behave properly, under the gaze of more than a few watchful members of the congregation. They were on public display, and so they had to get used to the idea of living up to the whole set of moral expectations inherent in Judaism. Their father reminded them that their ancestors were watching. *Don't ever do anything that would shame your ancestors.* If the children chafed under that yoke, the rabbi's stock answer was that it was just something that came with the turf. But he didn't limit his expectations of piety to his own children. One spring, almost all of the rabbi's confirmation class rebelled: They decided to skip class in favor of an important baseball game. Hearing about the plan, Rabbi Folkman sat down at his typewriter and wrote a personal note to each student's parents, warning that anyone who missed the class would fail to be confirmed. He sent the letters special delivery. Not a single student skipped.

From his earliest years, Judah was an admirer of his father's sermons, fifteen-minute homilies that would number more than two thousand in Jerome's career. In the rabbi's thoughts Judah found both answers and also questions he might never have thought of asking. His father was known within the community as a liberal rabbi, open to new ideas and eager to discuss them—with his congregants, his friends, his students, his children, his children's friends—and to see how they meshed with conventional wisdom. He taught his children there were no real intellectual boundaries—so why be restrained by borders that didn't exist? "Maybe that's why Judah has this ability to think outside the box," a childhood friend, Richard Wolfe, observed many years later. Such enlightened thinking arose from the rabbi's own experiences dealing with deep, soul-wrenching problems presented by members of his congregation. He was always on the front line, trying to help people cope with death, illnesses, the conflicts of raising children, and the stresses of living as American Jews. His views were constantly honed by his weekly struggles to come up with sermons that were honest and thought-provoking. He was in the spotlight every week and had to live up to the responsibility.

One Saturday when Judah was nine, the rabbi spoke about the German campaign to erase the Jews from Europe, raising an interesting question about the meaning of Albert Einstein's arrival in America as a refugee. "I would sit there and listen to the delivery," Judah Folkman remembers. "He kept asking the philosophical questions that were on the minds of the whole community. One was about the pogroms. If you've got a good God, He shouldn't allow that. My father said, 'Maybe He has a plan to move us all around in order to balance power.' It was a weird idea, but clearly, if Einstein comes here, atomic energy is developed here, not there." If nothing else, such talk drove home to the young Judah Folkman, if only on an intuitive level, the inseparable relationship between science and society.

Rabbi Folkman had other notions about educating his children, beyond books and school, beyond dinner-table discussions and Saturday-morning sermons. He wanted them to experience real life. So when he thought they were ready, usually around age seven, he began giving them what he considered a special privilege: accompanying him on his Saturday hospital visits. It was set up as a reward: If he or she had been well behaved, each child got a chance to go. When Saturday came, father and child would drive over to the hospital, then go from room to room, seeing one sick person after another. "This is my son," the rabbi would tell the patient and his family. "He will sit over there and be quiet." Then the rabbi would comfort and console the patient, and pray, sometimes through the barrier of an oxygen tent. During these visits, Judah always listened carefully to what his father said to the sick and registered the compassion with which he said it. The impression was indelible.

The rabbi had a particular reason for taking his eldest child along on his rounds, of course. Because he assumed that as the first-born son, Judah would also become a rabbi, this early exposure to his father's work was to be part of his education. But as time passed, the hospital visits had an unexpected effect on Judah. He knew his father's expectations, but when he was ten, after three years of silently following his father around the hospital in Grand Rapids, he quietly decided he didn't want to become a rabbi. Rabbis don't open the oxygen tent, he realized; doctors do. Rabbis offered kindness and consolation, but could they really help the patient get better? It was doctors who actually came in and laid hands on these people. And so it was that Judah Folkman decided what he wanted to do with his life.

Judah wanted to tell his father what he'd decided, but as excited as he was, as sure as he was of his decision, he was worried about his father's reaction. He expected an explosion, or at least a long lecture. What he got taught him something new about his father. "No?" the rabbi said when Judah told him he didn't want to follow in his footsteps. "In that case, you can be a rabbi-like doctor."

Rabbi Folkman's calm understanding came as a surprise to Judah, and over time he came to realize the wisdom in his words. He was telling his son, in so many words, to make the most of his choice, to devote himself to the task of making his ancestors proud. Another such moment came on the day of Judah's confirmation. Rabbi Folkman always prepared a private blessing for each of his bar mitzvah and confirmation students, to be whispered in their ears as he congratulated each of them. Judah was one of the last in a line of fifteen students, and as his father came closer, he wondered what his blessing would be. When he got to his son, the rabbi offered the simple exhortation "Be a credit to your people." A cliché, perhaps, but somehow it would ring in his ears and in his head for the balance of his life.

Rabbi Folkman's encouragement of his career choice fostered Judah's growing enchantment with all things medical and scientific. In those years many children—usually boys—received microscope sets, Erector sets, or crystal radio sets as holiday gifts, meant to open doors that might lead to useful occupations. Childhood was not nearly as programmed as it was to become, and electronic entertainment consisted of after-school adventure programs on the radio—*Captain Midnight, Sky King,* and *Tom Mix*—sponsored by cereal companies that kept the post office busy with exchanges of box tops and a few coins for magic decoders and "atom bomb rings." But it was the basement chemistry set that was the icon of boyhood—the Nintendo of its time. It was an incubator of scientific curiosity whose time would pass as the world changed.

By the time he was a teenager, Judah was already an old hand in the laboratory. His lab started with a standard Gilbert set but gradually evolved into a sophisticated arrangement of beakers and test tubes and Bunsen burners. A scientist who was a member of the congregation in Grand Rapids showed Judah and David around his lab. Judah asked about supplies, and the man told the boys where they could get their own. "So here were two kids who could barely get their noses over the counter going in to buy chemicals like sulfur," David recalls. Before long—and for years to follow—strange packages of chemicals and odd devices often arrived at the front door. Judah didn't quite blow up the basement laboratory, but there were always bangs and thumps plus bad smells wafting upstairs.

Judah's basement experiments proved one thing very early: He was nothing if not persistent. It didn't take much to get him interested in an experiment. And once he was engaged, it took a lot to pry him loose. He once persuaded a member of the congregation whose company worked with crude oil to give him some samples. Judah had heard that if crude oil could be distilled down to paraffin without solidifying, it could make a valuable lubricant. The catch was that it was extremely hard to prevent paraffin from solidifying. Judah tried it over and over but kept failing. "It's not working," his sister, Joy, told him finally, after he'd spent months trying. She thought he should give up. Judah kept at it, and kept at it, and still failed. It wasn't just that he wanted the experiment to succeed. He wanted to understand why he was failing. He wanted to know how things worked.

He also wanted the right equipment. When Judah was preparing for his bar mitzvah, his grandpa Benjamin, the real estate man, decided to give him a special gift. Not a fountain pen, not money—a jeep. World War II had just ended, and the military was selling surplus equipment to civilians. In Michigan, a fourteen-year-old could then get a learner's permit. Judah's younger brother and sister thought a surplus jeep was just about the greatest gift imaginable. "Joy and I thought it would be totally cool if Judah would drive us to school and we could climb out of that jeep," recalls David. "But Judah said he would much prefer to have a thousand-power microscope, with three objectives." Grandpa Benjamin was happy to drop the jeep idea and presented Judah with a Spencer microscope. The younger children watched in consternation as Judah happily carried his gift down to his home laboratory. "Joy and I wondered if there was something wrong with our brother," David says.

Judah became an unusually focused young man. His mind was now set on doing everything he could to reach medical school. But he did have other interests: He took up the trumpet, eventually putting together a little combo that David joined when the regular clarinet player was out. He became quite a good dancer. And his father, the rabbi, taught him how to fence. Jerome Folkman had taken up the sport while in college; he kept a couple of épées in the house and taught his elder son. "Parry! Parry! Thrust!" his brother, David, remembers Judah saying. But these were just diversions from Judah's passion for learning. One winter, the custodial staff of the junior high school went out on strike, forcing the school to close because there was no one to shovel coal and keep the heat going. Judah couldn't imagine closing school, and he volunteered to shovel the coal and stoke the fire. He got his friends to help out, and they were able to keep the school open. In summer, Judah headed over to a nearby medical clinic and volunteered his services in the electrocardiography department, helping technicians paste together patient records. Anything to get closer to becoming a doctor.

IN 1947, JUST BEFORE JUDAH was to begin high school, the Folkmans moved south to Ohio, the rabbi having been hired to head a large synagogue that served the affluent Jewish community in the section of Columbus known as Bexley. Jerome Folkman quickly became a popular rabbi at Temple Israel, and the family's house on Maryland Avenue was frequently full of visitors— members of the congregation, the mayor of Columbus and other prominent citizens, and, once a year, dozens of couples the rabbi had married. These annual reunions grew out of the role he had carved for himself. Soon after the move to Columbus, he returned to school, enrolling in a doctorate program in sociology at Ohio State University. He was developing a specialty in family counseling, work that he loved and that would eventually lead to an appointment to the Ohio State faculty. Teaching courses on marriage and family, he was on the way to becoming nationally prominent in the field. (His first book, published in 1955, was *The Cup of Life,* a kind of handbook for newlyweds.) He frequently delivered talks to audiences beyond the congregation, observing that the signs of social change were coming fast in America in these days after the war. He was starting to see more families destroyed by divorce, and he used his pulpit to warn that an early sign of a failing civilization is the destruction of families.

The rabbi's own family was going strong. His children remember a home with lots of repartee, jokes around the dinner table, parents who loved having their kids aim affectionate jibes at them and who quickly returned the favor.

As the children got older, their parents began holding what came to be known as the family culture hour. Each Saturday afternoon just before the Sabbath ended, one member of the family would have the chance to talk about a topic he or she was studying or was merely interested in, a tradition that would last for decades, long after the children were grown and had families of their own.

By the time Judah began attending Bexley High School, his interest in science had gone well beyond reading textbooks and tinkering with chemistry. In school, Judah became well known for practicing dissecting small animals in his basement. Then, as part of a class experiment, he used an electric motor to pump blood through the hearts of rats and kept the experiment going at home. For his entry in a school-sponsored science contest, he wanted to see how long he could keep a rat's heart going using cow's blood obtained from a slaughterhouse. In the basement he and a friend, Sandy Hepps (who would go on to become a surgeon himself), set up an apparatus powered by the small electric motor and a bicycle pump. He used Joy's toy oven as an incubator and attached tubes to carry blood and saline solution around in the system. And it worked: The boys were able to keep the heart going for days. Judah stayed up through the night and even cut some classes to keep it going. Then one day his mother and sister were upstairs when lightning struck, causing a power surge. A few minutes later, to their horror, Judah emerged from the basement drenched in cow's blood. "Mom almost fainted," Joy recalls, though it should also be said that Mom did nothing to discourage Judah's experiments. She even allowed him to store excess blood in the refrigerator. The Ohio Academy of Sciences applauded the effort, giving the teenagers a prize in the annual competition.

"He was much more mature than the rest of us," remembers class president Bill Creager, who went on to the U.S. Naval Academy. "We were screwing around, wasting time. I was interested in cigarettes, beer, and girls. He was totally focused." Remembers another of his friends, Jack Jeffrey: "I was somewhat in awe of Judah."

Judah may have been a science nerd, but his friends and classmates recognized something deeper: a certain humanitarianism not commonly found in a teenager. Judah was a dedicated Boy Scout, and in the summer of 1947 he attended the first world Boy Scout Jamboree, in France. The trip abroad was a telling experience. His siblings recall hurrying to the rail station in Columbus to greet Judah on his return, but they hardly recognized him when he stepped off the train. He had shed sixteen pounds during his overseas adventure. As Judah told it, the Scouts had set up their camps in areas still ravaged after the war, where they were constantly visited by desperately hungry children. Judah just couldn't eat with all those hungry children watching and wound up giving them most of his food. His scientific ingenuity was also a help. "The army had given us some hamburger, which was awful," he remembers. "They had also given us Coca–Cola, tons and tons of it. So we experimented by mixing Coke into the raw hamburger. When it was cooked, the heat caramelized the Coke, and it tasted terrific."

Back home in high school that fall, Judah was anxious to find an activity outside school that would get him closer to medicine, as he had when he worked in the medical clinic in Grand Rapids. He went down to the Ohio State University Hospital, the big teaching institution in Columbus, and volunteered to work as an orderly. Despite his youth, he felt at ease on the wards, having spent years trailing his father on his Saturday rounds. The job wasn't overly demanding. As an orderly, Judah would help patients get to and from their rooms, wheel gurneys through the hallways, and run errands for doctors and nurses. It gave him his first real look at life inside a hospital—the pain and fear of patients and their families, the joy of recovery—and his first exposure to the workaday world of a physician.

While wheeling a patient into an operating room one day, Judah was stopped by Dr. Robert Zollinger, a highly accomplished surgeon and teacher who ran a surgical training and research laboratory in a small building next to the Ohio State veterinary school. Zollinger was keen to spot young, talented students and bring them into the fold. He believed the best way to develop fine surgeons was to identify them early and get them into training right away, giving them years to practice and perfect their techniques. Zollinger argued that age twenty-five was far too late to pick up the knife.

"Why are you working in a hospital?" Zollinger asked Judah. The fifteen-year-old said he wanted to be a doctor. How about a surgeon? Zollinger asked. He had noticed the hardworking teenager's enthusiasm and self-assured manner.

Judah said he didn't know about surgery. He was thinking ahead but not *that* far ahead. Zollinger told Judah he should stop wasting his time as a lowly aide and do some real work in his canine lab. He could start learning what it was like to be a surgeon right next to the residents. Judah grabbed the opportunity and began spending afternoons and some weekends in the lab. Although the work in Zollinger's lab wasn't difficult at first, it was very different from what he'd been doing at the hospital. And he felt special to be singled out by Zollinger.

Zollinger was a heavyset, balding man who tended to look over the tops of his glasses and bark out instructions that were often accompanied by sardonic asides. "My residents do too much breeding and not enough reading," he'd say of those who seemed a little too preoccupied with their social lives. He was a gruff, demanding taskmaster who thought nothing of humiliating residents who didn't measure up. If one of them made a mistake during surgery, Zollinger would order him to move away from the operating table and stand in the corner of the room. Many residents lived in fear of their teacher, but they could not deny his stature. Zollinger was president of the American College of Surgeons, and he'd even had a medical disorder named after him: Zollinger-Ellison syndrome, a rare kind of ulcer caused by acid produced by pancreatic tumors.

Zollinger liked young Judah and treated him with a kindness that would have seemed foreign to the residents. Recognizing the boy's promise, Zollinger assumed the role of mentor, and the residents took their cue from him. They let Judah pass them surgical instruments during training operations on dogs and pointed out at each step what they were doing—and what they were avoiding. Eventually they showed him how to tie surgical knots, and Judah responded enthusiastically. He was so determined to master the skill that he took up stitchery, working to improve the dexterity of both hands. His mother gave him towels to practice on: He would put two towels side by side and stitch them together with a thread, as if closing an incision. Judah practiced nearly every night and eventually became ambidextrous, able to do sixty or eighty knots a minute. There was hardly a towel without knots in the Folkman house.

In 1950, as he neared the end of high school, Judah had some important decisions to make. He wanted to get a good start on his medical career by applying to an Ivy League school for his undergraduate studies. He was convinced that a bachelor's degree from Harvard or Yale, or maybe Princeton, would make it a lot easier to get into a good medical school, preferably Harvard. But Dr. Zollinger had another view. He wanted Judah to go to Ohio State and keep working with him in his lab. Judah wasn't sure about the idea. Ohio State couldn't compete with the eastern schools for prestige, and he was convinced the best medical schools wouldn't look twice at someone with an ordinary academic pedigree. He'd been told—and it was true—that no graduate of Ohio State had ever gotten into Harvard Medical School.

But Zollinger countered with a promise: If his young protégé went to Ohio State and continued working in the surgical training lab, he could arrive at medical school, whether Harvard or some other place, with experience far beyond that of his classmates. He could learn anatomy and participate in research. In fact, he'd probably be the only first-year medical student who could already do surgery.

Folkman applied to Harvard anyway—and he didn't get in. So he took Zollinger up on his offer and resolved to do whatever it took to become the first Ohio State graduate to make it through the doors of Harvard Medical School. He drove down High Street to the huge campus of OSU, made his way to the registrar's office, and signed up for a double major in chemistry and English. He figured Harvard would be more apt to notice him if he got superior grades in not one but two majors, and if he also spent his summers in school and graduated in three years. He didn't even wait until fall to get started, enrolling in summer classes and later taking proficiency tests to bypass some basic courses.

Ohio State, unlike Harvard or the other elite eastern colleges, was a quintessentially football-mad midwestern state university, an original land-grant university whose academic and research programs tended to be obscured by the school's annual bid for the Big Ten championship against the archrival University of Michigan and a trip to the Rose Bowl. Almost everyone was invested in the university's football fortunes. COME BACK AFTER THE GAME, signs in shop windows were apt to advise on Saturdays in fall, and the football team was even on the minds of Rabbi Jerome Folkman and his wife, Bessie, who never missed a Sabbath at Ohio Stadium. "Dad would wear his stadium clothes under his [clerical] robe, and would head for the stadium right after the Shabbat service," recalls David Folkman.

Judah, however, had other things to do. Fraternities and sororities were an integral part of the Ohio State culture, but Judah was a reluctant participant at best. He was so uninterested in the fraternity he joined that he was almost booted out for nonparticipation. Ironically, only his top grades saved him from expulsion. Without them, the fraternity's grade point average would have been so low it would have been decertified. Folkman much preferred Zollinger's dog lab to the frat house, reporting for duty each afternoon at two. By the end of his freshman year he was doing surgery. If a resident called to say he couldn't make it, he would ask if Folkman could fill in. Judah learned anatomy on the fly and soon became adept at abdominal operations.

He was even doing research. For three years he worked with two of Zollinger's surgical residents who were trying to find a way to minimize damage to the human liver during gastric surgery, an injury that occurred when blood flow to the organ had to be temporarily shut off. Experimenting on dogs, Judah and the two residents, B. H. Burch and D. W. Traphagen, found a way to cool the liver, extending to twenty minutes the time that blood flow could be cut off without causing organ damage. Judah's inventiveness was critical: He designed and created a paddlelike device with chilled fluid flowing inside that rapidly cooled a substantial part of the liver. The system worked so well on the dogs that it was used in the hospital's operating room and was eventually described in a published paper. Thus Judah, at age nineteen, became a coauthor on his first academic paper: a monograph titled "The use of aortic occlusion in abdominal surgery with a report of two human cases," published in the journal *Surgery* in his senior year. Soon after the paper was published, Judah got a letter from a researcher at New York Hospital asking him to come spend six weeks in the summer working on liver biology and blood flow in its lab. And would he please bring along those cooling paddles? Judah gladly accepted the offer.

By then, Judah, nervous but self-assured, had already traveled to Boston and settled into a chair in Dr. Howard Frank's office at Beth Israel Hospital. Soon to graduate cum laude from Ohio State, Judah faced his first interview with a member of the admissions committee of Harvard Medical School. Folkman had filled out the four-page application and written a long autobiography that he feared was dreadfully dull. But the Harvard gatekeepers found it compelling enough to send him on to the next step. Now, Dr. Frank had before him a would-be medical student who had already spent time in the operating room and had even invented a surgical device. Impressed, Frank led him off to meet Dr. Herman Blumgart, a senior staff member who was another member of the admissions committee. Blumgart was pleased to meet Judah. He was one of several Harvard professors who had received letters from a colleague who had once been a leading surgeon in the Harvard system of hospitals. "Take this man," Dr. Robert Zollinger advised. "He can operate!"

The committee wanted to take him, but there was one hitch: Judah was just nineteen, a year younger than the minimum. But his credentials were compelling, so an exception was made, and just before New Year's Day, 1953, the telegram arrived on Maryland Avenue in Bexley. The professor's strategy and the student's hard work had paid off. An Ohio State man was finally headed for Harvard Medical School, and his name was Judah Folkman.

Chapter Three

———

IT SEEMS APPROPRIATE somehow that the three Folkman men—the rabbi and his two sons—all graduated on the same June day in 1953. Judah received his bachelor's degree from Ohio State, and his brother earned his diploma from Bexley High School. But it was their father who carried the day. He climbed to the podium in Ohio Stadium and not only accepted his doctoral degree but also delivered the commencement address.

Two months later, Judah and David left home, again on the same day— and this time in the same car. David, also an exceptional student in high school, had accomplished what his brother had not: He had been accepted by Harvard as an undergraduate (as well as by Princeton and Yale). Both Judah and David benefited from a college fund set up by their well-to-do grandfather in Cleveland, and the two of them made the fourteen-hour drive from Columbus to Boston in Judah's yellow Ford convertible. Judah delivered his brother to Cambridge, then crossed the stone bridge over the Charles River, heading for the medical school.

What Folkman found before him was an institution entrenched in tradition. In a sense, all of America's medical schools were still mired in the nineteenth century. They admitted very few women and very few minorities, especially blacks. Though a major revolution—the use of antibiotics—was under way, new vaccines were being developed, and World War II, followed by the Korean conflict, had led to improved surgical procedures, it was still a time when doctors made house calls. Transplanting organs was still science fiction. The medical school curriculum had not changed dramatically in the preceding half century. Students started early with anatomy, studied infectious diseases, diagnostic techniques, surgery, gynecology, pediatrics, and psychiatry. They looked in people's ears, asked them to stick their tongues out and say "aaaah," inspected the retina of the eye, and pounded knees with small rubber mallets. They listened to heartbeats, took pulses, checked blood pressures, and took urine samples. Genetics, nutrition, and, especially, sexual function were discussed rarely, if ever.

The Harvard medical school, of course, was more steeped in tradition than most. The school was less than a decade younger than America itself, and its first class had consisted of just a handful of students under the tutelage of a three-member faculty. In those days, courses consisted of formal lectures— for which students bought tickets, rather than paying tuition—for several semesters, after which students apprenticed with practicing physicians for several years. Because there were no hospitals, there was no clinical training beyond the apprenticeships.

It was do-it-yourself medicine. One of the three original professors, Benjamin Waterhouse, who had been trained in universities and hospitals in Europe, received a document in 1798 telling of Edward Jenner's successful vaccinations for smallpox. Waterhouse, the professor of "theory and practice of physic," was the first to introduce the vaccine in the United States; he boldly demonstrated it on his own family. After being further tested in Boston, smallpox vaccination gradually gained acceptance in the United States. The second founder of the medical school was Aaron Dextor, professor of "chemistry and materia medica." The third of the original professors, John Warren, was a skilled surgeon and teacher who soon moved the medical school from Cambridge to Boston, for the sake of convenience. In Boston, the faculty found it easier to see their private patients and also treat patients in the dispensaries and military hospitals that were being established in the city. Warren's son, John Collins Warren, led the effort that established the Massachusetts General Hospital in 1811. The hospital was founded as a haven for the poor at a time when anyone with money was served at home.

By 1870, nearly a century after its founding, the medical school had begun to transform itself into a major institution. Admission standards became stiff; written exams were required; the departments teaching basic sciences and clinical practice were established; a three-year degree program was started; and the old apprentice system was dropped. Harvard Medical School became one of the professional schools of Harvard University, and in time it set the standard for medical education in a university context. The medical school campus moved to Longwood Avenue in 1906, and its five marble-faced buildings were erected surrounding the Quad. At the time, much of the surrounding land was vacant or being farmed, which offered room for many of

Boston's major hospitals to settle in and grow, creating what later became known as the Harvard medical area. Here, Harvard physicians introduced the use of insulin to the United States, invented the iron lung to support polio patients, grew the polio virus in culture, and developed the external cardiac pacemaker.

Judah Folkman was keenly aware of the history of the school he had long aspired to enter. But having made it through the gates, he felt a surge of inadequacy once inside. The place and the people exuded brilliance and sophistication. It was the very pinnacle of medical education in America, and here he was, a midwestern boy from a state school, arriving without the breeding that obviously accompanied many of his one hundred classmates. He looked around and saw honors graduates from Harvard and Yale who seemed so well read and well informed, so damned smart. They were articulate and self-possessed. They could debate like fiends, were often fluent in three languages, and seemed to know everything—or to think they did. Some arrived with freshly minted Ph.D.'s in chemistry, biochemistry, or biology. A few had been Rhodes scholars. Others had spent their entire lives on the Harvard track, starting early in the Boston public school system's famously elite Latin schools, which were sort of a Harvard farm system.

The Latin schools, one each for boys and for girls, resembled private schools because they ranked high among the best prep schools in the country. High percentages of their graduates went on to Harvard and Radcliffe. On those campuses, a status mark was the green book bag of the Latin schools; those who carried them were rarely shy about clueing outsiders in to their significance. All four classes of the medical school had meals together. One day a fellow student, one with a green book bag, casually let it drop that he was a summa graduate in chemistry and had studied with the professors who wrote the textbooks Folkman had used in Ohio. Folkman couldn't recall any of his former professors writing textbooks. He began to worry that maybe the instincts he'd had in high school were right: Maybe it had been a mistake to stay in Columbus. In truth, he was far from the only one who felt deficient in these surroundings, but it wasn't something most people would admit. So Folkman assumed he was the only one who didn't belong. The insouciance and one-upmanship of his classmates gave him the queasy sensation that he was in deep trouble—that despite knowing how to cut livers out of dogs and having come up with a gizmo that got him published in *Surgery*, he might not be able to cut it at Harvard. Maybe all those professors on the admissions committee had made a grave mistake. He worried that they had only let him in as a favor to their old friend Robert Zollinger.

Whatever Folkman's insecurities and Zollinger's actual influence, the mentor's enthusiastic backing opened a very important door: Folkman won immediate entrée into the cutting-edge biomedical laboratory of one of Harvard's most ambitious and enterprising surgical researchers. Dr. Robert Gross, chief of surgery at Boston's Children's Hospital, was another recipient of one of Zollinger's "Take this man!" letters. He heeded the advice, wasting no time summoning Folkman to help with his latest project. First-year students rarely got directly involved in research, at least not until they'd found their way around the medical school and sorted out who was doing what. But Zollinger's strong recommendation was enough to catapult Folkman past his classmates, no matter what color their book bags were, no matter their pedigrees. Gross asked him to work in his lab afternoons and weekends, whenever he could fit the time into his schedule. And Folkman made sure he found the time. He lived in Vanderbilt Hall, right across the street from the hospital's Carnegie Building, where Gross ran his lab on the second floor.

Gross was a leading light of Harvard medical research after World War II. With its close affiliation with Boston's major hospitals—Mass General, City Hospital, and the two Brigham hospitals—the medical school had in the previous decade become enormously proud of its accomplishments with anesthesia, heart operations to rescue "blue babies," and the beginnings of kidney-transplant research. On the other hand, the medical school suffered from stuffiness and a condescending attitude toward those who weren't inside the Harvard system. It was almost Germanic in some ways, with major professors firmly in charge, administrators doing their bidding. But for those involved, it was also exhilarating to work and grow in the presence of world-class physicians when, for the first time, the world of science was strongly penetrating the practice of medicine. Advances in chemistry led to new drugs, and groundbreaking diagnostic procedures were devised. And thanks to atomic physics, radioactive isotopes were used in hospitals and laboratories to see what had never before been visible: the inner workings of the human body. Just as important, for the first time government agencies began to take on the burden of supporting biomedical research, joining foundations and groups like the American Cancer Society in pushing medical experiments.

At the time, Harvard and its affiliated hospitals were the Establishment. They set the standards, both in Boston and nationwide, spawning the Massachusetts Medical Society and its world-famed medical journal, the *New England Journal of Medicine.* In fact, Harvard could well be described as the nation's first true medical center; it was more than just a collection of large hospitals. It was a mecca for minds and wills.

Robert Gross, a native Minnesotan, had come through Harvard Medical School by way of Carleton College in the 1930s, before the residency system was devised to slide new doctors into specialties. While waiting for a surgical position to open up, Gross had taken work as a pathologist at Children's Hospital. He did it to earn a living, but the job had an unintended benefit. In combating the deaths of babies and small children, he found his life's work: By the early 1950s, trying to find ways to save children born with serious heart defects had become the driving force of his career.

When Judah Folkman arrived, Gross was then struggling to develop a safe technique to correct inborn malformations of the heart muscle. Some babies were born with holes between the heart's two ventricles; others with misconnected major arteries that literally turned them blue from poor circulation. The first condition, called a ventricular septal defect, was one of the most serious congenital heart problems in babies, and it was usually fatal. Nobody had yet come up with a safe way to save the affected child, but Gross was determined. No matter how long it took.

His quest was hampered by a fundamental problem: When he tried to repair the defect surgically, he couldn't see what he was doing. There was too much blood. This meant he had to perform dangerous, experimental heart surgery blindly, his hands submerged in blood as he tried to sew the gap between chambers closed. Worse, the surgery had to be done in an area that was perilously close to the nerve fibers controlling the heartbeat. Unable to see what he was doing, Gross could cut those nerves—a disaster for the babies. Severing the pacing nerves left the heart crippled, unable to pump at more than twenty or thirty beats per minute, instead of the normal seventy-two. The condition, called heart block, was irreversible, and it hastened the child's death. Gross needed to find a way to do the surgery safely—to find a way to see what he was doing. What he needed was something that didn't exist: a reliable blood pump that could temporarily take over for the heart and leave the way clear for surgery. Gross loved tools and loved to fix things around the lab; he had a chest-high tool kit that was painted gold and monogrammed with his initials, REG. So he set out to design and build his own heart pump.

Judah Folkman happened to join the lab while Gross was struggling with the invention in his machine shop, and he saw the obstacles Gross was trying to surmount. The device had to pump enough blood, gently enough, to keep an infant alive while the heart was being repaired. It had to oxygenate the blood and keep it flowing. And it had to be reliable. Gross's working version was huge, the size of an office desk mounted on wheels. Other research physicians around the country were also at work on their own blood pumps, but unlike his counterparts, Gross was intent on keeping it simple—he wanted to be able to operate his machine manually if there was a power failure or if the motor quit during an operation. His task was even more daunting because he was one of the few trying to do these operations on newborn babies, with their tiny hearts and fragile lives.

It was a constant and often frustrating process of trial and error—mostly error. Gross and his machinist, Fred Savage, would build one version, then modify it and modify it some more. To pump blood, they tried a roller system that gently squeezed a plastic tube, akin to the way toothpaste is pressed out of a tube. That didn't work very well, so they tried a piston pump. They tried various methods of moving the blood through devices to pick up oxygen from the air without causing it to clot. When Gross decided the machine was ready, he began testing it on dogs. But in its early versions the machine failed miserably. The blood was touching metals that tended to make it clot, causing blockages that could be as dangerous as the condition Gross was trying to correct. When they shifted to plastic, the tubing cracked, or it jammed and stopped the pump. In one case, air bubbles got into the dog's brain, killing the animal. Gross decided a bubble filter was needed. He and Savage devised one using steel wool, but they found that the metal damaged blood. And so it went.

Dozens of dogs rolled through the lab, supplied by a company that bred and raised animals for research purposes. Gross used dogs that were about the size of babies, and he treated them as he would infants: After surgery they would be put into intensive care and monitored all night. Folkman sometimes spent nights at their bedsides, watching their IV lines and vital signs. Eventually the blood pump began working well and some of the surviving dogs became the lab team's pets. Gross's favorite was a German shepherd named Airplane. One morning, Gross called Folkman and told him to get dressed up. Gross wanted Folkman to accompany him, Dr. Paul Dudley White, who was President Eisenhower's cardiologist, and Airplane to the Massachusetts statehouse. The two physicians, the medical student, the dog, and a young heart patient who had been saved appeared before the state assembly in opposition to an antivivisection bill. Where would this patient be without dogs like Airplane putting their lives on the line? they asked. Their picture made the next day's *Boston Globe*. "My job was to make sure that Airplane didn't defecate in the statehouse," Folkman recalls. "I came equipped." The bill was voted down.

When Gross decided in late 1953 that the blood pump was finally ready for use on humans, he still preceded each operation with a warm-up session on a dog in the lab. "He would rehearse in the morning," Folkman recalls, "and then I would have to get out of school and skedaddle over there, help him wheel the pump across the bridge from the Carnegie Building to the Children's Hospital operating room, and he'd do a patient in the afternoon." There was a frantic scramble to get ready. All the parts of the pump had to be quickly and thoroughly cleaned and sterilized. And then the chaotic atmosphere would dissolve into silence. Gross insisted on a perfectly quiet operating room. If there was any talking, it meant something was going wrong. But in the early days with the blood pump, there was a lot of talking. Several infants in the first group of patients died.

The nature of the surgery proved to be as much of a problem as the pump. Gross never knew exactly what congenital defects he would find when he opened the baby's chest on the operating table, and sometimes they turned out to be beyond repair. In some cases there was more than one hole, and he just couldn't close them all. In others, even with the blood pump working, he couldn't prevent accidental damage to the nerves. In normal babies, the nerve bundle passes within the wall between ventricles. But in these endangered patients, the nerve bundle was displaced by the hole between the chambers. Gross couldn't tell to which side of the hole the nerves had been rerouted, so sometimes while trying to sew up the hole he inadvertently looped the suture around the nerve bundle. The fibers, cinched tight, would stop signaling, putting the baby into heart block.

By now, Gross had made Folkman an important member of his team. He was so impressed by his intellect and drive that he included him as much as possible. When his infant patients died, Gross sometimes asked Folkman to accompany him to the hospital's chapel to help console the parents. The young medical student was very adept in the lab, but Gross wanted him to see the other side of medicine, the human side. What Folkman saw in Gross, meanwhile, was a dedicated research surgeon who desperately wanted to reach the day when these grim visits to the chapel would be unnecessary. Face-to-face with the parents, Gross was extraordinarily comforting, and if there was a message he wanted to impart to grieving parents, it was that their children had not died in vain. He would hold their hands and explain that their baby's condition was more than medicine was equipped to handle. But it was good that they had tried. Without surgery, the baby would certainly have died. So the operation was a last resort—but also a first step. Gross and his team were learning, trying surgery that few in the world would even suggest, but which Gross hoped would one day routinely save babies.

The quest was so intense that Gross constantly tried to come up with ways to improve. Early one Saturday morning, he called Folkman and told him to meet him in the pathology department. On a shelf were dozens of bottles containing the hearts of babies, preserved in formaldehyde. Gross and Folkman took the tiny hearts out, washed them, and put them on trays, four or five to a tray. Then they took the abnormal hearts to Gross's lab and examined each one with a magnifying glass, looking inside and out to see where the nerve bundles were actually located in malformed hearts. They drew what they saw, then studied the drawings. They noticed that the nerves were usually rerouted below the abnormal hole, rather than above. With that bit of knowledge, Gross was better able to avoid catching the nerve bundles in the loops when he tightened stitches.

MEANWHILE FOLKMAN ALSO PLOWED along with his medical studies, digging in especially hard, still afraid he wouldn't be able to keep up. He was known for taking detailed notes during lectures and for asking incisive questions. "He was totally and completely a workaholic," remembers a classmate, Richard Freiberg. "When I would go out on a Saturday night, I knew I could come back and find Judah still studying and go down there and agitate him." Harvard's tradition of alphabetical seating put Folkman and Freiberg next to each other in classes, and they became unusually familiar: Each had to practice drawing the other's blood and putting tubes down the other's throat to learn these most rudimentary procedures. "We had no idea what we were doing," Freiberg recalls. "We were each other's guinea pigs. I remember very well that Judah had a very strong gag reflex. The tube kept coming right back out again."

The two students got to know each other well, but not so well that Folkman shared many of his insecurities about the Harvard ethos. It wasn't until nearly half a century later that Freiberg, an orthopedic surgeon in Cincinnati, heard that Folkman had secretly felt inadequate in their first year at Harvard. "That's the only failure of judgment I've ever heard him have," Freiberg says. "Everyone knew he was smarter than the rest of us."

From the beginning there was one class Folkman found a breeze: anatomy. With his experience in the dog lab back in Ohio—not to mention the exploding blood in his family's basement—he had not the slightest qualms about cutting up a cadaver. Folkman was in his element, unlike many of his classmates, some of whom were so repelled by the carcass that they refused to even come forward at first. Some got sick on the spot. Folkman, meanwhile, was intimately familiar with all the tools needed for dissection, as well as the look and smell of the tissues and internal organs. He would routinely finish a task in twenty minutes, while the rest of the class labored gingerly for an entire week. Three of his classmates managed to slice open their own fingers while trying to open their subjects' abdomens; others were so squeamish they could barely go skin deep. And at every few tables there was someone who absolutely refused to dissect at all. The reluctant student would sit on a stool, reading the instructions for the rest of the team, not touching anything.

Thus Folkman's skills were in great demand in anatomy class. Each day, the students—four per cadaver—had a list of body parts they needed to find and identify. It was arduous and exacting work, especially when the assignment was to locate specific nerves, show where they came from, where they went, how the muscles were attached to them, and how they worked together. Anyone who failed to complete the list during the day had to come back at night and finish the task. More than a few students quickly fell behind the dissection schedule and began coming to Folkman for help. At first he instructed his classmates at his own dissecting table, but then he began making rounds, dispensing guidance and answering questions. Before long, the anatomy instructor asked Folkman and two other students to be prosectors, helping demonstrate procedures for the rest of the class.

"Early on it was known that Judah was a very unusual and amazing character," remembers classmate John Remensnyder, now a plastic surgeon. "It was known that Zollinger had allowed him to scrub up for some operations on patients while he was still in college, or even high school. He had already participated in operations. We all knew about that, and it was quite amazing."

For his part, Folkman was struck by the disparity in ability among the students. All of them had to be academic stars of one sort or another just to get into Harvard, but it seemed clear that only some had the right combination of physical skill and intellectual stamina to think about careers in surgery. The others, though brilliant, clearly should avoid knives and other sharp instruments, Folkman thought. Maybe they should consider careers in psychiatry or neurology.

When it came time for their first formal training in the school's dog-surgery course, Folkman and Freiberg—who had also practiced some surgery on dogs before coming to Harvard—both zipped through a procedure so adroitly and so quickly that they were already sewing up when the instructor came around. The teacher became furious—he was sure they had faked it. "He was a very excitable man," Freiberg remembers wryly. So excitable that he had a habit of kicking laggard students in the behind. The instructor also had a memorable way of teaching his students to scrub for surgery: He would put masks over their eyes, smear lamp black and oil all over their hands, and then demand they wash it off completely, which was nearly impossible.

That was one way for an instructor to make an impression on students. Another way was through the power of exquisite teaching. One who left a deep impression on Folkman was a physiology professor, Dr. Clifford Barger, who lectured one day on heart block. Folkman, of course, knew all about heart block—everything but what to do about it. With Gross's encouragement, he had been thinking about the problem, and after class he asked Barger if he thought the condition might be overcome electrically by a device that could regulate heartbeat. Barger sat down, considered it a moment, then said, "That's a great idea."

Even at this early stage in his formal medical training, Folkman was thinking well beyond the classroom. He noticed that when lecturers mentioned medical discoveries in the course of their teaching, they made a point of explaining the history of the breakthroughs. The blood-thinning agent heparin, for example, had been discovered by a young man in Baltimore who was working for a biological supply company while waiting for admission to Johns Hopkins Medical School. Folkman decided there was no reason why a medical student could not figure out how to defeat the vexing problem of heart block.

Folkman noticed something else: His insecurities were fading. His work as a prosector in the anatomy lab led him to the realization that one of the things he did best and enjoyed most was teaching. His classmates, meanwhile, couldn't help but notice how completely involved Folkman was in every aspect of every course he was taking and that he still somehow found time to make Gross's dog laboratory his second home. They concluded that he was both a brilliant member of the class and also one of the two wittiest; it was a toss-up between him and Bob Krooth. Folkman's sense of humor often showed up when he was taking his meals among the medical school's four-hundred-member student body in the Vanderbilt dining hall. Puns, gags, and practical jokes helped relieve the inherent pressures of course work.

Like everyone around him, however, during the first year Folkman was more than a little concerned about how he was actually doing academically. Medical students at Harvard did not receive grades until the very end of the year. Tests consisted of long essay questions that would come back with comments but no scores. Those who were failing were discreetly notified; everyone else had to wonder whether they were at the top of the class, at the bottom, or somewhere in the wide middle. Some would emerge from test sessions bragging how they'd just aced the exams. But Folkman wasn't that confident. He felt, as he later put it, like he was climbing a mountain in the fog. He couldn't gauge his progress, and it tended to make him more impatient with his own inadequacies, real or perceived. Before one anatomy exam, he crammed hard with Richard Freiberg. They sat for hours asking progressively tougher questions, each trying to catch the other in a blunder. Finally, Freiberg asked Folkman to identify "gomphosis." Folkman fell silent, then finally admitted he had no idea what the hell it was. "It's the joint between the tooth and the jaw," Freiberg told him. Folkman was furious with himself. "It really upset him," Freiberg remembers. "He didn't like to be one-upped at all."

The moment of truth came on the last day of that first grueling year, when the class standings were to be posted in one of the major lecture halls. It was a long list of names appearing in order from the top student down. Anxiously approaching the list, Folkman quickly spotted his name—he was second, behind only Dorothy Hellman, one of three women in the class. (The brilliant Hellman suffered a serious neck injury in a sledding accident a few years later and died while still quite young.) Finishing so near the top of the class gave Folkman an enormous boost in self-confidence. He no longer had to worry that he wasn't smart enough or wasn't qualified to stand among the country's most elite students. The good grades also freed him to think bigger. Now he could afford to spend even more time doing something he loved: facing the challenge of work in Dr. Gross's surgical laboratory over at Children's Hospital.

GROSS WAS HAVING some success fixing congenital heart defects—he saved some babies who certainly would not have survived otherwise—but he was still losing other patients on the operating table or soon after surgery. The failures made life at the hospital difficult for Gross. He would come back from a tumultuous meeting and say to Folkman, "We *have* to make this work." Gross kept the details to himself, but the clear inference was that his colleagues were uncomfortable with his work and were putting pressure on him to stop doing the risky surgery. Indeed, most surgeons would have given up after losing one patient. But Gross kept going, even though he'd failed to save many. He believed that in the long run there was little to lose—since his patients were already under a death sentence—and everything to gain.

Gross was reserved, precise, and immaculate, his white lab coat always perfectly pressed, his hair always neatly groomed. He would appear on the ward in a wide tie with a little diamond stuck in it. He used few words and didn't waste a minute. But his seemingly cold exterior concealed an unstoppable inner drive. Folkman came to realize that Gross was never satisfied simply practicing the medicine of the day. He was always thinking ahead, always searching for new treatments at a time when children born with serious heart defects were dying because so little could be done to rescue them. So for Gross pushing the envelope of pediatric surgery—defying peers and superiors, operating in the midst of turmoil because of it—was nothing new. In fact, he had already worked for years under a serious handicap at Children's Hospital: His predecessor and mentor, Dr. William Ladd, actively despised him because of one career-defining incident.

Back in the late thirties, fifteen years before Folkman met him, Gross was working on an experimental technique to save newborn babies in whom a special blood passage had failed to close off normally at birth. A link between the pulmonary artery and the aorta at the top of the heart must be open during fetal life because the lungs are under water, and oxygen comes through the umbilical cord. But immediately after birth, a special muscle clamps the connecting vessel shut, allowing the newly inflating lungs to take over the chore of breathing and supplying oxygen. But in a few babies, the fetal channel fails to close, creating an eventually fatal condition, patent ductus arteriosus, that leaves the baby with poor circulation, and the heart has to work too hard.

Having seen victims of patent ductus in his earlier work as a pathologist, Gross had concluded that the opening could be closed surgically. He first tested his idea on dogs, and it worked. Ladd, though, warned him not to try it on a human. The chief of surgery at Children's, widely regarded as the father of pediatric surgery, thought the risk was too high. He feared that opening the infant's chest would cause the lungs to immediately collapse, perhaps fatally.

But Gross, convinced he could do it, wasn't to be stopped. He waited until Ladd left for a monthlong vacation on Cape Cod, which left Gross, for the moment, in charge of surgery. When a suitable case came in, he gave himself permission to do the daring operation, and in a remarkable feat of nimble, smart, and dangerous surgery, he succeeded. The little baby was saved. Then the only thing Gross had to worry about saving was his career.

When he returned from Cape Cod, Ladd was, as Gross expected, furious. The operation had succeeded, but what if it hadn't? Gross had directly disobeyed his superior—that was the only thing that mattered to Ladd. The two men had been close friends and colleagues for years. They had collaborated on one of the most important textbooks in the field, *Abdominal Surgery in Infancy and Childhood*. But anger overrode all of that. Gross responded to Ladd's fury by walking out, essentially going on strike. He spent the next few months sitting at home in rural Framingham, waiting for Ladd—or anyone—to call him. But Ladd let him sit. Gross, assuming he was out of a job, began making plans to leave Boston and take a position at Johns Hopkins Hospital. But before he could leave for Baltimore, he got a call from Children's Hospital. Gross was such a gifted surgeon that he was the only one on staff who could treat many of the desperate cases that were coming in from all over the world. No cardiac surgery had been done since he left. The leadership begged Gross to come back. Gross did return to surgery, but he and Ladd never repaired their relationship. Ironically, years later, after his former mentor's death, Gross was awarded the William Ladd Professorship in Surgery at Harvard Medical School. And he eventually succeeded Ladd as chief of surgery at Children's.

So that was the intense, high-stakes, and often combative medical milieu into which Judah Folkman was stepping. To Folkman, the moral was unmistakable: Advancing medical science takes brains and ingenuity, of course, but also persistence and fearlessness, and sometimes a willingness to take personal risks. "If the surgery had failed," Gross told Folkman, "my career would have been over. I'd have been a farmer."

As medical school wore on, Folkman identified more and more with Gross and his passion for pushing the boundaries. He tried to emulate him and often thought about how he might make a contribution to Gross's work, including the hole-in-the-heart condition.

Folkman collaborated with Dr. Elton Watkins, a thoracic surgeon working in Gross's lab, and together they devised a way to punch a hole between the heart chambers in a dog, almost exactly mimicking the condition seen in babies, so that Gross could practice sewing the defects up. Then, on his own, Folkman decided to take the next step: coming up with a likely way to close such holes in the absence of a reliable blood pump. Ultimately he sliced a deep slit down through the wall separating the two ventricles. Then, using a long needle to pull a small, stiff sheet of polyethylene down into the wall, he closed the hole between the chambers. The procedure was a success with dogs. The plastic held, the wound healed over it, and the heart worked properly.

Gross was so impressed with Folkman's ingenuity and skill that he encouraged him to submit a paper about his new technique at the annual meeting of the American College of Surgery, a prestigious gathering of leading surgeons in Chicago. The gathering featured presentations of new findings in surgery that were later published in a thick volume. If the forum's selection committee accepted his paper, Folkman would make history. No mere medical student had ever been selected to come to Chicago and discuss his work. Though the research had been done under Gross, he insisted that it carry only Folkman's name. And months later word came: The paper had been accepted. Folkman was about to give his first formal scientific talk.

Gross was thrilled—in his reserved way—and invited his protégé out to Framingham to help him prepare. After dinner Gross led him out into the apple orchard next to his house. "You stand there," he told Folkman, and then began walking away. He kept walking until Folkman could barely see him.

"Okay, give the paper," he yelled.

Folkman began, then stopped. "Why am I saying this so loud?" he called out. "There will be a microphone."

"Well, the microphone might fail," Gross called back across the orchard. He was a scientist who believed in what was later named Murphy's Law: If something can go wrong, it will. And if it does, he told Folkman, finish your talk no matter what. If the slide projector dies, just turn up the lights and tell the audience what they would have been seeing.

In Chicago, Folkman took the podium and looked out at the audience. He saw Gross in the front row, looking like a proud parent. Gross was ready to help, but the presentation went off without a hitch, and the audience gave the twenty-year-old medical student with his polyethylene contraption an enthusiastic reception: What a clever idea. What a bright young man.

Returning to earth in Boston, Folkman knew that the procedure he'd come up with may have been plenty clever, but it would be just an interim solution at best—a somewhat crude stopgap that would be obsolete as soon as someone came up with a workable blood pump that allowed surgeons to see their work and perform true open-heart surgery. Naturally, Folkman kept his attention focused on Gross's blood pump. He and Elton Watkins tried to sort out whether it could be improved. With Gross's encouragement, they brought dogs into the lab and got down to basics: How rapidly could the pump be run, and for how long, before the blood was too seriously damaged? How much blood needed to be circulated? Sometimes the blood failed to pick up enough oxygen, and they could actually see their subjects turn a dog's shade of blue. And gradually they began seeing some success: They overcame the clotting problem by using heparin, the blood-thinning agent that had been discovered by the premed student in Baltimore. They labored for months to come up with the right doses.

Another problem that frustrated Gross's team's attempts to close inter-chamber holes in children's hearts was that often when Gross started to operate, the heart would go into arrythmia, irregular beating that could be deadly. Between the incidents of arrythmia and those of heart block, Gross had ample reason to explore whether there was some way to restore near-normal heart-beat. In 1955, he and his team moved to attack the problem.

Gross couldn't do it all—operate, teach, develop the blood pump, and work on the heartbeat problem—so he asked Folkman, his boy wonder, to take on the heartbeat project. What they needed was a precise electrical stimulating system capable of mimicking the flow of electric signals that maintain normal heart rhythm. Gross was not convinced that the project would ever bear fruit, but he saw that Folkman was excited by the idea, and he was curious to see what the young man from Ohio might come up with.

Folkman wasn't exactly starting from scratch: The fact that electric pulses could be used to drive the heart artificially was already known. And he was heartened that Dr. Barger, the physiology professor, thought that using electrical impulses to overcome heart block might be a great idea. But others had tried and failed to come up with a practical and reliable way to drive the heart. A pioneering invention had been developed two years earlier by Dr. Paul Zoll across the street at Beth Israel Hospital. But Zoll's pacemaker, as it was called, was then unrefined and undependable. It consisted of big plates that doctors loaded up with voltage and then placed on their patients' chests. Repeated electric shocks through the skin could jump-start a heart and keep it going for a while—sometimes.

Babies who were crippled by heart block were occasionally put on the Zoll pacemaker, but the shocks were painful with every zap. The babies were crying and had to be sedated, a terrible ordeal for them and for their parents.

Still, Zoll and his collaborators had used the cumbersome system for several years. It was all there was. As ambitious as he was, Gross was not confident that his team could do any better, at least in the short term. And Folkman, though anxious to attack the problem, knew very well that this one was beyond him. He realized that he needed to go across the Charles River to the concrete campus of the Massachusetts Institute of Technology, a place he knew would be crawling with bright young engineers who could help.

Folkman showed up one day at MIT's division of industrial cooperation, where businesspeople could come for help in solving technical problems. He found his way to a professor, Kurt Lion, and described his research project. Was there someone around his age, a graduate student with creativity and time, who could help him? Folkman really didn't want to work with a senior faculty member, who wouldn't devote much attention or enthusiasm to the project. Lion thought immediately of a talented graduate student, biophysicist Fred Vanderschmidt.

Folkman explained to Vanderschmidt that he wanted to pick up the pulse that had been blocked and use it to stimulate the two lower chambers of the heart to return to the correct beating rate. What was more, he wanted to do this *internally,* with a device that would fit inside the chest.

"Well, if you want to do that, you have to know something about the nature of the signal," Vanderschmidt replied. "You have to know the characteristics of the source. You have to measure the voltage, then you have to put resistors across the measuring device to determine the resistance." Folkman listened, took some notes, then left. Vanderschmidt was confident he'd never see him again.

But a few days later, Folkman was back again, and he had the data. Vanderschmidt was amazed. "It was the most remarkable experience I've ever had working with someone who has a medical background," he said years later. Soon the two young men had built a crude prototype, a large and unwieldy device. When it was done, ready to be tested, it was Vanderschmidt's turn to load up and cross the Charles River. He showed up at Children's Hospital with his new contraption, walked into the operating room of the dog lab, and promptly fainted.

Once revived, the MIT expert watched Folkman begin hooking up the device they'd created. Folkman had severed the nerve in a dog's heart to simulate the same kind of heart block babies sometimes suffered during surgery. After the cut, the two upper chambers of the dog's heart, the atria, were beating away normally, but the two lower chambers, the ventricles, were lagging

far behind. Folkman took a very fine wire and sewed it into one of the normally beating chambers of the atrium. Then he measured exactly how much
voltage was coming out each time it pulsed. The signal was fed into their
battery-powered prototype, which responded to pulses from the atria by
sending a corresponding signal to the lagging heart chambers.

To their glee, their primitive system soon worked flawlessly. Each time the
atria beat, the ventricles followed in perfect rhythm. Their invention har-
nessed electricity from one part of the heart to pace the other. "You could literally turn the dog on and turn the dog off," Vanderschmidt recalls. "When
you turned it off, he would lie down on the floor and not be able to move. But
when you turned it on he got up, was frisky, licked your hand, just like a regular dog."

Folkman and Vanderschmidt had come up with the first pacemaker that
might work inside the body, but it was much too big and cumbersome for
practical use. Their next task was to make the pacemaker implantable, for if
they closed up the dog's chest without the pacemaker, the animal would go
back into heart block and eventually die. They had to come up with a system
that would fit inside the animal's chest, and a baby's.

Vanderschmidt got to work miniaturizing the system. Because he was
at MIT, he had ready access to the latest electronic technology, and in the
mid-1950s one of the very latest marvels was a tiny device called the transis-
tor. Benjamin Folkman—the grandfather who had wanted to give young
Judah a jeep for his bar mitzvah but ended up giving him a microscope—had
provided Folkman with one thousand dollars to help him do research. Folkman decided to use the money for transistors, special wires, and a machined-
metal case. With those ingredients Vanderschmidt quickly reengineered the
pacemaker, reducing it to the size of a pack of cigarettes. The first time
the new version was tried on a live animal, it was worn outside, strapped
to the dog's chest for demonstration. Switched on, the pacemaker allowed
the dog to walk. Switched off, he slumped to the floor. The first time they
showed the pacemaker to Gross, the dog passed out as soon as the device was
switched off.

Thus the MIT graduate student and the doctor-in-training had created
the world's first implantable heart pacemaker. Following a Harvard policy that
eschewed seeking patents, Folkman simply published the results (accepted by
the 1958 Surgical Forum) and left his invention in the public domain, where
it was quickly noticed by Minnesota Mining and Manufacturing Company,
better known as 3M. The company sent a couple of engineers to Children's

Hospital, where Folkman showed them the prototype, sending them off with a copy of the plans. Despite its obvious value, Folkman never even thought of patenting it. That just wasn't done at Harvard in those days; it would have been too commercial, too crass. A few years later, the implantable, battery-powered heart pacemakers would become available commercially, one version made by a company called Medtronics. The device, of course, became ubiquitous and earned millions of dollars in profit, but Folkman and Vanderschmidt and their institutions did not reap any benefit. Indeed, the only people at Harvard or MIT who got anything out of the pair's pioneering work were faculty members who required pacemakers themselves.

Folkman did profit in another way, though. He made his inventions—the development of the pacemaker and of the surgical method for correcting the ventricular septal defect—the focus of his medical school thesis. His achievements helped him to graduate magna cum laude and to win four major medical school awards: the Boyleston Medical Prize, the Soma Weiss Award, the Borden Undergraduate Research Award in Medicine, and membership in Alpha Omega Alpha, the medical school equivalent of Phi Beta Kappa. But most important, the research work and his time with Gross nurtured what was already becoming Folkman's professional weltanschauung. It put him at the center of leading-edge medicine, and taught him that this was exactly the place he should be. Gross wasn't the one who eventually perfected the blood pump (a team at the University of Pennsylvania and another in Minnesota beat him to it), but because of the pump and his wisdom, the pediatric surgery he pioneered would eventually become routine. Gross's grand dream would be realized, and nobody appreciated the sacrifices and the payoffs, or took the experience as a life lesson, more than Judah Folkman.

FOR A GRADUATING MEDICAL STUDENT avidly seeking an internship and residency, there were many fine institutions to consider but few to really aspire to, especially for someone intent on training to become a first-class surgeon. The crème de la crème of these was the leading Harvard-affiliated hospital, Massachusetts General. The venerable teaching hospital whose symbolic heart was its historic Ether Dome, an operating-room-in-the-round at the top of the original building where the use of anesthesia was first demonstrated in 1846, carried priceless prestige. More than a century after the anesthesia demonstration, medical students everywhere still coveted a Mass General internship. Each year, applications came not only from the top of the Harvard graduating class, but from hundreds of high achievers from the best medical schools throughout the country.

Judah Folkman suspected he had a good shot. His grades were excellent. He had strong recommendations, particularly from the eminent Dr. Gross. And his early accomplishments in research seemed unbeatable. But he knew the competition would be fierce. That year, 1957, Mass General was offering twelve internships, and the special few who were selected could plan on a unique six-year training program that would be an enormous springboard for their careers. Mass General was unusual in wanting its interns to cooperate rather than compete. So unlike those at other hospitals, new interns didn't have to concern themselves with the next rung on the ladder. Once they got in, if they did well they were all but assured of staying on through residency. Of course, the selection process reflected those high stakes. It was called an interview, but it was more like a marathon inquisition. On the specified day, the applicants, hundreds of them, converged on the hospital, and then one by one, each was summoned to a small room to be grilled on difficult medical questions by a panel of leading doctors.

When Folkman's name was called, he reported to the appointed room and found three professors waiting for him. They showed him a set of X rays and asked him to identify four visible fractures. They asked him questions of fact: What was the five-year survival rate for women with untreated breast cancer? Folkman guessed wrong. "Dr. Folkman," one of the interviewers said, "if a workman fell off a scaffolding and landed on his feet, what would you do?" Folkman said he would X-ray the patient. And what would you X-ray for, Dr. Folkman? He said he'd look for damage to the vertebrae. Where, exactly? Folkman picked the wrong spot; he was too high up the backbone.

Despite his two imperfect responses, Folkman realized he had made the first cut when he noticed that most of the candidates who'd arrived in the morning were gone. While waiting in the library for the second round, he looked up the answers to the questions he'd missed—20 percent was the survival rate for untreated breast cancer. Then he sat down, fidgeting and nervous like everyone else. Finally he was ushered into a room where eight professors began a more intense round of examination: questions on fine points of actual and hypothetical cases, questions about anatomy, drugs, surgery, causes of diseases. The interrogation seemed relentless, endless. Then it was back to a waiting room for the tenacious few who survived the second round.

Folkman was among them, and now he prepared for the third level, an interview with the final committee. It was seven o'clock, getting dark, and he was exhausted. He sat before the really big guns, the chairmen of all the hospital departments—general surgery, vascular surgery, urology, neurosurgery, gynecology, a dozen altogether. The session was led by Dr. Edward Churchill, Mass General's surgeon-in-chief. The questions began to fly, with Folkman in the hot seat. Immediately, he realized that the points on which he'd been weak in the earlier sessions were now being thrown back at him. It was a trick they used to see if the candidate was quick enough, resourceful enough, to make the grade. If he or she made a mistake, how quickly was it corrected? That's why they'd had the candidates wait in the library. Was this a doctor who could learn—who *wanted* to learn? Folkman realized he'd done the right thing by researching the questions he'd missed while waiting for the next round.

He was in.

Three weeks after graduation, Folkman arrived at Mass General at six A.M. to begin his internship. Instantly, he felt a flashback to those first weeks and months of medical school four years before: He felt inadequate, wondering if he would make the grade. He had become a star in the classroom and in the lab. But now he would be seeing patients, real people who would be putting their lives in his hands. Folkman was awed by the proficiency of the residents who worked above him. He observed the chief resident, a doctor with six years' experience and thousands of cases under his belt. And he had trouble imagining the day when he might possess such competence and self-confidence, able to cope with anything, always cool, always in control.

But mostly he felt tired. His group, all training to be surgeons, was first assigned to the emergency room and outpatient services, and the hours were beyond grueling: thirty-six on, twenty-four off, then do it all over again, week after week. Most hospitals might have one or two cases an hour, or even a night, but in Boston's best-known hospital the emergency room had six or seven patients going all at once: people with gunshot wounds, burns, broken bones, or head injuries. The doors would suddenly swing open and another case would be wheeled in on a gurney. All kinds of people, all kinds of problems, all kinds of attitudes, and they all had to be served immediately. When caseloads spilled over, the interns might be called in on their day off. During one early stretch, Folkman didn't get a day off for weeks. Occasionally there would be a letup, but then another emergency would come bursting through the doors. The residents had little patience for interns and peers who didn't measure up. One attitude was always drummed into them: This is Massachusetts General Hospital. You are here because you are the best. That means you perform at the highest levels. You do not whine. Every intern and every resident, in every hospital in America, went through years of similarly exhausting training, but it seemed that at Mass General everything was that much more arduous. Folkman could see that he had joined the medical equivalent of marine boot camp. But he never doubted the rewards would be worth the sacrifice.

After two grueling months in the emergency room, the interns moved on to a rotation in general surgery, assisting at first, then getting more deeply involved. Next came neurosurgery, when the interns spent virtually all day on their feet observing in the operating room. Then there was obstetrics and gynecology, where they saw the results of botched abortions, endometrial bleeding, and troublesome pregnancies. Such problems and pressures made Folkman doubly glad he had taken advantage of extra classes offered his first year in medical school. Each Saturday morning there was a major clinic in the amphitheater at Peter Bent Brigham Hospital, featuring a lecture by one of the great surgeons of Harvard, who would usually bring along a patient who had been successfully treated. Then the students would be invited to come back in the afternoon and watch the same procedure live from a glass-partitioned room above the OR, the esteemed surgeon describing the action through a microphone. The program was optional but Folkman squeezed every ounce of benefit from these and similar opportunities. His classmate John Remensnyder noticed that Folkman kept a large notebook, and after every operation he observed or participated in, he would write down his thoughts. One day Remensnyder asked to see the notebook. "It was pretty darned good," he remembers. He starting taking notes himself.

Each week at Mass General there was a "deaths and complications" meeting that required attendance by interns and residents, along with some senior staff. Together they would examine each case that was brought up, assessing whether errors had occurred and if so, whether they could have been avoided. Was it poor management of the patient? An error of diagnosis? Poor judgment? Bad technique? If an error was detected, the group had to decide which of the doctors was to blame: whose name should be written next to that error and who had to bear the responsibility for what went wrong. Folkman learned very quickly that mistakes happen even in the best hospitals, sometimes dreadful mistakes, and that there is no running away from them.

As the interns' training progressed, there wasn't much respite. By then, Folkman was living in a small apartment on Marlborough Street, near the hospital, though he actually slept more in the spartan quarters at Mass General where the interns could grab a few hours' rest. As it happened, Judah and his siblings were all now living in and around Boston. David had graduated from Harvard the same month Judah finished medical school, and he was now in his first year at the Harvard School of Business. Their sister, Joy, was attending Wellesley College, about twenty miles west of Boston.

Joy graduated in 1958 and had married one of Judah's classmates, a future cardiologist named Arthur Moss. It was a match that Judah had a hand in making. One night when he was still in medical school, Judah had invited his sister to have dinner. Moss stopped by their table briefly and a few days later called Joy for a date. Joy consulted her brother. "Who is this guy?" she asked. "Oh, he's the one I had picked out for you," Judah answered. "I was meaning to get the two of you together."

A year after he and Joy were married, Moss was drafted into the navy, a development that would turn out to be one of the most significant events in Judah's life. With the couple getting ready to head for Pensacola, Florida, Joy was worried about leaving her big brother, who had survived his internship and was now in his first year of residency, all alone with only his medical training to keep him occupied. She wished he had a girlfriend. Maybe she could even return the favor of introducing him to someone. She thought of Paula Prial.

Joy and Paula were classmates at Wellesley, though they didn't know each other very well because they lived in different dorms. But Joy knew enough about Paula to think that Judah might like her. She was very bright, at the top of her class. She was very talented, a music major with a beautiful singing voice. She was attractive, and she was Jewish. Joy also heard that Paula had recently broken off a romance, so she was free at the moment. Joy gave Judah her classmate's phone number on a scrap of paper, which he stashed in his hospital scrubs and fished out just before tossing the gown into the laundry. Judah and Paula went out to a late dinner in the Terrace Room at the Statler Hotel, so late that Paula couldn't finish her meal—so Judah did.

Joy's instincts were right; Judah and Paula did hit it off. But they found it hard to maintain a normal relationship. There was no way that Paula could compete with Judah's ties to Massachusetts General Hospital. He'd often cancel dates or show up three hours late. His intense focus on his studies hadn't gone over very well with girls he had known during medical school, one of whom, a Wellesley student, had gone to great lengths trying to spend more time with him. She started by matching up Judah's friend and classmate

Richard Freiberg with one of the pretty girls she knew at Wellesley and arranging double dates. Freiberg, knowing a good deal when he saw one, then pressured Folkman to go out. Sometimes it worked. Sometimes not.

Paula Prial was considerably more understanding. "Oh, you're just like my dad. He's always late," she said the first time Judah, very late, finally showed up making profuse apologies. Her father, Dr. David Prial, had long been a family doctor practicing out of the family home in Fall River, a small industrial city on Massachusetts's southern coast. Prial was a Russian immigrant who arrived in New York as a teenager before World War I, attended Columbia University, and then went to medical school in St. Louis before settling in Fall River. In this little city populated by many Portuguese and French Canadians, Dr. Prial's daughter grew up knowing that her father was one of the most beloved and respected men in town. The price was inconvenience. It was part of being a doctor's daughter, just as the expectation of model behavior was a requisite of being a rabbi's son.

Sometimes it would be close to midnight by the time Judah made it to Paula's apartment in Cambridge, and he and Paula would go over to the drive-in and sit in the car and eat hamburgers. They filled each other in on their first twenty years and talked about where they were headed. Judah made it clear he wasn't going to be like Paula's father, much as he admired him. He wanted to stay in academic surgery, teaching and doing research, though he didn't know where he'd wind up. He doubted Harvard would offer him a position when he finished his residency, but he was confident he'd land a good job somewhere. "After six years of training at Harvard and being board certified, there will be offers," he told Paula. "And if not, Dr. Churchill, the chairman of surgery, will get on the phone and find me a job." That was how it worked.

And Paula? She had gone to boarding school as a teenager and been accepted to all three of the Seven Sisters colleges she applied to—Wellesley, Vassar, and Radcliffe. In choosing Wellesley, she said, "I went for the scenery." She wanted to sing and to teach music, and Judah understood that immediately. It was one of the things she liked about him. "He was a little different," she recalls. "He really cared about what I was doing." She gave him a paper about a churchman who had codified Ambrosian chants, which Judah read and seemed to understand.

Judah found Paula to be a nearly perfect match. He loved her sense of humor, he loved her good advice and her talent, and he loved the way she looked. "She was also smarter than I was," he remembers. Paula seemed her own person and was clearly not going to be overwhelmed by Judah's burgeoning career. Paula was enrolled in a master's program in music at Radcliffe just as Judah began his second year as a surgical resident. One night some months later, Judah arranged to have a night off and told Paula to get all dressed up. They were going out for an elegant dinner at the Ritz-Carlton, the fanciest date they'd ever had, and he was determined to make it special. Mass General would not take precedence this night. But then the phone rang, and Folkman heard the voice of Oscar DePriest.

DePriest was a year ahead of Folkman in his residency at MGH, and he was calling with an emergency. His dog had been hit by a car and was unconscious. DePriest thought the dog had a blood clot in his brain.

"His tail is going to one side," DePriest said, very distressed, hoping he'd get help from the best dog surgeon he knew.

"Oscar, I've never heard of that," Folkman said.

"You've got to come and operate, Judah," DePriest said.

Folkman heaved a big sigh. He didn't want this night to be ruined, but he knew he had no choice. DePriest had been the one who had taught him day and night—a sergeant to his private, as he considered it—so loyalty and protocol dictated that he now head for the hospital, dressed in his best suit, and operate on DePriest's dog. Paula, also dressed to the nines, came along and pitched right in. Ever the trouper, she squeezed the anesthesia bag.

Folkman cut into the dog's brain and found the blood clot. The surgery was progressing well but Paula saw that Judah was uncharacteristically grumbly. They were both used to the intrusions of medical emergencies, so Paula asked Judah why he was in such a bad mood.

"Actually," he said as he worked on the dog, "this isn't exactly what I had in mind for this evening. I was going to propose to you tonight."

Oh, Paula thought.

A few hours later, cleaned up after saving DePriest's dog, Judah made it official. He got on his knees and presented Paula with a diamond ring.

As a resident, Paula's future husband was by now a major step closer to being a full-fledged surgeon. Returning to the emergency room, no one told him what to do. When he was on night duty, the decisions and diagnoses were his. Victims of car accidents, heart attacks, diabetic comas, suicide attempts— the cases were his responsibility. He had to mend a hand blown apart by a firecracker, extract a peanut lodged in a child's airway, open a chest and massage a heart to get it beating again. He would call in a senior assistant resident for more serious emergencies such as an appendectomy. Just a year later, in 1959, the position of senior assistant resident was his, and he was the one residents called on. He was one of the teachers, a status he had once despaired of ever attaining. Along the way, a few of his peers dropped out of the surgical residency program, opting for something a bit less taxing like obstetrics or ophthalmology. A few even left medicine altogether, unable to stand the pressure and the endless hours of work. But Folkman was just getting started.

Or so he thought. It wasn't long after he began his year as senior assistant resident that he came home to find his latest letter of acceptance. It was from the United States Navy, bearing an offer he couldn't refuse. Judah Folkman had been drafted.

Chapter Four

———

LATE IN JUNE 1960, Judah and Paula Folkman rented a trailer, packed up all their possessions, and headed south out of Massachusetts. They had been married less than a week, the wedding in Paula's synagogue in Fall River having been co-officiated by her new father-in-law. They planned a brief honeymoon in Washington, D.C., then a train ride to Miami Beach, before Judah had to report for naval duty—a short side trip on the way to a long side trip. He hoped his military obligation would go quickly.

True, Folkman would be doing biomedical research at the National Naval Medical Center, not the most unpleasant work for a young lab-oriented doctor ordered to spend two years in the service. And he appreciated the chance to start his marriage under less intense conditions than those he was leaving behind in Boston. But the call to navy duty had come just as he was finally getting deeply into surgery, something he had anticipated since high school. He was already counting the 730 days until he could return to Boston to resume his residency. He would not realize until much later that this inconvenient interruption in his career would thoroughly and fundamentally decide his future. Nor could he foresee that his particular assignment, ostensibly to solve a logistical problem for an aircraft carrier, would lead him to a moment of discovery that decades later would perhaps change the world forever.

Having deferred his service obligation for nine years—through college, medical school, an internship, and halfway through his residency—Folkman had gotten his draft notice six months earlier and was summoned to an interview with the Office of Naval Personnel in Washington. There he learned that it wasn't just that his number had come up; his conscription had a purpose. Walking into a small office with nothing but a desk with a Coke bottle on it, Folkman met a naval officer who asked him about his research at Harvard. The officer scribbled notes on a little piece of paper and said enough for Folkman to realize that the government was specifically targeting draft-age doctors who had serious biomedical research experience, a very elite group.

A few days later, at six forty-five on the morning of July 1, Dr. Fred Becker, a pathologist-in-training from New York University, reported to the front desk of the Naval Medical Research Institute in Bethesda. "There was this tall, rather odd-looking navy officer arriving at the same time," Becker recalls. "We both walked up to a petty officer at the door and simultaneously said, 'I'm reporting in.' "

The petty officer looked them over and asked, "For what?"

"For research," each said, again almost simultaneously.

"Listen, nobody gets here this early," said the duty officer. "You'd be better off coming in about eight-thirty because you have to report to the captain. So why don't you just go have some breakfast?"

The two men said they'd already had breakfast.

"Well, have another. The navy officers' mess has everything you'd ever want, and it's only fifty cents. And could I make a suggestion, sirs? You both have your medical insignias on upside down."

The two new navy doctors fumbled with their medical pins, then started over to the officers' mess. "By the way, I'm Fred Becker," said the man from New York.

"I think I've heard of you at Harvard," said the other. "I'm Judah Folkman."

"I've heard of you, too," Becker replied, and said yes, he had a Harvard connection. He'd served his internship in a prestigious program called the Thorndike Service at the Harvard-affiliated Boston City Hospital.

As the two young doctors sat chatting in the mess hall, each confided to being a bit bemused about finding himself in the navy. But they agreed they should try to make the most of it and made loose plans to try to do some biomedical experiments together if they had enough time away from their main assignments, whatever they turned out to be.

Becker, like Folkman, was an accomplished scholar at a young age. A native New Yorker, he had been a premed, prelaw, and creative writing major at Columbia University. Then, as a medical student at NYU, he was chosen to study under Dr. Lewis Thomas, a renowned researcher who became as famous for his books—*The Lives of a Cell* and *The Medusa and the Snail*—as for his medicine. After his internship in Boston, Becker had returned to New York to become one of the first fellows in a program set up by Thomas that was to become the model for many of the country's best pathology training programs. By 1959, realizing his draft deferments were just about exhausted, Becker followed Thomas's suggestion that he enlist, requesting a position at the National Institutes of Health. But the slot he wanted was filled, and Becker ended up in the navy instead, at the Naval Research Institute in Bethesda.

Both Becker and Folkman knew they were lucky to be there. They could have been sent to sea or to some naval base half a world away. But they'd been inducted at a time when the government was taking a renewed interest in scientific research of all kinds. It had been only three years since the Soviet Union had sent the first artificial satellite, *Sputnik,* into Earth's orbit, a startling event that the United States took as a signal that a new and highly competitive scientific age had arrived, and that the stakes were high. It was the height of the cold war, and a flood of money soon began to accompany the government's new interest in physics, chemistry, biomedicine, rocketry, electronics, and atmospheric science to support America's quickly developing military and space programs.

The navy was off to a rough start in space. The nation's first attempt to orbit a satellite, the navy's Vanguard mission, had blown up on the launchpad. The service was also testing spacesuits by sending men aboard balloons to altitudes as high as a hundred thousand feet, and one volunteer came down at sea and drowned. Meanwhile, it was also the dawning of the nuclear submarine age, and the navy was working on all aspects of keeping people alive and well for long periods in close conditions underwater.

Once they'd checked in with the navy captain, Folkman and Becker got their assignments. Becker was given two projects, both related to the space program and so secret that he couldn't even talk about them with his colleagues down the hall, including Folkman. One of his projects dealt with radiation biology—the navy was anxious to know more about the Van Allen belts, zones of radiation above the Earth's atmosphere that astronauts might encounter—and the other concerned the physical effects of severe vibrations on living things. "They were afraid that a human being might be shaken to death aboard a rocket," Becker recalled.

Folkman's first task was considerably less intriguing and unrelated to the space race or cold war politics. Because of his experience in Boston, he was assigned to assist a cardiac surgeon in the operating room, helping run a blood pump that had been designed and built by doctors in Bethesda. So one or two days a week Folkman would sit on the floor in the operating room and make sure the pump worked during critical surgeries. The pump wasn't used often, leaving him plenty of time to work on assignments in the navy's medical research institute.

The institute, a collection of brown-tiled labs occupying several floors of a building near the big naval hospital, was born during World War I, and it had a distinguished history, producing pioneering work on shark repellents, blood preservation, radiation, and plastics. It had lost some of its momentum since World War II, but the government's renewed commitment to research had invigorated the place with a fresh sense of purpose. The lab setting was a natural for Folkman—he was the latest in a long line of Mass General doctors filling the same position—but the atmosphere was anything but academic. It was a strictly military operation, staffed by navy medical technicians. Some of the career corpsmen had served in World War II and in Korea and been assigned to Bethesda as a reward, and they returned the favor with hard work. They scoured the lab every night, even if it didn't seem to need cleaning.

Folkman and the six other doctors and scientists assigned to the lab were not natural soldier types (although Folkman had taken some ROTC classes at Ohio State and joked that he had "gotten an A in tank") and their status as researchers allowed them a relatively casual military life. Right after reporting in, the group was taken to the Marine Corps training camp in Quantico, Virginia, and given a short course in shooting guns. Then once a week they were instructed by an intelligence officer—"a real tight-ass," recalls Becker—who lectured them on military secrecy. Although they had to dress in naval officers' uniforms every day and prepare their labs for regular inspections, their actual military activities were minimal. For Folkman it didn't go much beyond practicing sit-ups and push-ups at home to make sure he would pass the physical fitness tests. He and Paula, who had found a job teaching music at a nearby junior high school, lived in a two-bedroom apartment within walking distance of the medical center. Only occasionally did he have to participate in military events outside the medical center. Once he had to wear his dress whites, even strapping on a ceremonial sword. Paula thought Judah looked quite spiffy, although when they saw a picture later, they realized that he'd put the sword on backward.

Folkman, of course, was much more comfortable handling pointed medical problems, and it wasn't long before he set to work on his first assignment: teaming with his new friend Becker on a high-priority biomedical project they had been briefed on shortly after arriving in Bethesda. The United States had proudly launched and commissioned the USS *Enterprise,* then the ne plus ultra of aircraft carriers. Nuclear powered, manned by nearly four thousand sailors, and capable of waging warfare in any ocean in the world, *Enterprise* was a huge, gray floating military city that could carry enough stores to stay at sea for a year at a time. It seldom needed to come in to refuel; food, mail, and aircraft fuel could be supplied at sea by tankers. In fact, only one weakness kept the carrier (as well as the nation's new nuclear submarines) from being completely independent at sea: the need for fresh blood.

The big aircraft carriers had four operating rooms with a precariously supplied blood bank. The ship had thousands of captive donors, of course, and ship assignments were made partly on the basis of blood type, so that each ship had a good supply of each. But the navy was anxious to figure out how to avoid using crews as living blood banks that would have to be tapped in emergencies. At the time there was no way to store blood for more than a few weeks—after twenty-three days the red blood cells started to break down. The navy research lab had been working on alternatives for years. Another Harvard physician, Charles Huggins, had preceded Folkman in the lab and developed a way to freeze blood using glycerine as a preservative. But he hadn't been able to figure out how to thaw the blood safely and remove the glycerine.

Assigned to the project by their commander, H. C. Sudduth, a naval officer with a medical degree, Folkman and Becker were asked to explore whether something other than fresh whole blood could be found and safely stored for long periods, for use as a substitute for blood in emergencies. They decided to see what could be done with hemoglobin, the iron-rich substance within red blood cells that, in addition to giving blood its red color, has the critical ability to pick up oxygen as the blood passes through the lungs and then release it as it moves through the body's tissues. Could that vital substance be dried and then reconstituted to make it capable of both supporting life and remaining viable while in storage? They requisitioned various hemoglobin solutions from a medical-products company for testing. Some they tried had been put through a drying process similar to the method that yields evaporated milk and instant coffee. It was prepared in powder form so it could be stored aboard ship indefinitely, then be reconstituted with saline water. In this dawning age of modern conveniences, this was instant blood—just add water. But would it work as well as blood?

Folkman and Becker considered injecting the hemoglobin-rich solution and about ten other preparations into live animals, but they realized the only valid way to test them would be to drain all the blood from the animals and replace it with the substitutes. Impossible. Folkman had another idea. He thought of Dr. Alexis Carrel and Charles Lindbergh. Carrel, a French surgeon and biologist who died in 1944, won a Nobel prize in 1912 for his work in suturing blood vessels, transfusing blood, and transplanting organs. In 1938, he published *The Culture of Organs* with the famed aviator Lindbergh, whose sister-in-law had died from failure of a heart valve. In the book, Lindbergh and Carrel described how they had invented a mechanical heart—a glass chamber through which nutrients and oxygen were pumped—that could keep organs and tissues alive in culture. Carrel had kept alive one specimen, tissue from a chicken's heart, for thirty-two years in his lab at Rockefeller University in New York. Judah Folkman had read *The Culture of Organs*, and remembered that one of the organs that had been kept alive with the Lindbergh-Carrel blood-pumping system was a rabbit thyroid gland. Folkman filled out a requisition form for live rabbits.

The thyroid gland seemed to offer a good way to test the blood substitutes. It would be easy to extract—the rabbits would be left with another gland so they would even survive—and it would be easy to watch. He and Becker could gauge the hemoglobin preparations' effectiveness by adding some radioactive iodine to the mix and then seeing how much thyroid hormone the gland produced and how much of the iodine appeared in the secreted hormone. Becker could further assess the health of the glands by examining the tissues under the microscope.

Folkman devised a plastic, boxlike system with a small, enclosed transparent chamber to hold the rabbit thyroid. The reconstituted liquid blood substitutes were pumped through a series of plastic tubes into the gland and out again, down to an oxygenator, and finally back through the gland. The apparatus—part Lindbergh, part Folkman—struck his bemused but impressed partner as something of a Rube Goldberg contraption, but it worked. The gland was perfused—kept alive with fresh, oxygenated fluid running through it. Becker checked the gland daily, cutting out a bit of tissue and examining the cells under his pathologist's microscope to see whether the fluid was helping the gland thrive or was slowly killing it. The better solutions kept the thyroid alive for three weeks, an impressive length of time for an organ living in a plastic box.

As they tested each of their fluids, Folkman and Becker took notes, compiled their data, and filed their reports. Because both men were efficient and ambitious, the task turned out to be simple and direct, completed far ahead of schedule. They reported which of the hemoglobin solutions seemed most promising. Their mission accomplished (though the creation of useful artificial blood would still take years to achieve), the two men were anxious to get back to their medical careers and they naively asked Commander Sudduth if they could go home. Permission was denied, of course; both had a year and a half to serve. The two young doctors were told to perform their regular chores—Folkman's was running the blood pump in the operating room—and find something to do.

They decided to work right in their lab. The blood research apparatus still worked. The rabbit thyroids were still going strong. "We thought the gland looked beautiful, dripping into this little chamber," Folkman recalls. Still thinking about the hemoglobin preparations they'd been testing, they wondered how far they could go with them. It was clear they could keep the perfused thyroid gland alive for weeks at a time and that it seemed to be functioning approximately as it would in the animal. But what else could they do? And what else could they learn? One research approach would be to test different compounds—say, poisons—to see how much toxicity the thyroid tissue could stand. Another would be to try to measure how sensitive the thyroid was to atomic radiation, a serious subject at this moment soon after the dawning of the atomic age. But instead of those ideas, Folkman and Becker decided to see if the perfused tissue was capable of sustaining growth. Could the thyroid gland, sitting in its small chamber, support new cell growth, for instance, and even repair a wound? If cut, would it grow cells to mend itself? The answer was clearly no: Folkman made a cut, and all the thyroid did was bleed all over the testing chamber.

What they needed was something they knew could grow vigorously. What about cancer cells? Both knew that malignant cells grow like crazy. So what might happen if they implanted some cancer cells directly onto the bed of thyroid tissue? Would the perfused gland allow cancer cells to grow and spread, even in tissue culture? It was an enticing question, and not only because it would stretch their blood-substitute experiments. Cancer was still a major enigma, so mysterious that no one was even sure whether it was a single disease or a hundred different ones. It was clear that tumor growth involved abnormal, ultrafast cell division, and that cancer was extraordinarily hard to defeat for reasons no one yet knew. Like many medical researchers, Folkman and Becker were fascinated by the question at the core of any discussion of the disease: What is it that controls the biological behavior of cancer cells? In fact, they had discussed cancer during their first conversation, over breakfast in the officers' mess early that morning back in July. Becker had a particular interest in liver cancer because as a pathologist he saw a lot of it; many forms of cancer metastasize to the liver and kill the patient. And even this early in his surgical career, Folkman had seen all kinds of tumors, each one confirming cancer's standing among humanity's greatest medical puzzles. He and Becker were both well aware that treatment of cancer was a dismal proposition. The most effective approach, which wasn't terrifically effective, was to surgically remove the tumors and hope they hadn't yet spread. Chemotherapy was in its early infancy, with few drugs available and even less understanding of their effects. Radiation biology, meanwhile, had only recently been conceived; much of the data was still shrouded in cold war secrecy. So what the two young doctors-in-training had was an opportunity to play a little, to explore some frontiers without worrying about the pressures of academia as they explored the deep and uncharted enigma of cancer. The navy wasn't interested in tenure.

Still, Folkman and Becker worried how they might justify their idea to their superiors. Cancer wasn't their assignment. They didn't figure the spit-and-polish military was ready to indulge mere scientific curiosity, and they contemplated doing the experiments on the sly. Finally they decided to describe their idea to Commander Sudduth as a continuation of their studies of blood substitutes, which it was. But it hardly mattered. Sudduth said, "Sure—work on anything you want. Just don't tell anyone."

To begin, Folkman and Becker had to get hold of some cancer tissue. They decided to use mouse melanoma cells—the fast-growing skin cells responsible for the most deadly, metatastic form of skin cancer. They would probably grow profusely and also could be easily seen because they were black. Becker knew a few of the pathologists working on cancer across the street at NIH, including a famous cancer biology researcher, Dr. Thelma Dunn, and he went over to get some mouse tumor samples. Folkman, meanwhile, ordered more rabbits. When they came in, he removed a thyroid and Becker transplanted the tumor cells into it. The cancer cells took hold almost immediately. The gland and its new burden of tiny tumors were kept alive by a constant flow of hemoglobin. The tumor cells grew for several days—more confirmation, it seemed, that the blood substitute was viable. Folkman and Becker found this fascinating because the fluid was not blood. There were no red cells, no white cells, and many normal blood factors were missing from the lab-prepared hemoglobin solutions.

But then they noticed something very odd and very remarkable. They saw that all of the little tumors suddenly stopped growing as soon as they reached a certain size, about one millimeter in diameter, less than the size of a pencil point. That was entirely strange because living tissues don't usually act that way. In biological systems, pieces and parts don't grow to exactly the same size; there's always a variation across a certain range. There should have been a few big tumors, some small ones, and a range of sizes in between. The strange phenomenon they saw suggested there must be some sort of gate, some physiological barrier or control mechanism, allowing all the little tumors to grow but only so far.

"They should be growing," Becker said to Folkman. They both expected the tumors to grow until they filled the entire chamber. *That* would have been a dramatically successful experiment, showing that the blood substitute could support such unfettered growth. *This* was something else—but what? Why did they all stop growing? And why at that particular size?

Their first hunch was the most obvious. Maybe they'd just killed the tumor cells, ruining the experiment by somehow mishandling them so they lived only briefly. After all, despite their mystique, cancer cells were far from indestructible. Killing them was easy if you bombarded them hard enough with deadly chemicals or radiation. "Great—hemoglobin would be a good treatment for cancer," Becker said offhandedly. "We're trying to make something that's not toxic," Folkman reminded him, still focusing on the blood-substitute project and fully aware that the key to cancer treatment was killing off cancer cells without killing the patient. Both were aware that the infant field of chemotherapy relied on a standard called the maximum tolerated dose (MTD), which involved giving cancer patients the strongest jolts of poison they could withstand, without killing them. Doctors were working on ways to kill as many tumor cells as possible and then allow the patient to rest for a few weeks or months before follow-up doses were given. Most cancer research focused not on how cancer cells grew or behaved but on how best to kill them. Researchers began to screen vast arrays of chemicals in search of effective but not deadly poisons to use against tumors.

But were the cancer cells in their glass chamber really dead? Was anything dead? Becker took sections of the thyroids and could see under his microscope that they were in fact alive, and so were the tumor cells. Pondering this, he and Folkman decided to see what would happen if they transplanted the little black cancer cells from the cultured gland into live animals. Would the new, more natural environment get them growing again? Becker quickly extracted some of the little melanoma dots and then implanted them into live mice. The results were startling: The tumor cells instantly awoke. They blossomed, growing rapidly into such massive, aggressive tumors that they soon killed the mice. But why? Why did these small tumors all stop growing at the same size in the well-perfused rabbit thyroid gland, yet grow like wildfire in live animals? What made the difference? It wasn't something immunological, since the cells did stay alive on the thyroid. Was there some kind of substance that controlled growth, some kind of growth factor present in the animal's body that was absent in the perfused gland?

On close examination, Folkman and Becker realized they were seeing something fundamental: The tiny tumors, alive but dormant in the thyroid gland, didn't have any obvious connections to a circulatory system. "Then Fred does the histology"—the cell analysis—"and we both look at it and see that the tiny tumors in the thyroid don't have any blood vessels," Folkman recalls. "And the big tumors in the animals are filled with little blood vessels." In fact, almost immediately after the black tumor cells had been taken from the rabbit gland and injected into the mice, networks of capillaries began growing very rapidly, apparently sprouting from surrounding tissue that was already well supplied with blood. Thus the expanding tumors were quickly engulfed by a nurturing bed of new blood vessels.

What did it mean? Neither Folkman nor Becker could say for sure, though they sensed they had observed something very important—especially Folkman. It was Becker's sense that this little experiment and its results had lit a fuse within his partner. "I thought it was interesting," Becker recalls. "Judah thought it was terrific."

By now Becker had come to regard Folkman as a marvel, someone whose mind worked every second. He remembered the day, not long after they'd reported for duty, when the hard-line intelligence officer at Quantico lectured on secrecy. Becker looked around at the doctors and scientists, all military neophytes listening to a lecture on the cloak-and-dagger methods the Russians might use to spy on their work. "We sat there kind of stunned—what the hell could we give away? We didn't know anything. But I glanced over, and there was Judah taking notes on intelligence methods. He was the one person who was really paying attention. I remember I once called in a plumber, and Judah even took notes about what that guy told him about cleaning the drain. He learns from all of this and thinks about these things. Every time he runs into something of interest, he goes back to the lab to see if it's applicable." In one instance, Folkman heard a news report that a civilian diving crew had been killed when their small submarine became tangled in cables hanging from a sunken ship. Folkman heard that the atmosphere inside their tiny submarine contained a high percentage of helium. He also knew that helium carries heat away very rapidly and surmised that the crew had died because they simply got too cold. He went into the lab and fashioned a blanket that used helium to control body heat during surgery. "He's always asking, What does it mean and is it useful?" Becker says. "And he's never cowed by the probabilities being against him."

Another young medical draftee, Dr. David Long, a cardiac surgeon from the University of Minnesota, had joined the navy lab early in 1961, just as Folkman and Becker were starting their experiments with the tumor cells. Observing from his corner across the room, he was struck by how clearly Folkman saw that the results revealed a previously unknown biological phenomenon. "He knew it right away," says Long. "He could grasp things, he could see right through them. He was standing there, and he told me what was happening. And I believed him."

Long soon began his own collaboration with Folkman and saw firsthand his extraordinary ability to seize on a scientific moment and turn it into something important. Both men were using plastics—silicone rubber tubing, or "silastic"—in their experiments, and they noticed that some of the special biological dyes they used stained the tubing, while others left them clean. Curious, they conducted experiments in their spare time over the course of a year and found that oil-solubility was the key. The dyes that dissolved in oil crept right through the walls of plastic tubing, in essence slowly leaking out. Folkman and Long realized that what they might have on their hands was an important new way to deliver drugs, hormones, or other agents. To test their idea, they loaded small amounts of various drugs into three-quarter-inch-long silicone rubber tubes, and sealed the tubes with silicone rubber cement. The little tubes were then sterilized and implanted into animals' hearts. The tubes successfully released the drugs at slow, steady rates for very long periods.

But were there any side effects? One day Folkman asked Fred Becker to look at some tissue samples he'd extracted from hearts. "What are you doing with hearts?" Becker asked. Folkman told him that he and Long had been working on an idea to implant silicone rubber cylinders that could slowly release drugs. Becker looked at the sections under his microscope and saw no inflammation. Folkman and Long prepared a paper on their findings, later published in the *Journal of Surgical Research,* and the navy filed for patent protection for the idea. Years later, Becker realized that in his spare time, almost as a hobby, Folkman had created a major new biomedical industry: the world of implantable capsules. Its most famous application would be a long-term contraceptive known as Norplant.

Working alongside Folkman in the navy's laboratory, Long, like Becker, came to regard him as an indefatigable source of scientific intuition. He noticed that Folkman could name every Nobel laureate in medicine and describe the history of their work in detail. At first Long thought this was some sort of infatuation—like a baseball fan memorizing Hall of Fame names—but then he realized that Folkman was actually studying methods of discovery. "He was examining the thought processes, the invention processes, of these truly brilliant people," Long says. Folkman, in fact, had read the papers of the Nobel winners, trying to discern a common approach. "What came through," he said years later, "was open-mindedness, enormous curiosity, and obsessive persistence."

Folkman decided he had seen something new and important in the dramatically different ways that tumors grew in the two distinct environments, something worthy of that curiosity and open-mindedness. It was indeed a bold view in the context of the times. Even noticing blood vessels and how they grew was unusual; few scientists would have considered it a fruitful area of general study, let alone focusing on cancer. Finding the right chemicals to kill tumor cells was the hot topic that attracted researchers and the people who financed them. As for the physiology of blood vessels in general, it would have been hard to find anyone who considered it anything but a closed subject, unworthy of exploration. There were arteries and veins, they carried oxygenated blood to all the tissues and waste-laden blood away through the heart, into the lungs, and out again. Simple. Direct. Case closed.

With Folkman as lead author, the three young navy researchers prepared a brief report on their organ-culture work and submitted it to the Surgical Forum. But the paper, just four hundred words long when it was published in 1962, described only part of what the team had observed. It simply reported how they had grown tumors in an organ-culture system, saying nothing about what was most interesting: how the tumor cells all stopped growing when they reached a certain size—perhaps hinting at how certain biological "on-off" controls worked—and what happened when the same cells were transplanted into the mice. And nothing was said about the most intriguing observation of all: the important difference they'd noticed about the growth of new blood vessels and their relationship to tumors. Unwilling to go too far too soon, Folkman included only the most veiled reference to what he was actually thinking. "This technique," he and his colleagues wrote, "may prove to be useful in other areas of cancer research, for example, as a method of studying cell adhesiveness and metastatic potential of various tumors."

Of course, Folkman didn't know exactly where the discovery would lead or even when he would get back on the trail. He had years of training in clinical medicine and surgery ahead of him. But he knew this: In this most unlikely setting, working among young doctors in navy uniforms, an irresistible puzzle had been placed before him. It was an enigma that might indeed require obsessive persistence to unravel, but as Folkman prepared to return to Boston, he knew he was taking unfinished business with him. "This is where I'm going," he told Fred Becker, fully aware that it was a destination in the distance, beyond what his mind could see.

Chapter Five

———

FOR JUDAH FOLKMAN, RETURNING TO BOSTON in mid-1962 was like being doused in a cold shower. Reentering the intense life of a surgical resident in the demanding environment of Massachusetts General Hospital was a jolt to his system after two relatively leisurely years in the navy. In fact, the hours and pressures he faced, especially during a tour of duty in the emergency room soon after his return, made Mass General seem more like the military than the navy had. It was a form of combat, and he was like a midranking officer, taking orders from senior men, barking them out to those underneath. The battles were round-the-clock and often chaotic, and the images remained forever in his memory:

A patient is brought in vomiting blood all over the floor. They assign you that patient and you have to get an IV into the vein immediately. But you can't find the vein. If you're too slow, the senior resident says, "Get out of the way!" and does it himself. So you have to perform—fast. You need blood, and you have to let them know you need blood, now. You have to get some blood back in—you don't want the heart to stop because that will cause brain damage. And you're still trying to work out the diagnosis and decide whether to head for the operating room, while three other cases come in, patients with gunshot wounds, or alcoholics with liver disease, or auto accident victims. You can't control what's coming in. You're constantly deploying people. Then you're supposed to decide whether you need more help. Many times you've got to free a doctor up to go to the next patient. You have to do triage, decide who has to be served first. So you're going all the time. It's like a fire department with many fires and only three fire engines.

The pressures didn't ease much when Folkman moved on to the operating room. He was on duty at five-thirty every morning, planning, researching, and performing operations throughout the day, seeing patients, guiding interns. "Always under pressure," he remembers. "You have to avoid mistakes. You're learning, doing some tremendously complicated procedures. By six o'clock you get through, but you've still got to see patients in the wards. And when there are night surgeries you may finish up at midnight, and half the time you've never even had lunch."

Not that any of this came as a surprise. Folkman had been determined to become a surgeon almost since the day he had first met Robert Zollinger while still in high school, and he was well aware that each step in the process would be harder than the one before. Nobody cared if you were tired. Eating and sleeping were your problem. Years later, state legislatures would outlaw such relentlessly grueling regimens, but in the 1960s, doctors in training expected and got the worst. As Dr. Michael Gimbrone, who went through the same program a few years after Folkman, put it: "It was sort of an Iron Man thing. You were given more responsibility than you would have thought legally possible."

The experience allowed Folkman to hone his natural gifts. He became a true artist with the scalpel, each successful operation confirming the almost unconscious thought that had pushed him into the operating room in the first place: that, in contrast to a doctor with a chronically ill patient who treats and treats and treats that patient without ever really making him well, a surgeon could do something for the patient and it would stay fixed.

Folkman was also keenly observant and a natural mentor, so he was simultaneously learning and teaching. He picked up cues and clues from everything, even in the hectic atmosphere of a busy emergency room, and he was ready to share everything he learned. As a senior resident, he decided to put together his own guide for what doctors should do in medical emergencies. He asked all his colleagues in residency to write down, on index cards, every situation they had personally experienced where a patient would have died within thirty minutes if nothing had been done to intervene: cardiac arrest, anaphylactic shock, transfusion reactions, airway obstructions, and so on. At first, he got not one response. Then, as a joke to his woefully underpaid brethren, he offered to pay a quarter for each life-threatening emergency. Then the cards started to come, and they kept coming—three thousand of them in all, many more than he could dole out quarters for.

"I put them all on the floor, all three thousand of them, and I went through them," Folkman remembers. "There was every kind of emergency you could imagine. But only fourteen that occurred over and over again." For these, he wrote a quick guide to saving lives. For example: Blood pressure is going down but pulse is going up. What does that mean? One of two possibilities: The patient is losing blood or having heart failure. Experience shows that nine times out of ten, it is blood loss. But what about that one case in ten that is heart failure? Folkman's rule: Look at the neck veins. If there is no blood pressure, but the neck veins are standing up, it means the heart is failing, because the blood is pouring into the heart and can't come out. Simply put, high neck veins means heart failure; no neck veins means blood loss. But what if it's the latter, and no blood is visible? That means it's internal bleeding—either inside the gastrointestinal tract or outside it. When he asked students how they would figure out which one it was, they usually said, "Take an X ray." His reply: "No! Listen to the abdomen. If there's blood inside the gut you'll hear a rumble like you've never heard before, because the blood is stimulating the gut to get it out. But if it's outside the gut, say from a ruptured spleen, it will cause paralysis of the gut and you'd hear no sound. So in two seconds you could find out where it was."

Folkman wrote a set of terse guidelines for each of the fourteen situations, and his colleagues soon began asking for mimeographed copies. They dubbed his collection "The Bang Bang Book." "If you know these fourteen, you'll look brilliant," Folkman told his colleagues. Before long he turned the information into an informal evening course for interns about to become residents. The class wasn't an official part of the curriculum, but it was always standing room only.

A few months after his return to Boston, Folkman was sent on the road. The rotation system sent residents to work for months at a time in hospitals in the Boston suburbs whose house staffs often lacked the advanced surgical skills of the Mass General residents. It was a good deal both for the local hospitals, which got much-needed help with tough cases, and for the residents, who got a chance to perform challenging surgery away from the "mother ship." A rent-free house was part of the deal, but so was a job description that included being on call twenty-four hours a day.

Folkman's first such rotation was to the hospital in Salem, north of Boston. "About the third week I was there—I'll never forget it—there was a forty-year-old lady, a Polish woman, who came in with a horrible duodenal ulcer," he recalls. "They started to operate on her but got to a point where they couldn't close it." The duodenum is the first part of the small intestine, and it can be hard to close safely. If a surgeon closes it too narrowly, foods might not be able to pass through it. As Salem's surgeons struggled with the problem, Folkman was finishing a procedure in a nearby operating room, and the staff surgeon asked him to take a look. They were about to close their patient up without finishing the operation—every surgeon's nightmare—and send her by ambulance downtown to Mass General for a second operation. But Folkman said to wait. A great gastrointestinal surgeon, Dr. Claude Welch, had recently invented a procedure to cope with that duodenal problem, and Folkman thought he could perform the surgery. He had studied Welch's research paper and had even watched him demonstrate the operation. "I've seen him do it," Folkman told the Salem surgeon. "You use a soft rubber tube, you put it in, and you close the duodenum around the tube very loosely and put the tube out to drainage. You wait two weeks in the hospital, and then you slowly pull the tube out." The local surgeon trusted Folkman and allowed him to perform the procedure on the patient. The operation succeeded, and news of the tour-de-force achievement soon spread throughout Salem Hospital—more important, it spread back to the main hospital in Boston.

Although the residents were not always aware of it, their skills were constantly being assessed by senior members of the Mass General staff. It was a silent evaluation process that would influence the direction of their careers. Two of the twelve senior residents would be selected as chief residents in surgery and stay on for a seventh year. For the ten who didn't make it, the announcement signaled the end of their training, a vaguely anticlimactic conclusion to this long and grueling road to surgery. There was, of course, no shortage of exciting career opportunities for any doctor who had finished a Mass General residency, but to be named chief resident was confirmation that a doctor was the best of the best and that the sky was the limit. The recipients of the honor were likely to achieve board certification sooner than the rest, and being chief resident was a career springboard to a top position at almost any major medical center in the country. It was not unlike the competition for "Top Gun" at the navy's highly competitive combat flight school in southern California. These are the pilots you want at the controls if you're in trouble. If there was any doubt about the value and prestige of being named a chief resident at Mass General, all one had to do was gaze on the wall on which hung photographs, never to be removed, of every chief resident in the hospital's history.

It was a mysterious selection process. There were no interviews, no obviously objective criteria. And as far as anyone could tell, it was more or less the decision of one man: Edward Churchill, the chief of surgery. The senior residents could only guess how much influence the staff surgeons had on the outcome, though one thing they did figure out was that some of the rotations (those to hospitals in Salem, Lynn, Middlesex, and to major wards in the main hospital) involved more responsibilities than others. "So people began to understand that they were on an inner track or an outer track," Folkman recalls. "Salem was on the inner track, and Middlesex was on the inner track, and some of the guys didn't get there."

Folkman knew he was on the inner track, and realized that pulling off the Welch procedure on the patient in Salem did nothing to hurt his chances of being named chief resident in surgery. But he had never been given to fits of overconfidence. Nor, on the other hand, did he tend to shortchange himself. He knew exactly what his strengths and weaknesses were and didn't let sentiment cloud his judgment. "I've never met anybody who had a better understanding of himself," remembers Fred Becker, his navy colleague. Becker, who had returned to New York after his two years in Bethesda, came up to Boston to visit Folkman and Paula around the time of the selection process, and one day the two young doctors strolled alongside the Charles River, discussing their careers. Folkman had figured out who his main competitor for chief resident would be, and he was worried: He thought the other senior resident might be a little more dexterous than he was. "Here was this unbelievably brilliant guy, a super surgeon—I would have had Judah operate on me any day, any time—and I'm listening to him analyze himself." Becker was not in the least surprised when Folkman later called with the news. "Of course, Judah was chosen," Becker said.

Folkman, flushed with excitement and pride at the appointment, was also well aware of the immense challenge before him. As he puts it, "The chief resident is the busiest doctor in the hospital—period." He would be in the hospital almost all the time, and despite the word "resident" in the title, he would function more as a senior surgeon than as a doctor in training. In fact, he had more experience than many older doctors at other hospitals. By this point he had already performed thousands of operations, from appendectomies to tumor removals. He had dealt with head injuries and spinal injuries, had tried to reattach arms, had rebuilt faces, unblocked intestines, and removed ulcers. Now as chief resident Folkman was not only directly on the firing line, he was in charge of the army, working directly under Dr. Churchill. Operating room assignments, personnel issues—virtually everything having anything to do with surgery was his responsibility. Other doctors' problems now became his problems. Their mistakes were his mistakes. And in between, he performed his own surgeries. With his position came a few perks. He had his own operating room, with his own staff of nurses. And he asked an orderly he knew, Paul Wesley, to be his personal operating-room assistant.

On any given day, there were fifty or sixty or seventy patients on the wards, including terribly sick people, dying people, patients waiting to go into the operating room, and others being wheeled out. It was a time before intensive care units were well developed, so concentrated in one ward would be people in comas and others with perforated ulcers, extreme diabetes, ruptured aneurysms, or severe auto accident injuries. It was Folkman's job to decide who got surgery and when, and who would perform which operations. He had to be sure the right doctors were doing the right procedures, that inexperienced interns didn't operate before they were ready, and that when they were ready they worked with the right senior resident. "You had all these personalities," Folkman remembers. "Some people are whiners, always whining because there is too much work. And there were also some who were so happy just to be there."

Being in a top leadership position for the first time, Folkman now had the added burden of guiding and sometimes disciplining younger doctors who were having trouble coping with the extreme pressures of hospital training. A few years later, after his chief residency was over and he was running a major department, he would even have to remove a junior resident who took his frustrations out on patients. "He was tired and he was surly," Folkman remembers. "The nurses were complaining; there were mountains of complaints. I had a talk with him, but he didn't change. So we actually had to remove him. Eventually he was moved to plastic surgery, where there were no big emergencies. He just couldn't handle it."

Being chief resident was a heady assignment, but the prestige was not without its limits. Although he had only one main boss (Churchill, the chief of surgery) Folkman often had to defer to various visiting professors, who came in to do surgery, and occasionally to private surgeons, some of them very well known, who treated elite patients. These patients—"the Gold Coast trade," as the medical staff called them—were usually cared for in wards in Baker House and Phillips House, where the hospital rooms were so large and luxurious that some even had grand pianos. "You'd make the rounds, and there would be Cary Grant, or someone like that," Folkman remembers. And suddenly the chief resident was not quite so chief or quite so esteemed. He was there to serve the famous person's famous doctor. "You were their boy,"

Folkman says. It was actually a throwback to the time in the nineteenth century when surgeons operated in people's homes, and the young doctors were considered the surgeons' helpers.

Folkman followed protocol, but he was more than a mere helper. On one occasion, he was making rounds with Dr. Edgar Willock, the hospital's great vascular surgeon, when they stopped at the bed of a man on whom Willock had performed a major blood vessel operation. But just as Willock and Folkman were talking to the patient, the man's heart stopped, and he collapsed on the spot. Willock was shocked—the patient had been ready to go home—and suddenly the room was in pandemonium. At the time, most patients would have died under these circumstances, even in one of the world's greatest hospitals. Indeed, Willock fully expected the patient to die. But Folkman quickly cut the man's chest open and massaged his heart, getting it going again. "We closed him up, and he was perfect." Ripping open a chest and massaging a heart by hand was a new procedure, and to men of Willock's generation, Folkman as much as anyone personified an emerging new age in medicine. His actions were right out of "The Bang Bang Book."

DAILY CHALLENGES, NIGHTLY HEROICS, relentless pressures—and yet, it all seemed almost straightforward compared to what was going on in the home of Judah and Paula Folkman. To make his grueling schedule half livable, Folkman and Paula had rented one of the new Charles River Park Apartments, which had just been built across the street from the medical center. When the midnight calls inevitably came, Folkman could slip over to the hospital in no time at all. Paula, meanwhile, had found work of her own in Boston, using her music training to land a job as an editor and proofreader for the large Boston-based music publishing company, E. C. Schirmer. It was a job she could do at home as she and Judah began their family.

Laura Folkman was born in 1964, and to her parents' great distress, she had cystic fibrosis, an inborn disorder that would forever make her health precarious. She would be terribly vulnerable to even ordinary infections, while serious complications such as intestinal blockages and pancreatic insufficiency were possible. The irony of the situation was not lost on Laura's parents. Folkman remembered his days as a medical student with Robert Gross at Children's Hospital and how he had sat beside Gross as he tried to console the parents of children born with serious illnesses for which there was little or no treatment. *We're working on it,* Gross would say. Now Folkman was one of those parents.

Still, Laura was born with immediate access to the very best in medicine, so her parents were spared some of the feelings of helplessness and vulnerability that commonly accompany the illness of a child. "I took really good care of her," Folkman would say years later. And Paula added: "*We* took fabulous care of her, as a matter of fact." They quickly picked up every hint of infection and treated them early. The Folkmans kept a special enclosure, a mist tent, ready for Laura. And they had the best experts at Children's to help with her treatment. In one instance, Laura was running a very high temperature, and her father brought her into the hospital to see Dr. Harry Shwachman, a pediatric pulmonologist, the "father" of cystic fibrosis diagnosis. Shwachman stabilized Laura with an IV but was worried about keeping her in the hospital for two weeks, as was customary. Laura might pick up another infection from one of the other cystic fibrosis patients already there. Instead Shwachman arranged for all the IV equipment to be taken home, where Folkman himself could get Laura through to recovery.

Cystic fibrosis is known as a recessive genetic disease, striking only when each parent contributes a mutant copy of the gene to the infant. Neither Judah nor Paula had had any inkling that either of them—let alone both—were carriers of the defective genes. Until an affected child was born, there was no way to know they carried the gene, beyond having a family history in which cystic fibrosis cases were already known, and neither the Folkman nor the Prial family was aware of any history of cystic fibrosis. Now the Folkmans had to decide whether to have another child, despite a one-in-four chance that this child, too, would inherit the disorder. For the first time doctors were beginning to make progress in caring for young cystic fibrosis patients—but that progress had limits, as Laura's experience showed. The Folkmans had long and frequent discussions before deciding, despite the odds, to have another baby.

Kenneth Folkman was born a year after Laura. And the news was bad again. In fact, it was worse: This baby, too, had cystic fibrosis, and the complications were even more severe than Laura's. Kenneth was born across the street from Children's Hospital, at Richardson House in the famed Boston Lying-In Hospital, and it was soon obvious that he was suffering from intestinal blockages that would require immediate surgery. Folkman quickly called in Dr. Robert Gross, his old mentor, who arranged for an operating room at Children's Hospital and an ambulance to bring Kenneth around to the back of Children's. The rules prevented them from simply walking the baby across the street, but Gross didn't want to waste a minute when it came to Judah and Paula Folkman's baby son. He strode over to the birthing hospital himself, wrapped Kenneth in a blanket, signed him out, and personally carried him across the street for surgery. The surgery cleared the intestines, but it was not enough to save Kenneth's life. Soon after, the baby's lungs failed, and, only a few weeks after his birth, he died.

For the more fortunate Laura, constant loving care did pay off. Her parents succeeded in nurturing her safely through childhood, and they ultimately decided to have a third child. Their daughter Marjorie would be born in 1969. To her parents' profound relief, she escaped cystic fibrosis.

Being the father of sick children put Folkman in a special position, one that helped shape the doctor he was becoming. He was more aware of what it is like to be on the other end of all the diagnoses, tests, and treatments he had trained to deliver. It only deepened a conviction that already came naturally to him: his belief that compassion is as elemental to being a great doctor as is brilliant technique. Folkman regarded his interactions with patients as something far beyond an occupational obligation. He strove to be the best and the fastest at every procedure he performed, but he also remained acutely aware that a living, breathing person lay on the table in front of him. He devoted full attention to fine-tuning his ability to read every patient's body language and emotions; he held the children and listened to their parents; he knew the patients' names and histories; he saw them day or night. He tried to build trust and always felt a certain pride when patients started introducing him to their relatives as "my doctor." It was at that point he felt he had attained trust, the patient's unspoken certainty that he or she wouldn't be abandoned. "Gradually you learn," Folkman later reflected, "and you begin to *give hope.* You don't promise things, but the worst damage is destroying hope. It's very easy to destroy hope, and very hard to get it back. Raising false hope is a big fear all physicians have, but patients don't really ever punish you for it."

Folkman's counterpart, chief resident of medicine Dr. Jay Sanders, remembers standing with him at the bedsides of patients who were on the brink of death. The young doctors struggled to decide whether to try something— a new procedure or medicine, anything—or to let go and allow the patients to die with some measure of dignity. Often Folkman would try to treat both the patient's disease and his or her emotional needs. He could see when a patient was terrified, asking God why this had happened to him, and was in dire need of peace and comfort. He could see when a patient's family was terrified as well. Not all doctors were able to confront the challenge of easing their patients' fears, but Folkman felt he would be incomplete as a physician unless he tried. He had plenty of mentors helping him become a brilliant doctor, but there was only one who could really teach him how to be a more humane one. He didn't tell many of his colleagues, but he began to call his father. "He told me in a shy way that he would call his dad and go over the case, and then come back and work with the patient," Sanders recalls. Folkman was determined to become exactly what his father hoped he would on that day in the hospital in Michigan when Judah was just ten. He was becoming a rabbi-like doctor.

His father's sage advice became especially important in a case when Folkman had to place a life-and-death decision in the hands of a patient's family. He faced a bitter division. Some relatives wanted to give up and turn off the respirator that was keeping the patient alive; others adamantly argued against it. "Listen to the person who takes care of the patient" is how Folkman remembers his father's advice. "Always, the ones who are furthest away are the loudest. They never called while he was well, and they're trying to make up for it now. So what you do is sit down with that person who cared for the patient, who cleaned up the vomit, gave the medicines, and did all the hard work. You ask that person, and you really hear it from the heart. You just be quiet. And then out comes half an hour of feelings and memories and wishes."

Folkman felt that such emotional interactions were so important that he sometimes shared his father's advice with residents and interns. After a while, when faced with especially difficult, heartrending cases, some of Folkman's colleagues would turn to him and ask: "What would your father say?"

Folkman applied the same openness to his relationships with his subordinates. His style was to bring people along rather than beat them into submission, as some chief residents were known to do. To adopt the medical-star personality of some surgeons would have been wholly unnatural to him. "Everybody loved Judah; he wasn't a 'surgical' personality," Sanders said. The one time he had lost control, he'd learned his lesson—from the big man, Dr. Churchill. It had happened years before, when Folkman was barely out of medical school.

"I was just a second-month intern, when you're very nervous because you don't know a lot of things," Folkman recalls. "My patient was eighty-five percent covered with burns. Usually, more than fifty percent and you were dead, and this patient did eventually die. But you never know whether you can get him through. There wasn't a burn unit like there is now, so we were out on the ward and I had only one IV. He had only one available vein left because he was burned everywhere. I had this IV protected, and the bottle was dripping and somehow while I was operating the nurse had let the IV run down, so it clotted. I was very upset, and I bawled her out on the ward. I said, 'Just look at what you've done!' Within four hours, there was a call to come and see Dr. Churchill. Now Churchill had been a brigadier general in the war, so the message said, 'Come in dress uniform,' which meant get out of your scrubs, get dressed, and come see him." Churchill had once been assigned to work in Europe with General George S. Patton, and had been in charge of surgery for the army in Europe for four years. At Mass General, Churchill was every bit the surgeon in chief. "In his office, he had no chairs. So you stood in front of his desk. He said, 'Folkman. Do you see this stack of records?' He pointed to a pile that almost reached the ceiling. 'These are all residents waiting to get your slot. Now, over here'—he pointed to a much smaller stack—'these are nurses. We need nurses. We don't need residents. Now, in your class you're the only one who has a chance to make it to professor. So why don't you grow up and act like one now? Dismissed!' "

Folkman never again dressed down a nurse in public.

JAY SANDERS REMEMBERS the night well. It was the first time Judah Folkman first told him about his bright idea. Like Folkman, Sanders had been drafted while in the middle of his residency at Mass General. Instead of the navy, however, Sanders had been assigned to work for the U.S. Public Health Service in the massive medical research center, the National Institutes of Health. It counted as military service, but the surroundings were decidedly unmilitary: no uniforms, no saluting, and definitely no guns. With almost no prospect of having to fight anyone, Sanders and his fellow draftee-doctors called themselves "the Yellow Berets."

Sanders had returned to Mass General at the completion of his two-year hitch in Bethesda and put himself back on track for what was to become a vigorous and creative life in medicine. Decades later, he managed to simultaneously hold positions at Yale, Johns Hopkins, and the University of Miami Medical Center, while also serving as scientific director of the Commercial Space Center in Florida for NASA. He had developed a special interest in planning the health support systems for astronauts who would live aboard the planned space station, as well as for those who might one day land on Mars. But in the spring of 1964, Sanders was finishing his long residency at Mass General, celebrating the news that he, too, was one of The Chosen: He would serve as chief resident in medicine.

The two men, one a surgeon and the other an internist, became colleagues and good friends. There was something of a siege mentality at work: Just getting through the long, difficult days and nights often constituted a triumph, and they often got through together. They shared experiences and background. Sanders, too, was Jewish, and that year, 1964, they both found themselves on duty on the holiest night of the year: the eve of Yom Kippur. Under their care were some very sick patients, including a few who might not survive until morning. "We decided on that night we were going to find out whether God is Jewish or not," Sanders recalls. "You're supposed to fast for Yom Kippur and not do any work. So we decided that God wouldn't be out taking any patients. And if any of our patients died, it would prove that God isn't Jewish." None died that night.

Folkman and Sanders often went down to the cafeteria to grab a midnight meal. It was a highlight of the day, a time to relax for a few minutes and reflect on the day, or the week, or the future. Sometimes their conversations drifted to the subject of what might come next for them. What would they do at the end of their terms as chief resident? One night, Folkman told Sanders that in addition to becoming a surgeon he planned to do research. And the research he expected to pursue was something he had first noticed during his time in the navy lab. "He began to unfold this story for me," Sanders recalls. "He said he had come across this interesting finding, that you can grow tumor cells in culture dishes and they grow and grow, and then stop."

Although Folkman had been forced to put his pursuit of the phenomenon on hold for the last three years, he had still toyed with what it might mean— in his head, if not in a lab. Bolstered by an obscure piece of research he had found in the pathology department library, he was excited by the prospect that the experiments he'd conducted with Fred Becker were the beginning of something special. He told Sanders about his ideas. "I think the tumor is making something that causes the host to grow blood vessels and feed the tumor," he said. And what if there were also balancing substances that *inhibit* blood vessel growth? What if they could be found? "That could be the one bullet you'd need to get rid of tumors."

Clearly Folkman had allowed his mind to wander. He was not above waxing optimistic to his friend, who found the theory positively elegant. "It was extremely simple and very compelling in its logic," Sanders said. "I thought it was absolutely fascinating. And Judah said that was what he was going to pursue."

Folkman's chance to do research was approaching. As the end of his tenure as chief resident approached in 1965, he had choices to make. Where he went now would not be the decision of an admissions committee, or the United

States government, or the chief of surgery. Now well known as a star surgeon, the cream of the crop, he could virtually write his own ticket. He could go into private practice in a major city like New York and perhaps become one of those famous private surgeons raking in tons of money. But the scent of a big payoff after all those years of grueling training and a humble lifestyle held little appeal for Folkman. In passing, he thought of the other extreme, the Peace Corps. But he'd already given two years to the navy, and in truth, he was more committed than ever to the academic life, a career that would allow him to do what had always come naturally to him, ever since those what-did-you-learn-today conversations over the dinner table: *think, think, think.* He would teach, perform surgery, and when the time and circumstances were right, he would finally pursue his research—starting with the seductive question that had laid dormant since his time in the navy.

Folkman wanted to stay at Harvard but wasn't sure the medical school would offer him a position. He was wrong: The first offer he got was to remain at Mass General and become an instructor at the Harvard Medical School, certainly a plum job. Simultaneously, he was offered a job at the Harvard-affiliated Boston City Hospital, which also included a position as instructor at the Harvard Medical School. City Hospital was less prestigious than Mass General, but the man who made the proposal, Dr. William McDermott, pushed the offer with a point that rang true for Folkman. McDermott, a new Harvard professor who had just taken over the respected Fifth Harvard Surgical Service at City Hospital, advised Folkman that the best thing he could do for himself was to leave Mass General. You should never stay at the hospital where you were trained, he told Folkman. You will always be seen there as a resident, no matter how great you become. You'll never live that down. So you must move if you want to develop.

It was a hard decision: Turning down an offer from Mass General took real guts. "But, in fact, McDermott was right," Folkman reflected years later. "Of all the people who stayed there, nothing ever really happened to them. They all stayed in this cocoon; the really great contributions came from the people who left."

As a newly minted instructor, Folkman began teaching third- and fourth-year students who came over to City Hospital from the Harvard Medical School. He was also in charge of the surgical service at City, rotating duties with other instructors, teaching the chief resident, making rounds. Meanwhile, he became board-certified in surgery and in thoracic surgery. But not too long after his arrival at City Hospital, Folkman heard rumblings that changes were looming across town at Children's Hospital, and they centered around his former mentor, Robert Gross, the chief of surgery. It turned out that the hospital trustees had lingering concerns that Gross's concentration on cardiac surgery meant the hospital had for too long been paying insufficient attention to general pediatric surgery, and there was a movement to replace him. The timing was convenient: Gross was closing in on retirement age, so it was logical for the hospital to begin thinking about an heir apparent. Ultimately, in 1967, the trustees sorted things out by creating a new position for Gross—cardiac surgeon-in-chief—that would effectively usher in the future by placing him to one side. The man they chose as his successor, the surgeon who would lead the number one children's hospital in the world, was thirty-four-year-old Judah Folkman.

Despite his star status in surgery, Folkman was a highly unusual and controversial choice to fill the position of surgeon-in-chief, especially in the eyes of many of the top surgeons from all over the country who coveted the job and didn't get it. Not only was Folkman very young for such a distinguished position, but he would be making a quantum leap from instructor, the lowest rung on the academic ladder, to full professor. The normal tenure-track progression of instructor, assistant professor, associate professor, and then professor almost always took a decade or longer. Moreover, Folkman, while a gifted general surgeon, was not thoroughly trained and experienced in pediatric surgery.

Folkman was not without his own doubts. Shortly before being named to the top spot at Children's, he had turned down a similar offer at Beth Israel Hospital, another Harvard-affiliated institution in Boston. It was an impressive display of prudence over ambition: Folkman had felt he was not ready to be chief of surgery at a major hospital. But then Gross came to him just a few months later, urging him to make himself a candidate for the position at Children's. Folkman had the same misgivings about his qualifications, but after thinking it over and talking about it with Paula, he decided that demurring would be too great a disappointment—even an insult—to his mentor. He agreed to apply for the job.

Gross, of course, pushed his protégé's candidacy, but there was a limit to his influence. The decision was firmly in the hands of a committee of fifteen professors that included the likes of Dr. Francis Moore, chairman of surgery at Brigham Hospital, and Dr. Jacob Fine, the chair of surgery at Beth Israel, the hospital Folkman had just turned down. The committee interviewed a wide field of candidates and decided that Gross was right: Folkman was too impressive to pass up. He had performed spectacularly at Mass General, was doing the same at City—with scarce resources and meager staff—and he seemed a rare man of both accomplishment and potential, a great surgeon who was also a natural leader. "How will you improve the field of pediatric surgery by the time you retire?" the committee asked. Folkman hadn't come in thinking of specific plans, but his answer was instinctive and it struck a chord. He said he had a special knack for picking up clues and hints about diseases by careful observation of his patients. His goal was to take these clues into the research laboratory, seek answers, and try to bring new surgical procedures and treatments back to the bedsides of future patients.

Gross had done much the same, but in Folkman the committee members saw a potential for achievement and honor surpassing even that of his predecessor. They decided Folkman was special enough to make him the youngest professor of surgery in the history of Harvard University. A year later, the school would enhance the honor, creating an endowed academic chair and naming him the Julia Dyckman Andrus Professor of Surgery. Left unsaid but not unnoticed was the significance of his selection as a social development. Before being named the Ladd Professor of Surgery in 1947—a time when ethnic restrictions and quotas were still in force at Harvard, among other elite institutions—Gross had been asked to bring in his baptismal certificate to prove he was not a "hidden Jew," presumably because of the sound of his name. Twenty years later, his successor as chief of surgery was a rabbi's son.

Folkman plunged into his new job with characteristic devotion, determined to overcome his own insecurity, as well as the jealousies he knew were inevitable. Some senior doctors at Children's did not hide their resentment at being passed over in favor of a younger and much less experienced man, and they eventually left. But at the same time, Folkman couldn't deny one of the biggest knocks against him: that the head of surgery at Children's Hospital ought to have a strong background in children's surgery. Folkman had done some pediatric surgery at Mass General but did not specialize in it. Once more, Folkman's mentor had a helpful idea. With Gross's urging, the hospital arranged for its new chief of surgery to leave town for six months of intensive training with one of the world's most respected pediatric surgeons. As this surgeon later noted, Folkman was the first person Harvard ever sent *away* for training.

DR. C. EVERETT KOOP—"CHICK" to those who knew him well—had spent more than twenty years transforming a small, run-down hospital in

Philadelphia into one of America's leading children's medical centers. Later to become an influential surgeon general of the United States, Koop had throughout the fifties and sixties brought a special gutsiness and drive to his work, and he'd helped to elevate pediatric surgery to a new and noteworthy level. When Gross called him with the idea of sending Folkman down to Philadelphia, Koop was enthusiastic, flattered, and somewhat obliged.

Koop himself had once made a similar trip north, in the late 1940s, when he was becoming a pediatric surgeon. Koop, just like Folkman now, had been named surgeon-in-chief at his city's children's hospital and needed more pediatric experience himself. But unlike Folkman, who was taking over at a world-class institution, Koop was trying to improve a small, ill-equipped, century-old hospital in a downtrodden section of Philadelphia. His hospital arranged for him to go to Children's Hospital in Boston for six months and learn from the famous Dr. Gross. The timing of his informal fellowship, though, was not particularly good. He came to Boston at the height of Gross's problems with his boss William Ladd, who was about to retire and seemed to be focusing much of his energy on making sure Gross didn't succeed him as chief of surgery. Thus Gross was in a funk, and he was not a very outgoing man anyway; as Koop later related to Folkman, Gross rarely said more than two words a day to him during his sojourn in Boston.

Koop was determined to give Folkman a more meaningful experience in Philadelphia than he'd had in Boston. Although he was supposed to have worked with Gross, Koop was generally only allowed to be an observer. He seldom got to scrub up and join in surgery himself. Nevertheless, he managed to soak up enough from the experience to help build what was to become one of the finest pediatric surgery training programs in the country—the one Gross wanted Folkman to spend a year in. It took some serious rule-bending and arm-twisting on Gross's part. "[Gross] was very keen on having him come here with me," Koop recalls. "But Harvard wouldn't let him go for a full year. So we tried to cram two years' worth of work into six months. I didn't want him to go home and be embarrassed."

In one of their first conversations, Koop told Folkman he was going to introduce him as chief resident. "We have an open slot," he told his visitor. "We won't tell anybody you're a professor." It was a secret they kept until the day Folkman left. None of the staff in Philadelphia knew that the new chief resident was actually the surgeon-in-chief at a much more renowned hospital. "Nobody had any idea," Folkman recalls with mischievous relish. "The nurses, the other residents. They just thought I was a resident waiting in line."

Upon Folkman's arrival, Koop put him to work performing the most complicated kind of surgery—operations on newborns. "They're the ones operated on in the middle of the night," Folkman said. "You've got to get everything right, and it usually takes years to learn that." Surgeons had to perform some especially delicate procedures many times over before they could claim to actually know how to do them. Folkman was soon aware that an inordinate number of these tricky cases were showing up on Koop's doorstep. Koop explained that he had cultivated long-term relationships with doctors around Philadelphia and arranged for many of the difficult cases to be sent to his hospital. Pennsylvania was one of the few states that had osteopathic schools, so many of the state's doctors were osteopaths who were performing difficult operations on children. In more than a few cases, they were in over their heads. "Koop would tell the osteopaths that when they had these kinds of problems, they should send the patient to him. They would get into trouble and then the child would be shipped in," Folkman says. "So Koop was always getting these kids, who had half their appendixes out, and half they couldn't get out. He would solve it, do the operation, and send the child back." It was an oddly symbiotic relationship: The osteopaths helped Koop turn his hospital into one of the nation's leading training centers for pediatric surgeons, and Koop helped the osteopaths keep from getting sued for malpractice.

Late in 1968, knowing Folkman was coming down for his crash course, Koop called in some long-standing IOUs. He started calling doctors in southeastern Pennsylvania, saying he had a Harvard professor to train and asking them to keep him supplied with their toughest cases. "I want you to send every single baby here from January first to June thirtieth," he told the local doctors. That first month, there were twenty-five cases, and in February there were twenty more—virtually an operation a day. For his part, Koop found working with Folkman so exhilarating that he eventually canceled his travel schedule to stay and operate each night with the young doctor. "Judah was the most stimulating trainee I've ever had," Koop later said. "He never let me do anything without having a reason for it. He kept me on my toes constantly. He was extremely curious, and very grateful to be there and learn. We hit it off because we're the same kind of people." Koop shared the duties on the operating table with Folkman. If they performed a hernia operation, each would operate on one side. Then, after scrubbing, Folkman would write copious notes on virtually every moment of every operation—everything from which side of the table he'd worked from to what he'd had to do when something went wrong—and type them up each night.

Folkman was comfortable with the work, but one operation frustrated him. A young boy was in the operating room with undescended testes, and Koop was using a procedure he had invented to correct the problem. For Koop, it was a routine operation—he could finish it in seventeen minutes— but Folkman just couldn't finish it. "After an hour and three-quarters, we were still there, and I could see that Judah was depressed. The next morning he came in yelling, 'Fingernails! It's fingernails! That's how you do it so well. You have fingernails, and I don't.' He showed me how I would hold things down with my thumbnail."

One night, Koop had to tend to a special patient: Folkman's daughter Laura, now four. Folkman called him at four in the morning and brought Laura in. She was very ill, probably a result of her chronic problems with cystic fibrosis, but he wasn't sure what was wrong. Meeting the Folkmans at the hospital, Koop examined Laura and thought she had many of the symptoms of appendicitis: abdominal pain, spells of nausea and vomiting, low-grade fever, painful coughing. Koop hoped it was some kind of viral infection, because putting Laura under anesthesia to remove the appendix could very well do permanent damage to her lungs, exacerbating her breathing problems. It was raining that night, and the ceiling of the old hospital was leaking as the Folkmans sat with Laura until sunrise. "We sat there in lawn chairs because they didn't have beds for parents," Paula Folkman remembers. "The rain dripped on my head until I moved the lawn chair." By five in the morning, Laura appeared to be improving. "I don't think we have to operate," Koop said finally. Laura recovered, and Koop never did find out what her problem was. But his relief was palpable.

Koop was a great believer in house calls. He emphasized to his residents that they could learn more in five minutes at someone's kitchen table than in a long and detailed office visit. House calls were fast going out of style by the late 1960s, but Koop thought there was at least one group of patients for whom it was worth saving the tradition: dying children. He felt that children who were going to die should die at home. He made a practice of visiting their homes to see whether it was possible—"to see whether there was an alcoholic mother, or a demented grandparent." Koop had a lot of heartrending pediatric cancer cases, at a time when there wasn't much in the way of treatment (such as chemotherapy) that did much good. So he would bring morphine with him to help ease the children's pain. He made his house calls on Thursday nights, and he always took his chief resident with him. For these six months in 1969, that was Folkman, who recalls: "He would call [a parent] and say, 'I'm coming out your way. Could we have coffee?' It was amazing. God, we drove to Lancaster. He always fixed it so he'd get back by one o'clock in the morning. So every Thursday he'd say, 'Get someone to cover for you, you're coming with me, unless you're operating.' I learned a ton of stuff." Folkman, too, became a believer in house calls. Some years later, he attended a meeting for young surgeons and got up and asked how many of them had made a house call in the past five years. Only a few hands came up, and Folkman, in his usual gentle style, explained the virtues of treating the whole person, and how a house call was a good way to do that.

If there was one conviction of Koop's that took deep root in Folkman's medical soul, it was his refusal to surrender. "He would never, ever give up on a child," Folkman says. "The medical service would say let's withdraw, let's pull out the tube, let's stop the respirator. This child is going to be a vegetable. There's too much brain damage. But he would always say if the child's alive, he's potentially curable. He'd say there's a normal child under these dressings; we've got to work on it. He never gave up. And on the wall in his office he always has these letters that say 'former vegetable.' Those kids were fine."

Although Folkman had gone to Philadelphia to learn from Koop, Koop also found those six months a remarkably enriching period in his professional life. "People who spend time with Judah Folkman have their lives changed," he later said. "It changed my life. He's such an enthusiastic person that it's contagious. He stimulates people to be curious."

Koop's plan for Folkman had worked. He crammed two years of training into six months, and Folkman went home to Boston an experienced pediatric surgeon. "When I came back to Children's Hospital I could out-operate almost everyone there," he relates in a rare burst of immodesty, more as an acknowledgment of Koop than of his own prowess. "Koop had taught me so much stuff they had never heard of. They'd call me and ask, 'How would Koop handle this?' I'd say, 'This is how I'd handle it,' putting together what Koop had taught me with what Mass General had taught me." He soon felt a difference in the atmosphere. There seemed to be no more doubts about his qualification to be surgeon-in-chief.

And nobody balked when Folkman ordered all his residents to grow their thumbnails long.

Chapter Six

———

THERE IS AN OLD SAYING that only the lead dog in a sled team gets a fresh view of the world. In science there are lead dogs; only they can see what's ahead, and they often lead the team in new directions. Judah Folkman seemed destined to be one of those lead dogs—a researcher who would blaze new trails, leaving indelible footprints. To do this he needed a platform for the kind of independence every visionary in biomedicine, real or imagined, needed. Even in the early days of his career, years before the College of Cardinals of Boston's medical establishment made him a main man at Children's Hospital, Folkman knew that to pursue really daring ideas, he had to have his own lab. Not that he considered the idea that had lingered in his consciousness since leaving the navy excessively ambitious. The process of nailing it might require a good bit of ingenuity, but the idea itself? To Folkman, it was more a product of logic than daring.

After all those years of training in other people's labs—Zollinger's, Gross's, the navy's—and after putting his research ambitions aside altogether through the end of his residency, Folkman finally got his own little shop in 1965 at Boston City Hospital. Indeed, it was not much more than a bench or two. The hospital itself was described as historic, which meant old and run-down, and Folkman's lab was humble. It was a small space that was cut up into smaller spaces: several cramped rooms for an office, a sterile bench area, and a makeshift animal-operating room. Folkman's laboratory was tall and narrow, with windows set near the tops of the walls. The office was so severely sized and oddly shaped that some thought it resembled a phone booth—albeit one with books piled on the floor and up the walls. Sometimes Folkman felt as though he were looking up from the bottom of an empty swimming pool.

But at least it was a lab Folkman could call his own, and he was working in a part of the world in which research was not only encouraged but required. "Publish or perish" was axiomatic at Harvard, where the quality and quantity of the research being done, and the publications that resulted, outweighed even teaching ability in the struggle for tenure. If he were so inclined, a brilliant researcher who produced world-class results could ignore students altogether. Folkman was not of that ilk—he couldn't imagine separating research from teaching—but he fully intended to devote himself to something he had been forced to ignore: the mystery of tumors and their blood vessels.

He had left the navy with a seed of conjecture taking root in his mind. The way tumors inserted in rabbit thyroids triggered the growth of blood vessels suggested to him that cancer seemed to have an ability to somehow coax blood vessels to grow toward tumors and feed them—that is, to make a new life-support system. Each tumor seemed to set up a private flow of nourishment that kept it robust, thriving, and on the move. Without a blood supply, oxygen and nutrients had to seep through solid tissue. But they couldn't get in fast enough to support unimpeded growth, and metabolic waste products couldn't get away soon enough to avoid poisoning the cells. Vascularization—the forming of new blood vessels to support tissues—seemed to make all the difference in the tumor's world. A tumor without blood vessels was stuck—not dead, but dormant.

Though he'd had to put these observations and ideas aside when he returned to Boston to resume his medical training, the ultimate meaning of the Bethesda rabbit thyroid experiments had never been far from his imagination. Even during the long nights and frantic days of his residency at Mass General, he'd managed to occasionally stir and massage the idea, trying to fit together at least some of the smaller pieces of the puzzle, always with the big picture in the back of his mind. And the big picture, he postulated, was this: Cancer cells seemed to produce and emit some kind of growth-stimulating factor that triggers vascularization. What if that growth factor could be isolated and identified? Could it be used to spur the healing of wounds, or to alleviate other problems where more blood vessels were needed? And, most provocative, might there also be other substances that *inhibit* blood vessel growth? Could they be used as weapons against cancer?

It was a kind of intellectual growth factor that had spurred Folkman to keep thinking so boldly. Soon after returning from the navy, he had set out to search the medical literature to see if anyone had covered this terrain before. One day during a lull in the emergency room, he went to the pathology department library and found an eighteen-year-old paper in a bound periodical that excited him. In 1945, a researcher at the National Cancer Institute, Dr. Glen Algire, had published the results of experiments that had led him to believe—just as Folkman did now—that blood vessels are somehow drawn inexorably toward tumors. In their report in the *Journal of the National Cancer Institute*, Algire and three colleagues described how, in studying the biology of cancer, they had implanted little transparent plastic chambers in mice, then put tumor samples into the chambers. They found that blood vessels grew directly toward the tumors.

Eagerly leafing through the yellowed article, Folkman read Algire's description of a series of experiments that had allowed him to make some interesting observations about the growth of new blood vessels. Algire and his colleagues gathered a hundred mice and divided them into three groups. They made surgical wounds in the first group of mice to see how blood vessels responded to the injuries. They transplanted normal tissue into the second group. And they transplanted tumors from the mammary gland into the third group. Algire made daily microscopic photographs of the results. In the transparent chambers on the injured mice, new blood vessels could be seen growing toward the wounds after five days. By the ninth day, the area was filled with new vessels and the wound had healed. By then, many of the new capillaries had disappeared or blended into arteries. The group of mice with normal tissue exhibited a similar result.

But vascularization was even more striking in the mice carrying tumors: New capillaries started creeping in almost twice as fast, within just three days, and the number of vessels was double what Algire saw in surrounding tissues. And the process didn't seem to stop. "The rapid growth of tumor transplants is dependent on the development of a rich vascular supply," Algire wrote. "[A]n outstanding characteristic of the tumor cell is its capacity to elicit continuously the growth of new capillary endothelium [blood vessel cells] from the host."

Algire was especially intrigued by how much faster the new blood vessels grew toward tumors than toward ordinary wounds. And it naturally made him wonder what caused the difference. "If the capillary proliferation is a response to a specific substance, this substance, as produced by the tumor cells, is more rapidly effective than is that from traumatized tissue." He postulated in the journal that something coming from inside the tumor cells might be the factor responsible for what seemed to be a continuous production of lots of new tumor-feeding blood vessels, and the growth of those tumors. But while Algire appeared to be the first to suggest that blood vessels grow toward tumors, and that it might be a substance from the tumors that induces this growth, he had not tried to prove, as Folkman hoped to, that tumors absolutely *depended* on this process to grow.

In any case, Algire was like a lead dog—a lone dog, actually—whose footprints had almost disappeared. As far as Folkman could tell, not much attention had been paid to the findings, and there was no evidence that Algire, who had since died, ever followed up on the study himself. Folkman found a few other studies involving the use of time-lapse photography to document the growth of tumors implanted in hamsters and rabbits. These, too, indicated that tumors induced blood vessels to grow toward them. But again, the results didn't seem to spark further interest, even from the authors, some of whom were most excited about the technology that allowed them to film the action inside the tiny chambers.

One reason for such indifference to discoveries that Folkman considered extremely tantalizing, findings just crying out for more study, was a general lack of interest in the circulatory system as a research subject. Very little was known about blood vessel physiology and function, but to the research community it seemed that what was already known was quite enough. Although obviously important, the vascular system was considered just an intricate arrangement of pipes that carried blood to all of the body's tissues and then carried away wastes, including the carbon dioxide that needs to be exhaled. There wasn't all that much more to learn, the thinking went, so why spend time, effort, and money on a subject that offered little chance for real advancement, either of science or of careers? As for the developing war on cancer, blood vessels weren't even on the radar screen. Algire's finding came in a vacuum—two decades before cancer research was to become a burgeoning scientific enterprise.

So if Folkman wanted to study the relationship between tumors and blood vessels, he would have to invent an entire new field of research. A lead dog couldn't have a fresher view than that. He began to refer to his new territory as "angiogenesis," a loosely defined term coined near the turn of the century to describe the production and growth of new blood vessels—"angio" referring to blood vessels, "genesis" meaning origination. The term had first appeared in print in 1900, in a paper about the growth of adrenal glands by a doctor named Rudolf Steiner that was published in the *Johns Hopkins Hospital Reports*. It was used again in the mid-1930s by Dr. Arthur Hertig, a Harvard physician who was studying placental pregnancies. Now, in 1966, it showed up again—in a grant application to the National Cancer Institute from Judah Folkman. It signaled the beginning of what for Folkman would be a kind of double life. While it was obviously not unusual for top doctors to be involved in research, Folkman's devotion to a single idea was remarkable, especially for a surgeon.

In appropriating the term "angiogenesis" for his new one-man field, Folkman was applying an obscure word to an even more obscure and difficult subject. Almost nothing was known about when, how, why, where, and under what conditions blood vessels will grow or won't grow. The closely related phenomenon called "vasculogenesis"—construction of a circulatory system during embryonic growth—was being studied by embryologists, but there was essentially no understanding of what occurs in blood vessel physiology later in life. It had been assumed that once the circulatory system was formed and completed, little else changed beyond repairing the damage incurred by injury. With so little study preceding him, then, Folkman would have to learn all he could about blood vessels, starting from square one.

A few things were known: that blood vessels are lined with semipermeable tissue called endothelial cells, and that a blanket of muscle cells surrounds this tissue the way a tire surrounds and restrains an inner tube. This sheath of smooth muscle cells is capable of squeezing down or opening up the channel—the lumen—in which blood flows, altering blood pressure. Important substances manage to leak out of, and into, the walls of the blood vessels to meet the body's physiological needs.

After studying up on the subject, Folkman began to suspect that the vascular system was not just a plumbing system but actually a complex and very active organ in itself. Like other parts of the body, the circulatory system had its own unique architecture and biochemistry, its own repair mechanisms. It was clear that blood vessels were vital to all of human biology, and not only because they are the body's transporter of nutrients and wastes. Hormones course through the blood vessels to reach their targets. Blood helps transport heat into and out of organs. Folkman had a strong hunch that the story didn't end there. He had no trouble imagining that all kinds of vital secrets were locked up in those supposedly humdrum endothelial cells.

The circumstantial evidence had been accumulating in the back of his mind for half a decade. First, he had seen with his own eyes, in the original rabbit thyroid experiments in his navy laboratory, that a lack of blood vessels correlated with a lack of tumor growth. Then, during cancer operations performed during his residency at Mass General, he had seen signs that tumors may also lie dormant in humans if they haven't induced blood vessel growth.

Over and over again, Folkman saw that big tumors always had plenty of blood vessels; tumors lacking blood vessels tended to be very small and white, resembling, except for color, the dormant tumors he and Fred Becker had seen in thyroid glands in the navy lab. The Algire paper also provided support for his ideas. So now it was time: Folkman was primed for action as he opened his one-man lab on the bottom floor of the old Sears building at Boston City Hospital in fall 1965.

One of the first things he did in his new digs was to go back to the beginning and re-create the navy experiments. "I started again with the perfusion experiments," he recalls, "just to check it, just to repeat it." Just to be sure he wasn't fooling himself. He also repeated the test with a slight alteration, perfusing small sections of puppy intestines instead of rabbit thyroids. The results were the same: The tumors on perfused organs stopped growing while still small, and those transplanted into live animals got new life from blood vessels that grew toward them soon after their arrival. Squeezing lab time in between his heavy surgical and teaching duties, Folkman kept doing variations of the assays. And he set out to learn everything he could about solid tumors to give himself a firmer grounding in knowledge of his prey.

But after that, what? Folkman had boiled his thesis down to three strong possibilities and one major speculation. He thought that the lives of tumors depended on the growth of new blood vessels. He thought that the tumors actively stimulated this growth. He thought that the way they accomplished this was to secrete a substance that induced nearby blood vessels to sprout new branches which grew in toward the tumors. And most audaciously, he speculated that a substance capable of reversing the process—of stopping blood vessel growth and starving tumors to death—might exist. This last idea was essentially an inspiration, a leap of faith based on little but the knowledge that nature seldom does things one way: If there's one force pushing, there's usually another pulling.

All four of Folkman's ideas were challenging, even groundbreaking. All four were dismally short of supporting evidence. So the task he faced was to prove each of these difficult points to a community of scientists and doctors naturally inclined toward skepticism. Testing the new ideas and proving they had real validity would be especially hard because none of the potent tools that would later emerge in modern biology yet existed. For the most part, biology was still a descriptive science—taxonomy—in which researchers put much of their time and effort into finding, naming, and describing new species, or parts of new species, and the intricacies of living cells. Biochemistry—meaning the structure, properties, and activities of hormones, growth factors, and similar strange chemicals—was germinating but still far from mature.

For one thing, the means for separating individual biochemicals from complex body fluids were still primitive. The new field of molecular biology was very much in its infancy—the first gene had yet to be isolated—and researchers were still struggling to uncover how DNA, and its sister molecule, RNA, worked together within the living cell. In fact, it was not yet clear what role, if any, genes played in the cancer process. Some forms of the disease seemed to be inheritable, at least in part, but how that worked was a mystery. So the lack of fundamental knowledge was itself a barrier that Folkman would need to surmount. Three decades later, he would look back and remark upon how naive he had been about the mountain he was trying to climb: "I was too young to realize how much trouble was in store for a theory that could not be tested immediately."

FOLKMAN HAD BEEN WORKING virtually alone for nearly two years, repeating the early experiments over and over, thinking about where he should go next. In 1967 there came a knock on the door of his tiny lab late one afternoon. Michael Gimbrone Jr. was a second-year medical student who had heard that Folkman was experimenting with live organs and blood vessels; he had decided to visit the young surgeon after classes to see if he could get involved. Gimbrone was one of many admiring students—Folkman was already known as a brilliant and enthusiastic teacher with a dazzling career ahead of him—but it was one thing in particular that brought Gimbrone to Folkman's door. Like Folkman had been a decade earlier, Gimbrone was so fascinated by biomedical research that he had gone directly into lab work during his first year at Harvard Medical School. To Folkman's delight, Gimbrone said he hoped to take a one-year leave from school the following year to devote himself full-time to research in blood vessel biology.

The son of a criminologist, Gimbrone had grown up in a blue-collar neighborhood in the gritty industrial city of Buffalo, New York. In one important way, Gimbrone and Folkman were much alike: Each had decided early to become a doctor, and each had been influenced and encouraged by his father. A good part of Gimbrone's fascination with things scientific came from his father's use of science to detect crime and criminals. Michael Anthony Gimbrone Sr. had developed some of the early chemistry to detect latent fingerprints. "He also had a strong conviction that being able to help other people was an important dimension of human existence," Gimbrone Jr. says in an echo of Folkman's recollections of his own father. While in high school, Gimbrone enrolled in a summer program at the Roswell Park Cancer Institute, a cancer research center in Buffalo, which whet his appetite for the laboratory. For college, Gimbrone chose a major in life science at Cornell University. He continued to sign on for summer research positions at Roswell Park and also at the New York University Medical School, where he learned cell physiology. As a summa cum laude graduate in zoology from Cornell, Gimbrone was set for medical school, and he was accepted by Harvard in 1965.

Almost immediately after his arrival in Boston, he found a research home in the department of anatomy and cell biology. There he learned to use the electron microscope, an extraordinarily powerful tool that employs a focused beam of electrons rather than light to create images of extremely small objects. The potent microscope was only about a decade old at the time, so new that it was hard to find inexpensive knives sharp enough to slice off the ultra-thin tissue specimens it was designed to view. The Harvard laboratory did own an exotic and expensive diamond knife, but it was off-limits to all but ranking faculty members. "As a student, I wasn't even allowed to be in the same room with a diamond knife," Gimbrone recalls. "There was only one in the department, and it was kept in a vault." So Gimbrone and his colleagues resorted to breaking shards of glass off windowpanes to cut their specimens.

In the cell lab, Gimbrone worked under Donald Fawcett, one of the world's leading experts in ultrastructural anatomy and cell science, as well as the author of classic textbooks in the field. One of Fawcett's interests was the fine structure of capillaries, the tiniest blood vessels, and it was through Fawcett that Gimbrone picked up his enduring fascination with blood vessel biology. This made him a natural fit when, having heard about Folkman's organ-perfusion work, he arrived at the surgeon's City Hospital doorway seeking a yearlong research position. Folkman welcomed him and talked about his work, emphasizing that he believed he had spotted something new and important—something few people seemed interested in. Gimbrone agreed, based on his own studies of endothelial cells with the electron micro-scope, that blood vessels seemed far more complex than conventional wisdom had it. As Gimbrone recalls, "The term 'vascular biology' didn't exist. People didn't appreciate that there are cellular components that mattered a damn." And the number of researchers then interested in blood vessel biology "was small enough so we could all fit in one phone booth, depending on whether someone had eaten a big lunch."

Folkman couldn't help but recognize a little of himself in Gimbrone, and they clicked immediately. He saw that Gimbrone had both a special interest in the obscure area he was pursuing and the intellectual rigor to make a real contribution. "You could tell he would be a professor, even when he was a student," Folkman said many years later, after Gimbrone had indeed become a renowned professor of pathology at Harvard, running a research lab of his own. Gimbrone's leave from medical school was approved, and in 1968 he became Folkman's first lab associate.

As part of their early research, Folkman and Gimbrone began trying to grow endothelial cells in culture, hoping to learn what controlled them and how they differed from other kinds of cells. They failed to make the cells grow in isolation, but the work did yield an ultimately critical piece of the puzzle. Having noticed that blood vessels in perfused organs gradually deteriorated and disintegrated, Folkman set out to find out why. He and Gimbrone devised a series of experiments that might test the effects of various bloodborne substances. When they got to platelets, they saw that these particles, which help the clotting system plug up damaged blood vessels, seemed to protect the blood vessels from deterioration. They tested the idea by perfusing one set of thyroid glands from dogs with fluid containing platelets and another set with fluid lacking them. To help run the perfusion experiments with Gimbrone, Folkman hired an undergraduate student from Boston College named Joe Corkery, who, like Gimbrone, was eager for laboratory experience and willing to come in nights and on weekends to help keep the longer-term perfusion experiments going. Some tests had to be run twenty-four hours a day, and Gimbrone and Corkery stayed through the night, keeping each other up with coffee and ordering pizza.

The early results were promising: Indications were that platelets performed functions beyond plugging leaks in blood vessels, actually extending the vessels' lives. But before the data could be confirmed, Folkman got a tap on the shoulder from the Harvard administration. It seemed the novice grantee was spending too much of his grant money too fast. Pace yourself, he was warned, or you'll be out of money before the term of the grant is up. To Folkman, slowing down was out of the question. He and Gimbrone had another idea. Dogs were very expensive, so they changed to rats.

Changing species didn't change the results. With no platelets present, they found, the endothelial cells swelled up, became inflamed, and eventually died. But with platelets in the fluid, the cells remained intact. It would be years before they learned that the difference was caused not by the platelets as a whole, but by a protein they released—a "growth factor" that few scientists at the time, despite Judah Folkman's research, believed existed. Whatever it would eventually come to mean, the work was considered worthy basic science and was accepted for publication in the prestigious journal *Nature*, with Gimbrone as the first author. It would become the basis for his thesis and eventually help him graduate from medical school magna cum laude in 1970.

In the scheme of things, it was a small triumph. Folkman liked to think the data—suggesting some invisible growth-stimulating factor might be present in association with platelets—supported his overall thesis. But those on the receiving end of this argument found the connection much too nebulous. Nor were they much impressed by the perfusion experiments. They saw little value to the prevailing winds of cancer research. Exploring the life of cancer cells, and developing new and better poisons to wipe them out, were what everyone else wanted to talk about—not the intricacies of blood vessels that just happened to be nearby. Unfortunately for Folkman, many of these skeptics were ensconced on advisory boards of grant-making agencies and on the anonymous peer review panels of scientific journals. They found it easy to snipe at Folkman's contentions about angiogenesis and cancer, often repeating the damning, dismissive statement that became a mantra: "Your conclusions are not supported by your data"—the kiss of death for a research proposal or a scientific paper up for publication.

Only one journal published a word from Folkman on the subject of tumors and blood vessels. This was *Annals of Surgery*, which accepted an early paper on perfused organs. But the 1966 monograph did not propose the idea that tumors are actually *dependent* on angiogenesis. In any event, it was a surgical journal, a publication that few biological scientists would bother to read. Folkman couldn't get past the front door of any of the specialized journals to which he submitted his work. *Cell Biology* rejected him, and so did *Experimental Cell Research*. The *British Journal of Cancer* echoed the others: Your conclusions go beyond your data. *Reject*. Or: This is a "special case": the lack of blood vessel growth in an isolated thyroid gland is "not generalizable" to cancer as seen in patients. *Reject*. Though Folkman found the perfusion experiments fascinating, and he had taken the time to think through what he was seeing, the reviewers tended to dismiss them as "artifacts" of an experimental system. He wasn't using whole blood, so that could be why the tiny tumors stopped growing. He wasn't using the whole animal with all its hormones and enzymes, so maybe that was the problem. And why focus on blood vessel growth alone?

"I remember the skepticism of some of the reviewers, which taught me some perspective on the politics of research and science," Gimbrone says. "Judah was clearly not in the mainstream of research; his ideas were out in left field. Cancer cells were the issue then, and Judah's idea that the host and the tumor have a dynamic dialogue, and that one depends on the other in the sense of inducing capillaries to grow—there was no precedent for that."

As Folkman was only beginning to understand, a certain herd mentality existed in the research world, which could work in either direction—toward an idea, or away from it. The herd generally did not make an enthusiastic leap toward a new and alien concept, especially one that some seemed to regard as a bit facile. Moreover, there was a deep and enduring divide within biomedicine between doctors seeing dying patients and scientists studying fine slices of tumor tissue under their microscopes. The two groups spoke different languages, attended different meetings, communicated through different journals. Instead of blue-sky theorizing, hard-nosed experts demanded hard-nosed data—incontrovertible cause and effect, firm links between proven biochemical processes. Folkman had no quarrel with this as a general principle, but he detected something else at play: He and his theory had a public relations problem. He was focusing on normal blood vessel cells, while it was clear to almost everyone else that the problem was really deranged cancer cells. The goal of cancer research at that time was to find exploitable weaknesses in these cells—oxygen sensitivity, heat, radiation, chemicals, surgery. Some of those approaches—notably surgery, radiation, and chemotherapy—were already starting to work in a few patients. Normal blood vessel cells? What did they have to do with the abnormal cells of cancer? People weren't buying what Folkman was selling.

Folkman readily admitted he was venturing into territory where much more was unknown than known. He was just starting the journey, without a map or compass or a guide of any kind. Nonetheless, facing walls of skepticism and indifference, he pressed his conviction that he at least had good reason to follow this trail. "Judah had a clear notion that tumors secrete something. But he didn't have any idea how to prove that in 1968," Gimbrone recalls. "So his concepts clearly ran ahead of the data, and that attracted more criticism than was warranted."

Even at Harvard, Folkman's home turf, a place where he had flourished since his arrival as a medical student fifteen years before, there were some unkind whispers. Some of his surgical colleagues wondered why he was wasting his time on this angiogenesis thing when he should have been devoting himself exclusively to the operating room. Others were wary of Folkman's audacity, even offended by it. Never reticent about his ideas, Folkman was always willing to discuss his latest experiments and where he thought they might lead, regardless of his actual progress in the laboratory. Folkman's style was not boastful, but still it did not fly very well in the conservative research atmosphere of Harvard, or within the small community of people who were in a position to decide whether Folkman would be supported with government grants. They were not all that interested in letting him into the science club. "Science is an extraordinarily disciplined business, and occasionally people come along like Judah who break the rules, and people's rigidities," observes Dr. Fred Rosen, a longtime participant in research governance at the Harvard Medical School. "It happens with people who are very, very creative, people who have vivid imaginations."

Only later would it seem that Folkman was helping tear down a Berlin Wall between medicine and science, a brick at a time. In those years, "the idea of a physician being highly integrated with basic research and discovery would boggle people," says Stephen Atkinson, a Harvard Medical School business administrator in the 1970s. "In the halls of academe, being a surgeon is not a very high distinction. Judah flew against a lot of stereotypes"—but also reinforced them with his scattershot research style. "He was flying on a wing and a prayer. His grant proposals were being returned. He was getting no as an answer, but it wasn't just no. It was 'Have you lost your marbles?' "

Even if Folkman's idea seemed like the most logical, most reasonable thing in the world, it suffered from the boldness of its author, who was presumed to be an arrogant surgeon who lacked any credibility in the lab. Basic human resentment would block the way, then and for years afterward.

SOON AFTER HIS BIG APPOINTMENT to be surgeon-in-chief at Children's Hospital and his six-month sojourn with C. Everett Koop in Philadelphia, Folkman packed up all his equipment and schlepped it across town to his new home. At Children's he was given a two-room laboratory in the old Carnegie Building—where he had worked years earlier doing dog experiments with Robert Gross—and got his perfusion pumps, tubes, and chambers reassembled.

But now Folkman had to consider how far these few tools would take him. Though he had tried to advance his original navy experiments, he was coming to see that he had a long way to go before he would convince anyone that angiogenesis played a key role in tumor growth. Moving on from rabbit thyroids, he had perfused small sections of puppy intestines in an isolation chamber. He had also created a pouchlike chamber on a rat's back by pumping air under its skin in order to watch blood vessels approach implanted tumors. In both systems, he was able to monitor tumor growth in relation to blood vessel invasion, but neither system offered the clarity and the hard evidence he needed to support the angiogenesis thesis. As many of his colleagues rightfully pointed out, for example, it was difficult to prove that the squiggly red blood vessels growing toward the tumors weren't just the result of inflammation from the invasion of the tumor. That was the criticism Folkman heard most from colleagues at Harvard and from reviewers. After all, blood vessel growth was often seen in association with inflammation resulting from injuries. And the implantation of a tumor certainly qualified as an injury. But Folkman didn't see it that way. "One of the things that really drove Judah around the bend in those days was people saying, 'Oh, it's just inflammation,' " Gimbrone says.

Folkman believed he saw evidence to the contrary and not only under the microscope. One day, he came back to the lab at City Hospital after an operation, all in a lather. He grabbed Gimbrone, quickly erased the chalkboard, then began drawing a tumor. "See this?" he said. "I have this patient. . . ." It was a woman with metastasized ovarian cancer. The primary tumor Folkman found was rich with blood, while scattered around in her abdomen were tiny white blobs of tumor that had apparently not yet called in a blood supply. They looked just like the dormant tumors Folkman had seen in the lab. "There's got to be something," Folkman insisted, pointing to the growing tumor. "See this vascularity? The tumor *must* be releasing something."

Gimbrone loved the way that, unlike many researchers who toiled in isolated labs, Folkman took his inspiration from real life. "He was operating on people," Gimbrone later reflected, "and trying to understand what was going on." Every day Folkman shuttled between surgery and the lab, trying to make connections. Gimbrone and Joe Corkery would come to work by seven-thirty to begin the day's experiments while Folkman was in the main hospital doing surgery. They would anesthetize their subject, take out a thyroid, perfuse it, take their biopsies, and take their measurements. "Then Judah would come back," Gimbrone recalls, "and I'd have a sense that the experiment was a total failure, a washout. He'd ask, 'How did it go today?' and I'd be embarrassed to say. But he had this uncanny ability to step back mentally a foot or two and look at what had transpired. Then he would say, 'Isn't that interesting? There was X and X,' which would have nothing to do with the original design. It would sometimes be a transcendental leap in logic. It would take you a while to see what he was thinking, but it made you very resourceful. It was a tremendously liberating thing in terms of your ability to conceptualize."

Folkman needed all the resourcefulness he could get, for no matter how convinced he became about angiogenesis, it didn't change his dilemma. He could do a thousand perfusion experiments, he could do a thousand cancer surgeries, and they still would not yield enough solid data to demonstrate his contention that tumors depended on new blood vessel growth, and that they somehow had the power to make it happen. He needed to find a way to test the angiogenesis phenomenon in a living animal in a way that made it clear the response was not just inflammation. He needed tests that would show the phenomenon clearly, and that other researchers could confirm. The work in rats relied too much on subjective observations (it was too hard to quantify what was going on in the complex environment of a rat's back) and the thyroid experiments, he later remarked, "were scant evidence on which to propose a general mechanism of tumor growth." But he was stuck in what people had started calling a catch-22. Without more data, he wouldn't get grants. And without grants, it would be hard to pursue the data.

Hard—but not impossible. His search might proceed slowly, but it would proceed.

Michael Gimbrone left Folkman's lab after graduating from medical school in spring 1970. He moved on, with the benefit of his mentor's recommendation, to the internship program at Massachusetts General. Meanwhile Folkman decided that to keep angiogenesis alive he would simply have to invent a new science. He would have to create some of his own tools and find new measuring techniques. He would have to dream up precise tests that would yield credible results, hire bright people, and, not incidentally, keep scrounging up enough grant money to keep the lab running.

Folkman did succeed in getting some minimal funding from the National Institutes of Health—a "career development" award of twenty-five thousand dollars that just about covered the salary for him and one technician. Completely by accident, he learned that the grant was awarded grudgingly. At least one reviewer didn't want Folkman to have too much "career development." An accompanying document bore an anonymous, hand-scribbled, and very telling note in the margin: "This is the limit. We do not want Folkman to build an empire."

Chapter Seven

———

SEEING A BUDDING EMPIRE in Judah Folkman's small fiefdom took an active imagination. At the time, his most experienced collaborator was Ramzi Cotran, a pathologist who had his own lab at Harvard Medical School and who had agreed to work with Folkman on his tumor assays. There was part-timer Joe Corkery, along with a few other students and postdoctoral fellows who came and went. There was only one fixture: Folkman's assistant, Paul Wesley, who had been with him since his residency days at Mass General. Among Wesley's many duties was making sure the gold-handled surgical instruments Folkman had been awarded when he was named chief resident didn't get mixed in with the hospital's own instruments and disappear. In a busy operating room, it would be hard to distinguish one from another on a casual inspection.

As for laboratories, there are the gray or white lab benches, the same glassware, the centrifuges and electron microscopes, the young researchers hunched over their experiments, working a problem day after day for weeks or months. The most notable distinguishing characteristics are usually the cartoons, photos, and pithy quotations taped to walls and bench dividers, empirical proof that in a laboratory humor is a necessary aid in the struggle to hang on to sanity during the inexorable grind to produce research results.

The crucial difference between labs, of course, is the people who work in them. It doesn't take long before a newly established laboratory begins evolving an aura, depending largely on the boss's personality, his or her field of study, and the kind of people recruited as graduate students and postdoctoral fellows. Some laboratories follow the German style, with a dominant Herr Doktor-Doktor Professor rigidly in charge, while others are so loosely organized it's not exactly clear who is the boss, if there is one at all. A few research laboratories become so large and stuffed with research students that the leader is seldom seen except by appointment. And there is good reason why graduate students and postdoctoral fellows have long been known as academic slaves. Younger researchers-in-training get minimum financial support while doing most of the day-to-day, hands-on work. Generally, the lab's leader is in charge of guiding the research, resolving squabbles, and—most important of all—finding the money to stay open for business. An additional duty, sometimes honored in the breach, is for the lab chief to help steer his academic offspring into promising jobs.

It's also true that, as in any other sphere, there are varying levels of competence in the research world. Some labs are run under inspired leadership and produce luminous work; others perform adequately and turn out well-trained, if not brilliant, alumni. But more than a few university and medical research labs are run by people with enormous prestige but no understanding of leadership or how to inspire creative work. At any given moment, almost every major university will have a laboratory in which the atmosphere is so poisonous and rancorous that technicians and clerical staff flee, and students sometimes leave with their research careers in tatters. There are even occasional suicides as students break under the intense pressure to perform world-class research under tight deadlines—sad cases in which the admonition to "publish or perish" becomes tragically literal. Charm school and management training are not part of the scientific curriculum, so young graduate students and postdoctoral fellows may find themselves working for extraordinarily irascible and cantankerous senior scientists.

Generally the goal for young people pursuing graduate work is to win acceptance into a famous scientist's laboratory, propose imaginative research, win a grant to fund it, and publish the results in a respected journal. If everything comes together right, they move on to other jobs—perhaps even found labs of their own. And in rare instances, given support from a mentor, a sparkling research record, and sufficient papers being published, a researcher might get an offer of a faculty position within the university and a chance to get on the tenure track. Quite often, however, by the time a student is ready to move on, mentor and mentee are no longer speaking, sometimes because as the student has matured in the research, he or she has developed ideas of his or her own that threaten or even contradict those of the boss. Some bosses can stand it, others can't; disagreements over small technical points can turn into wars. The amount of vitriol expended can be astounding.

Judah Folkman was not a famous scientist in 1971, so postdoctoral fellows were not exactly lining up for positions. Nonetheless, he was under way, and despite his changeable staff and modest grant money, he was a man utterly focused on backing up a laboratory hunch with hard scientific proof. He wanted to respond to two points of criticism of his earlier work: First, that he had only experimented "in vitro" (outside the natural setting of a living body), and second, that the blood vessels he had observed growing toward tumors in rats were not the result of angiogenesis, but simply inflammation, the body's response to the wound created by implanting the tumor. To overcome both problems, he would have to come up with a living system in which new blood vessel growth, tumor growth, and the complex process of wound-healing could be clearly and separately documented. Were there parts of the body where blood vessels didn't normally exist? If so, he could see if tumors could induce new blood vessels to grow into such privileged sanctuaries.

Once again, Folkman found help in the archives. Back in 1941—four years before Glen Algire published his paper—Harry Greene, a pathologist studying immunology at Yale University, described how he had transplanted rabbit tumor tissue into the front chamber of guinea pigs' eyes. In his paper in the *Journal of Experimental Medicine,* Greene reported that most of the implanted tumors grew larger and larger, and were soon laced with blood vessels. In a few animals, however, he noticed that the tiny tumors remained suspended in a clear eye fluid called aqueous humor, never getting close enough to blood-rich tissue to connect to new blood vessels. These tumors failed to grow, even though they remained alive after more than a year. Greene harvested these tiny, dormant tumors and reimplanted them into the bodies of rabbits. And soon they were no longer frozen in time: They grew wildly after new blood vessels sprouted and reached them.

Folkman saw these results from a different angle than Greene. Greene was studying the body's defenses, and he was excited to find that the front of the eye was a rare place that appeared to be disconnected from the immune system. (This kind of work would lead to the discovery that corneas could be transplanted from one person to another without being rejected by the recipient's immune system.) Folkman saw something more in Greene's decades-old work: the immediate answer he was looking for. He could use the eyes of animals as his new experimental chamber.

There were good reasons. First, the front of the eye is naturally free of blood vessels, so it would be a fine place to test the idea that tumors go dormant without access to a blood supply. Second, the eye is transparent from the front, so any changes in tumor growth and the arrival of blood vessels could be clearly seen. By transplanting tumors from rabbits into the animals' own eyes, he could eliminate the possibility that an immunological reaction was confusing the results. "We were being criticized all the time for working in vitro," Folkman recalls. "So we said we'll just take a tumor that is in the animal already."

He started by transplanting minuscule chunks of tumor from the rabbit's body into the small anterior chamber of its eye, behind the cornea and in front of the lens. The rabbits were anesthetized, then positioned so their eyes were under the lens of a specially designed microscope. When Folkman peered down each day, he could see the tumors floating in the aqueous humor, slowly growing to about half a millimeter in diameter after two weeks. Left alone, without a nearby blood source, the tiny balls of tumor tissue could not connect up to the rabbit's circulatory system and couldn't continue to grow. But then Folkman extracted these tumors from the front of the eyes and reimplanted them farther back, allowing them to snuggle up next to the well-fed tissue of the iris. Within three days he saw that the tumor tissue became engulfed in new blood vessels. When that happened, the tumor began growing explosively. In fact, he calculated that the tumors expanded to sixteen thousand times their original volume.

Though he could not say he had dispatched the inflammation issue, Folkman regarded the experiment as a major step forward because it was his most successful work in a natural setting, in live animals. He had established, at least in his own mind, that given the chance, tumors called in a life-support system. But how? He was convinced—as Glen Algire had suspected twenty-five years before—that tumors secreted something that lured blood vessels to them. But his work thus far had made this idea little more than an intriguing hypothesis; he had not come close to finding tangible evidence for this most critical piece of the puzzle.

That summer, Folkman was happy to temporarily welcome back his protégé Michael Gimbrone. Gimbrone decided to return to Folkman's lab after his internship, delaying his residency in pathology to spend the 1971–1972 academic year doing the research he loved. Folkman, meanwhile, was on the move. In July, Children's Hospital opened its first dedicated research facility, a twelve-story tower named for Dr. John F. Enders, the Nobel prize–winning Harvard researcher whose discovery of a way to grow polio virus in a human cell culture system opened the door to the Salk and Sabin polio vaccines. As surgeon-in-chief at Children's, Folkman received the entire tenth floor of the new building as a large and modern lab. It was a far cry from the cramped spaces he had occupied at City Hospital and then at Children's. In fact, the new space seemed almost too roomy, especially when grant-making committees were due to come for a close look. "We'd get nervous when they came around for their census," Gimbrone later remembered. "We didn't have a lot of dollars and we had to get all our people in there and make sure they were doing things."

Folkman was anxious to get Gimbrone involved in the next phase of eye experiments, hoping to demonstrate even more clearly how differently tumors grew when they were very near a source of blood and when they were very far from one. To do this, he and Gimbrone decided to implant the little cancers into the very center of the rabbits' corneas, a place in the body that was devoid of blood vessels. Then, when the tumors became dormant, they would transplant them into other rabbits' irises, where they would be surrounded by blood vessels.

Getting the tumors into the center of the corneas was a difficult operation to perform, but Gimbrone happened on to some help at Boston's Retina Foundation. He attended a lecture there by Nahan Zauberman, an ophthalmological surgeon who was studying how some diseases caused capillaries to grow across the cornea in response to injury, blocking vision. Zauberman described how, in an attempt to cause capillary growth in the corneas of lab animals so he could study how to treat it, he had worked out a delicate way to poke plastic tubes into the cornea to deliver damaging histamines. After the lecture, Gimbrone and Folkman—who had never done eye surgery—asked Zauberman to teach them how to do the procedure so they could adapt it for their own use. "He knew how to split the cornea—nobody had ever done that—and he taught us how," Folkman recalls. "Gimbrone became a slick eye surgeon."

Once he had mastered the procedure, Gimbrone was able to cut a tiny pocket into the very center of a rabbit's cornea and then drop in a piece of tumor. The tumor grew very, very slowly for weeks, forming a flat, thin layer shaped like the cornea itself, but not getting very large. Once the tumor reached a few millimeters it seemed to become dormant, at which point Gimbrone extracted a small piece of it from the cornea and implanted it onto the blood-rich iris of a different rabbit's eye. Within days he and Folkman saw new capillaries sprout from the iris and begin growing toward the tumor sample. "We plunked that little bugger down in the iris," Gimbrone later said, "and [growth] went exponential."

Folkman loved it. He and Gimbrone took the results as the strongest, most visible evidence yet that tumors had to recruit new blood vessels in order to grow wild. Even years later, Folkman would recall the results of these experiments as one of the most important, thrilling achievements in his long history of angiogenesis research. It gave him a big boost in confidence, and he was now without any doubts that the new blood vessels did not arrive uninvited. In fact, he was so convinced that the tumors were secreting something that he felt justified in giving this mysterious substance—which he had yet to isolate, identify, or even prove existed—a name.

Trying to come up with an appropriate and catchy acronym, Folkman first tried vascular stimulating factor—VSF for short. Then he changed it to TEM, for tumor endothelial message. Finally he settled on TAF: tumor angiogenesis factor. Whatever the acronym, it was clearly a stand-in. As Dr. Isaiah Fidler of the M. D. Anderson Cancer Center in Houston observed years later, it was easy to scoff at the notion of naming a substance whose existence hadn't been proven. "If you have to call something a 'factor,' " Fidler says, reflecting the views, spoken or tacit, of many researchers who heard about TAF in these early years, "it means you don't know what you're talking about."

Folkman knew as well as anyone that he had a long way to go to identify the factor and that it could take years. But he had a plan of attack. He would start by using a painstaking chemical method called "fractionation," which was like slicing up an apple into ever-tinier pieces to find the one with the worm. In the case of TAF, he would try to separate the substance in question from the cancerous world in which it seemed to reside. He started with rat tumors.

Folkman carved the cancers out of the rats, then put the tumors into a pressure vessel. He pumped nitrogen into the chamber at high pressure, so the tumor cells would be forced to absorb the gas. Then he released the pressure suddenly. The abrupt change in pressure caused the nitrogen-filled tumor cells to burst and disintegrate, leaving a soupy collection of proteins at the bottom of the chamber. He called the fluid "tumor-conditioned medium" (TCM). It no longer had any intact tumor cells, but somewhere mixed into it there presumably was something that was important to the tumor—the protein he was calling TAF. The big task would be to separate it from the rest of the fluid. It was a problem roughly analogous to trying to separate the apple flavor from a gallon of apple cider—only much harder.

To begin, Folkman and his staff poured the material through a cylindrical glass tube filled with negatively charged starch beads that would attract some molecules but not others. It was a way to begin separating the complex fluid into slightly less complex fluids, since some of the molecules in the tumor-conditioned medium would stick to the starch beads and others would come out the bottom of the cylindrical column. The next step was to see which of these was active in promoting angiogenesis. The test was conducted on the back of a rat, with air pumped under its skin to form a viewable chamber. Folkman collected the fluid that had come out the bottom of the glass cylinder and dribbled it onto the white tissue surface of the rat's back. Then he watched what happened under a well-lit microscope. If this fluid failed to trigger angiogenesis, it meant that the active fraction—the one containing TAF—was still in the glass cylinder. When that proved to be the case, he removed the fluid containing these active molecules from the column, then poured it into another column, this one loaded with *positively* charged beads. Again he dripped the resulting substance onto the rat's back to see what part of the fractionated fluid retained the activity. He performed the process again and again, changing the conditions in the cylinder each time. After half a dozen steps, the tumor-conditioned medium had been whittled down from perhaps a thousand different agents—including proteins, water, and fragments of the cells' internal machinery—to a much simpler glob of fluid containing what Folkman guessed to be only fifty agents. At that point, the fluid had been reduced to a volume too small to continue.

Proteins—complex molecules, which are composed of chains of amino acids—are fundamental components of all living cells. They drive the hormones, growth factors, and structural elements that control what goes on in the living organism. Cells do their work by making and excreting proteins that act as messenger molecules, in effect telling other cells what to do or not to. At this point in Folkman's career it had only recently and imperfectly become understood that proteins are the products of genes, the central control elements of life. For each protein in an organism there is a specific gene in each cell's nucleus. Genes are turned on or off, depending on what the body needs and where it needs it. For example, if the body needs the protein called insulin, a glucose-controlling hormone, specialized cells in the pancreas begin making and releasing the agent, which keeps sugar use in balance. The living body is in essence a protein factory that maintains itself by making, altering, accumulating, and connecting proteins to one another.

The main problem with doing research to identify growth factor proteins

in 1971, however, was that most of the proteins in the body were still unidentified. (Many still are today.) Tracking down and identifying a protein was
extremely difficult, especially if it was present in only vanishingly small
amounts. Their very existence could be shown only by the results of their actions. The first known signaling proteins, present in amounts as small as billionths of a gram, could not be isolated with the existing technology. They
were shown to exist only because of the work they did, the changes they
caused in the function of cells.

So even if Folkman's starch beads and cylinders brought him closer to purifying TAF, he was still far away. The data was insufficient to publish; for
now, he would have to continue calling his angiogeneis trigger a factor. And
more than a few people would continue to say he didn't know what he was
talking about.

IN FALL 1971, FOLKMAN got his first chance to expose his theories directly to a significant segment of the Boston medical community. His audacity in trying to devise a general theory for cancer without strong evidence had
already rubbed some of his colleagues at Harvard the wrong way, especially
because he implied, in essence, they were missing the mark about cancer.
Folkman didn't have respected credentials in the field of research—he was
only a surgeon, after all, not even an oncologist—and he hadn't published
enough in peer-reviewed journals to lend his work credence. His reputation as
a Harvard surgical wunderkind was off-putting to senior scientists who were
steeped in their details. Folkman had too few details.

Still, some people were more intrigued than irritated. One of those who
thought Folkman's ideas deserved a forum was Dr. Louis Sherwood, the
young chief of endocrinology at Beth Israel Hospital who was in charge of re-
cruiting speakers for the hospital's Seminars in Medicine, a relatively informal weekly lecture series for doctors throughout the Harvard system. Each
year Sherwood also had to pick a dozen of the weekly talks for publication in
the official organ of the Massachusetts Medical Society, *The New England
Journal of Medicine*. He invited Folkman to speak. Folkman would finally be
able to present his favorite subject to an audience of medical colleagues. And
that audience might turn out to be much larger than the hundred or so doctors who usually showed up for the lecture.

After striding to the podium in the medium-sized auditorium one morning
in October, Folkman began outlining his ideas in typical technical language.

"The growth of solid neoplasms is always accompanied by neovascularization," he informed the group, as a way of introducing the notion that each tumor was independent and had to recruit new blood vessels from surrounding tissue in order to grow. "This new capillary growth is even more vigorous and continuous than a similar outgrowth of capillary sprouts observed in fresh wounds or in inflammation." In other words: Don't think inflammation is the cause. "It has not been appreciated until the past few years that the population of tumor cells and the population of capillary endothelial cells within a neoplasm may constitute a highly integrated ecosystem." Or: I believe that cancer has an elaborate life-and-death relationship with blood vessels.

Then Folkman moved on to the heart of the matter. "Tumor cells appear to stimulate endothelial cell proliferation," he said, "and endothelial cells may have an indirect effect over the rate of tumor growth." This was his thesis that tumors created a trigger to bring in new lines of support. And then, as a secondary effect, the endothelial cells grew to form the new blood vessels. He used the term TAF for the first time in public, conceding that the substance "has not been completely characterized," a significant understatement.

Folkman explained what he'd learned so far from the animal assays: Newly formed capillaries disappeared after TAF was withdrawn, indicating the substance had a specific mission and didn't cause permanent changes in blood vessel structure. He had fractionated several kinds of tumors, from both humans and mice, and in each case the growth factor had been isolated to a rough degree. "Therefore, TAF appears not to be species-specific," he said, "and its primary target is the endothelial cell."

Folkman had laid the groundwork. He proposed that tumors go dormant if blood vessels fail to grow and bring in more nutrients, and he suggested that it was the enigmatic TAF that allowed rapid tumor growth. Now he offered his most challenging idea of all: Maybe the process of angiogenesis could work in reverse. Maybe TAF could be inactivated or blocked by some opposing substance, stopping new blood vessel growth and preventing the cancer from expanding. Might it even interrupt the dangerous phenomenon of cancer's spread called tumor metastasis? He had a name for this hypothetical process, too: antiangiogenesis. And that, Folkman told his colleagues, was what he was after.

As he finished, Folkman looked about the room, well aware that it was filled with doctors who lived in a world in which the only ways to treat cancer patients were by poisoning, burning, and chopping out tumors. Folkman was asking them to think more imaginatively, to dig a little deeper, and to consider

more subtle notions. If we learn a few critical things about the interaction between the growing tumor and the patient's body, he suggested, perhaps it will
be possible to sabotage the tumor's life-support system and thus starve it to
death. Rather than the medical equivalent of bombing tumors back to the
Stone Age, Folkman proposed a form of clandestine subversion. "We are not
unaware of the difficulties involved," he acknowledged, offering ballast to his
enthusiasm.

"Although the evidence for these proposals is still largely indirect and
fragmentary," he said in conclusion, "it seems appropriate to speculate that
antiangiogenesis may provide a form of cancer therapy worthy of serious exploration." At the very least, even if antiangiogenesis therapy turned out to be
impossible and the entire concept was wrong, "careful exploration of its consequences may reveal something fundamental about the behavior of tumor
cells growing in a packed population."

Mindful of the dismissive response he'd gotten from so many journals and
grant reviewers, Folkman hoped his presentation might engage some of his
colleagues closest at hand. But the reaction was more like a polite yawn. The
group, primarily doctors treating patients day to day, seemed to view Folkman's findings as a laboratory curiosity that had little to do with the real lives
of cancer victims. "At that point we didn't think he could go very far," remembers Louis Sherwood, who had invited him. "It was an interesting biological concept, but it was very speculative." The talk closed with only a few
questions and little comment. Then the crowd of Harvard doctors headed
back to their wards and offices, leaving Folkman at the podium feeling he'd
had no impact at all. His ideas just did not jibe with the way doctors were then
thinking about cancer. They were too theoretical—really, too visionary—for
this group of clinical physicians. Folkman could not yet offer them a distinct
alternative to the standard therapies.

His talk appeared in the pages of *The New England Journal of Medicine* a
few weeks later, and again Folkman felt his colleagues' apathy. Maybe it was
because he hadn't submitted his presentation as a peer-reviewed article, but
once again it seemed to Folkman that almost nobody was much interested in
this idea that so consumed him.

SOON AFTER GIMBRONE'S RETURN to the lab, Folkman had told
him about his recent work and suggested he take a few weeks and think about
what might be challenging and useful to do next. One day during this brief

period of contemplation, Gimbrone ambled over to the Harvard co-op and came back to the lab with a little compass, the kind junior high school students use to draw circles in geometry class. "Okay," he told Folkman, "your hypothesis is that tumors secrete something to cause blood vessels to grow. How can we test that, and test it critically?"

Gimbrone had done a little research on the density of corneal tissue, and he had a plan. "Low molecular-weight substances will diffuse through the tissue more readily and over a longer distance than higher molecular weight substances," he said. "So here's a crazy idea." He took out his little compass and made a series of circles. What if they implanted tiny bits of tumor at various distances from the center of the cornea—he plotted out the points with the compass—and compared how fast and how far blood vessels traveled to them? If they were right that tumors released a factor that stimulated blood vessel growth, Gimbrone expected that at some distance from the edge of the cornea they would see signs of blood vessel growth being activated. If that happened, they would then have an indication of how far and how quickly the substance traveled through the corneal tissue. And that would offer confirmation that such a "diffusing factor" actually existed, as well as clues about its molecular makeup—clues that could eventually help isolate the stimulator.

Folkman thought this was anything but crazy. Like detectives trying to put together a profile of a suspect, they would try to learn something, anything, about the elusive substance they wanted to prove existed. They started by inserting little tumors directly in the middle of rabbits' corneas, as far away as possible from the nearest blood vessels. They calculated that if the suspected mystery agent consisted of large molecules, it wouldn't diffuse very well through the corneal tissue and might not even reach the outer edge of the cornea. Meanwhile, in other rabbits, they carefully implanted their small chunks of tumor farther and farther off-center, progressively reducing the distance between the tumor and the bed of blood vessels in the iris.

The experiments worked beautifully. Tumors that were implanted more than three millimeters away from the blood-rich iris triggered no angiogenesis. Those that were placed a little closer stimulated some blood vessel growth, but not enough to send sprouts all the way into the cornea to reach the tumor. But those planted within 1.2 millimeters of the iris attracted new blood vessels within a day or two. Folkman and Gimbrone could see capillaries penetrate the cornea and head straight for the tumors. And once they connected, those tumors grew enormously; after about a month they nearly matched the size of the eyes themselves. To Folkman and Gimbrone, it was more proof of principle that tumors were creating an agent that recruited the blood vessels they needed. Skeptics had told Folkman they seriously doubted that tumors secreted a diffusable substance, but by his lights, "This proved diffusion. Here's the tumor, and for the first time new vessels came in over a distance."

Folkman submitted a pair of papers on the cornea and eye experiments to the *Journal of Experimental Medicine* (the same journal had published Harry Greene's work that had inspired Folkman). Both papers were accepted; one marked the first time he had gotten the word "angiogenesis" into the title of a peer-reviewed article. But his elation would be short-lived. Soon after he published his findings, Folkman gave a talk at the Massachusetts Eye and Ear Infirmary, and at the conclusion a young postdoctoral student stood up and challenged his conclusions. In her own work, she said, she had once put a simple chemical, uric acid, into the cornea. And this had caused blood vessels to grow without any involvement of tumors at all. Gimbrone's findings on diffusion rates notwithstanding, it was enough to cloud his and Folkman's claims of seeing true angiogenesis. It was a serious assault on Folkman's idea, and he knew it. Yet again, he found he couldn't disprove the old inflammation argument.

It got worse for Folkman when the postdoctoral student published her small experiment as an abstract, which became Exhibit A against him. The abstract was cited repeatedly by people sitting on review committees as evidence that Folkman's angiogenesis research was unworthy of funding. The reviews were officially anonymous, but Folkman sometimes heard through the grapevine who had said what. Occasionally, the criticisms were written into the rejection notices. In one instance that hurt him to the core, Folkman heard that at a meeting of a grant-review committee, a respected pathologist had asked, "If uric acid can do it, what's so special about a tumor?" Folkman, he said derisively, was "just working on dirt."

The comment frustrated Folkman terribly, and he would never forget it. "We had all this beautiful work," he said, "and we couldn't defend it." Not yet, anyway. He was disheartened, but not defeated—and not about to abandon his theory. After all, wasn't it at least *possible* that dropping uric acid into the cornea caused a defensive reaction, setting off the secretion of the same kind of blood vessel growth factor that Folkman thought came from tumors? Folkman didn't have to think twice about it: He would explore that possibility. And he would keep at it until he understood the mechanism so he could prove his theory or disprove it himself.

Despite such determination, the setback was a strong dose of reality for

Folkman, and it prepared him for a long struggle. He acknowledged, in a way that he really hadn't before, that the phenomenon he called angiogenesis could take years to understand. At the moment, it seemed almost inaccessible to study. More visible processes—blood clotting, for instance, or nerve fiber growth—could be watched, dissected, and experimented with in laboratory dishes. But angiogenesis was much more cryptic. Disentangling it from common functions like inflammation and scarring would require new approaches, new tools, and deep new insights.

Folkman believed that those things would come. In the meantime, he would continue to pursue other tracks of research that might unearth new clues. He'd simply move on to his next idea. He did, after all, have a lot to prove.

Among Folkman's theses was that without angiogenesis, small tumors were unable to grow significantly because the dense tumor tissue acted as a barrier to the flow of oxygen and nutrients. Meanwhile, the poisons that naturally resulted from metabolism couldn't get out fast enough and ended up killing cells at the tumor's center. He considered this thesis consistent with a fundamental property of biophysics: that the rate of diffusion determines the rate of growth. Only the arrival of new blood vessels could overcome that diffusion barrier and allow growth of the tumor.

Folkman came up with a new plan to test this idea. He and his team suspended tiny samples of various tumor cells in a jellylike goo called agar in laboratory dishes. The agar was laced with amino acids, oxygen, fetal calf serum, and other nutrients the tumors needed to grow. But it had no source of new blood vessels. Would the tumors keep growing or stop at a certain size? Folkman watched as the tumor cells began expanding, forming small spheres afloat in the agar. Then, as he expected, the tumors all stopped growing. As dissection of the tumors later showed, cells hidden deep inside were dead and dying, presumably because the tumors weren't able to slurp up enough nutrients to sustain them, while waste products accumulated.

Folkman thought the experiment offered good evidence that tumors do need more than a small amount of basic nutrients to thrive. They need angiogenesis. Moreover, he realized these new results in the lab corresponded with something he had seen in the clinic. He had observed that some patients with eye cancers—retinoblastomas—had small, round tumors that floated in the eyes' clear liquid, the vitreous humor. These seemed to be tumors that had failed to connect with a blood supply. They were orphans, stuck in dormancy, just like the small experimental tumors growing in lab dishes.

All the while, Folkman remained preoccupied with the perennial inflammation argument, and one day came up with a new idea to counter it. A voracious reader of scientific literature, he happened on to a book by a Pennsylvania biologist, Joseph Leighton, in which he described his way of using an ordinary chicken egg to watch the behavior of tumors. Leighton cut an inch-square window in the shell of a fertilized egg, placed a tumor in it, covered the opening with Scotch tape, then put the egg in an incubator. Folkman saw immediately that this could be another way to track and measure angiogenesis in a live, natural setting. All he needed to do was make sure the growing chicken embryo was kept as warm as it would be in a nest under a mother hen. And it worked: Inside the egg, the tumors could be seen drawing in new blood vessels.

Folkman and his team named the experiment the chicken chorioallantoic membrane (CAM) assay. It would become one of his most valuable and enduring tools, especially after one of the lab members, Dr. Robert Auerbach, a visiting fellow on sabbatical from the University of Wisconsin, sorted out a way to improve the window-in-the-shell method of performing the experiment. Auerbach's vital contribution to the research was simple. He cracked the egg open, poured the combined yolk and albumen into a petri dish, put a lid on the dish, and then warmed it in an incubator until a chick embryo began to grow. After three days, the chick's tiny heart could be seen beating rhythmically under a low-powered microscope, and a network of thin red lines began meandering through the egg white and up around the yolk. When Folkman and his team put tiny pieces of tumor into the dish, it wasn't long before new capillaries began growing vigorously toward them.

Auerbach was only the first of a small parade of visitors who heard about Folkman through the cell-biology grapevine and spent brief stints in his laboratory, willing to risk a little time on the chance that Folkman might be on to something. Folkman was heartened to see that there were always a few scientists who would listen to his ideas and ignore the persistent warnings from colleagues that working with Folkman was a waste of time. Those who joined his lab either as postdoctoral fellows or as visiting scientists were the ones who wanted to see for themselves. They had actually talked with Folkman, who was extraordinarily open, friendly, and persuasive. It was a pattern that would be repeated over and over again in the coming years: A few young scientists would come to the lab to see the work for themselves, and they would get hooked on Folkman's ideas and enthusiasm.

As encouraging and exciting as the results of the CAM assay were to the experimenters, they were a virtual secret to all but a small circle of scientists, many of whom were wholly unimpressed. Thus Folkman's career was a paradox. He was still earning enormous respect as a pediatric surgeon; yet, for reasons he could not fathom, he was ignored, even scorned, as a researcher. His hunches about cancer could not seem to find intellectual or financial sustenance from the body politic of science, as if the process of growing a theory was itself a matter of angiogenesis, and Folkman's notion was floating in a sea of vitreous humor, unable to induce a pipeline of support that might help it sprout in the scientific imagination.

Folkman did have a few supporters. He would see Robert Gross in the hallways at Children's, and his old mentor would ask how things were going—not the surgery, but the angiogenesis research. And the Great Man at Children's himself, Dr. John F. Enders, whose name graced the building in which Folkman toiled, was happy to lend his encouragement, though with some bemusement. At one point early on, Folkman showed Enders a grant proposal and asked whether Enders thought he was giving away too much of his thinking. It was an uncharacteristic concern. Although scientists by nature tend to be almost ferally competitive—guarding their ideas jealously, never leaving notebooks open for view, seldom talking about unfinished work at meetings—Folkman was almost a blabbermouth, always sharing his ideas in the interest of furthering them, even sharing new research materials like the CAM assay. But there were limits to his altruism, and he was not immune to the competitive impulses so rampant in the profession. He didn't want someone exploiting the ideas in his grant proposals.

Enders sat down and puffed on his trademark pipe as he read the proposal for half an hour. Then he looked up and told Folkman he had nothing to worry about. "It's theftproof," he said. "No one will believe it."

There was one more esteemed elder who saw real promise in Folkman's work: a physician who himself had beaten back furious skepticism and personal contempt to advance the treatment of cancer like no one before him. As early as 1968, he had recognized in Folkman a creative mind that shouldn't be ignored, and he identified with his struggles. So when a public relations man from the American Cancer Society came to him one day looking for promising new research that might interest the public, the doctor, by now a figure of great renown and considerable power, had thought of the bright young surgeon. If you're looking for fresh ideas and engaging researchers, he told the publicity man, you really ought to go see Judah Folkman.

PART TWO

Chapter Eight

———

ALAN DAVIS WAS ON a hunting expedition the day he arrived on Dr. Sidney Farber's doorstep in Boston. It was fall 1968, and Davis was still learning the ropes of his new job on the press relations staff of the American Cancer Society in New York. He had been recruited from the medical school at the University of Utah, where he was on the PR staff, so he was not unfamiliar with the vagaries of medical and academic politics. What he didn't know when he accepted the job was that his new boss, Pat McGrady, the garrulous and popular spokesman for the society, was losing a power struggle with the doctors and administrators who ran the organization. Now, a year later, Davis had to take over one of his boss's most important jobs, and he was feeling the pressure.

McGrady had been with the American Cancer Society since the late forties, and he had invented what had become a major event for the organization: a yearly seminar for journalists, designed to raise public awareness of cancer. In its first few years after the Second World War, McGrady's annual press seminar was a traveling show. He rounded up a gang of reporters, crowded them onto propeller-driven planes, and ferried them around the country to visit leading cancer research facilities, where they sat through lectures on the hottest topics in the field, as selected by McGrady. But after a few years of herding cantankerous reporters through scary flights and tangled arrangements, the society decided it was easier to bring the scientists to the journalists.

By that time, the American Cancer Society—known for short as the ACS—was a mature organization, well structured, quite professional, and relatively well known. But it was not that way in 1913, the year the American Society for the Control of Cancer was founded by fifteen New York City doctors and business leaders. At the time, cancer research was totally obscure—the first virus that caused cancer in birds had just been identified—and cancer was not a subject for polite discussion. The disease was submerged in a climate of fear and denial and was rarely mentioned in public—even though it claimed seventy-five thousand lives a year in the United States alone. One reason it got so little attention was that cancer was overshadowed by infectious diseases. Antibiotics had not yet arrived on the scene. Thus the handful of founders who gave birth to the society faced a formidable task. They had to reach thousands of doctors, nurses, and laypeople with a troublesome message about a disease that very few even wanted to hear about. The founders' best weapon was publicity. They began producing articles for popular magazines and professional journals, and they published the monthly *Campaign* newsletter, filled with information about cancer.

The big push for public notice, backed by serious fund-raising, began in 1936, when Marjorie Illig, a field representative for the society and chair of the General Federation of Women's Clubs' public health committee, got a big idea. Illig proposed creating an army of her own, forming a legion of women volunteers who would wage a public war on cancer. Called the Women's Field Army, the thousands of recruits put on khaki uniforms bearing badges for rank and achievements, and set out in earnest to raise money and help educate the American public. Illig's effort was a huge success. Within three years, there were some 150,000 people active in the cancer control movement, and the cancer society joined the March of Dimes and a few others as one of the most formidable volunteer health groups in the country.

The society took on its modern form soon after World War II ended, reorganizing itself into the American Cancer Society in 1945. A year later, with the vigorous help of the philanthropist Mary Lasker and her friends, the ACS took in more than four million dollars, dedicating a quarter of it to research. The results came soon. Chemotherapy was used to induce temporary remission of cancer, lung cancer was linked to cigarette smoking, and the Pap smear was developed as a viable test for incipient cervical cancer. As such real achievements began to accelerate, the publicity system needed to accelerate, too. Pat McGrady's response was the press seminar, and it became an institution. The nation's science and medical writers came to the meeting each spring expecting a good show—cancer news worth reporting. And each spring, McGrady tried very hard to give it to them. And it was no coincidence that hordes of volunteers began going door-to-door for the organization's national fund drive soon after the press seminar got under way. There was a premium on getting as much cancer news as possible into print and on the air that week. Breakthroughs were preferred, but almost-breakthroughs were more than welcome, at least as far as Pat McGrady was concerned.

The press seminar had always been McGrady's baby. He had perfected the art of luring journalists to the meeting, by holding it at the end of winter in an appealing southern spot and never failing to deliver enough news for the reporters to justify the trip to their editors. By 1968, he had enjoyed twenty years of virtually free rein in choosing the speakers and deciding which stories to push. But recently some members of the ACS's governing board had been unhappy with his choices. There were complaints that McGrady's standards were not always scientifically rigorous. In fact, his detractors were not unjustified in calling some of the people McGrady brought to the lectern just this side of harebrained.

He invited a woman who claimed to have developed a vaccine for cancer. There was also the nun who said she could diagnose cancer (among other diseases) by simply looking at a person's blood. And McGrady was extremely enthusiastic about a compound called DMSO, a chemical derived from wood, which he was convinced would be the perfect delivery system for drugs because it passed right through the skin. (He also thought it could be a good treatment for arthritis.) According to McGrady, you could tell DMSO worked because "right after you rub it on your skin you get the taste of oysters in your mouth." McGrady did a lot of combat over DMSO, which was not approved for any medical use, and he eventually published a book called *The Persecuted Drug: The Story of DMSO.*

McGrady's attitude about guest speakers at the annual press seminar was to let reporters get a look at everyone involved in cancer research and decide for themselves who was worthy of attention. A crusty former reporter himself, he was extremely well liked by the members of the national medical and science press corps, and he had an uncanny ability to match the right stories with the right reporters, yielding reams of coverage for cancer. But by the late 1960s, the society was losing patience with McGrady's headstrong manner. The board moved to appoint an oversight committee of famous cancer experts to vet McGrady's selection of speakers for the press seminar. The three committee members—Jonathan Rhoads, chief of surgery at the University of Pennsylvania Medical Center; Richard Mason, vice president for research at the cancer society; and Sidney Farber, the distinguished pathologist at Children's Hospital in Boston—would presumably make sure there weren't any more nuns posing as scientists.

McGrady was not a bit pleased with this intrusion into his domain. He had no intention of going along quietly. Instead he turned over the next press seminar to the man he had recently hired and was grooming as his eventual successor, Alan Davis. Davis knew how important and tricky an assignment it was. He would have to recruit a flock of engaging speakers—scientists who not only had something to say but could also say it in reasonably plain English—and he would have to make sure they weren't so outrageous that inviting them would get him fired. He decided a prudent first step would be to introduce himself to the members of the new oversight committee and ask if they had any suggestions. He started with a visit to Sidney Farber up in Boston.

Farber was in every sense formidable. A tall and husky man in his mid-sixties with a white mustache and graying hair, he exuded dignity and command. He had a number of claims to prominence, perhaps the most notable being that he had revolutionized the treatment of childhood leukemia. But Farber had done more than that. He was a masterful physician, but he also cultivated a politician's spirit. He had close ties to the reigning figures of Boston, notably Richard Cardinal Cushing, the head of the city's Catholic diocese. In the 1950s Farber had been a powerful voice on a national level promoting the idea of government-supported biomedical research. He was instrumental in the movement that led to the establishment of the National Institutes of Health. And he had founded the famous Jimmy Fund, a charity to help children with cancer, a fund which was almost hyperactive in Boston. Years later, the Dana-Farber Cancer Institute, a preeminent cancer research and treatment institution, would be the enduring monument to his career, but there would be irony in its location right across Binney Street from Children's Hospital, a place where he had once been bitterly denounced as a poisoner of children.

Farber had pioneered the use of a leukemia therapy that would eventually become a standard cancer treatment, but whose mere mention once sent shivers down the spines of many doctors and parents. In the late forties, Farber had devoted much of his time in the pathology lab to developing the first chemotherapy agents, experimenting first on animals. After a special cancer ward was set up at Children's, he began using the treatment on children who had no other hope. But chemotherapy was then so primitive that it made many of the children feel far sicker, and Farber's insistence on using it drew bitter reprobation from many of his colleagues. Dr. W. French Anderson, who was to become an important genetics researcher but was then a house officer at Children's, remembers Farber clashing head-on with members of the hospital staff. "The fact was that chemotherapy for many, many years merely extended the dying for these kids," he says. "By taking these chemotherapeutic agents, which were poisons, these kids were absolutely miserable. They weren't being helped at all; they were just being kept alive. I was an intern when Children's Hospital made the decision to stop having interns on that service, because it was psychologically so traumatic for us. We all understood the rationale—that it could lead to a cure—and it did. [But] there was horrible suffering—for the kids and for their families."

The theory behind chemotherapy is that some chemicals might be able to attack and kill cancer cells, and appropriately enough, the theory has its origins in warfare. As reported many decades later by Graham B. Jones of Clemson University, some time after World War I the University of Pennsylvania's department of research medicine conducted autopsies on seventy-five soldiers who had been killed in an accident with mustard gas, a horribly disabling chemical weapon first synthesized in 1860. The examiners were surprised to find extreme reductions in the number of white blood cells (leukocytes) in the stricken soldiers' blood. Around 1930, according to historian Edward Shorter in *The Health Century,* Dr. James Ewing at Memorial Hospital in New York suggested mustard gas should be tested against tumors. It was too toxic to be taken internally but did have some effect when applied to skin tumors. In 1942 research on mustard gas resumed when Yale pharmacologists Louis Goodman and Alfred Gilman were asked by the army to study a chemically refined version called nitrogen mustard. After injecting the highly toxic compound into rabbits, Goodman and Gilman noted how quickly the animals' white blood cells disappeared. Hoping to see if they could give enough of the drug to kill a tumor without killing the host, they gave injections of nitrogen mustard to a mouse suffering with advanced lymphoma. Almost miraculously, the cancer regressed and disappeared. But when they stopped treatment, the tumor grew again and eventually became resistant to further treatment. What they had seen was drug resistance, which would become a vexing problem as chemotherapeutic drugs were developed in great numbers during the following decades.

The first doses of nitrogen mustard were given to a cancer patient later in 1942, when Goodman and Gilman persuaded a Yale colleague, surgeon Gustav Lindskog, to try it on a forty-eight-year-old silversmith who had advanced lymphatic cancer. After receiving the doses of nitrogen mustard, the man— the first recorded chemotherapy recipient—improved dramatically. His large, bulging tumors receded visibly, but like the mice he soon became resistant to further chemotherapy, and he succumbed to the cancer. It was a milestone but a secret milestone. In those war years any report with a link to chemical warfare was rigidly classified. Nothing was published about the experiment until 1946. But it did set the stage for Dr. Sidney Farber's first use of chemotherapy against childhood leukemia, in Boston.

By Farber's time, the goal of chemotherapy had come into focus: to find drugs that would kill dividing cancer cells without doing too much damage to healthy tissue. The problem was that cancerous cells weren't the only cells dividing. Among other tissue damaged by chemotherapy were the rapidly dividing cells in the gut, the bone marrow, and the hair follicles. Damage to these cells led to side effects so severe that they were frequently worse than the cancer itself. Extreme nausea, rampant diarrhea, and vomiting were typical, followed by hair loss, weakened immunity, and terrible discomfort. So the first cancer therapies were brutal. The patients who didn't die during treatment often wished that they had, and success rates, especially in the beginning, were dismally low.

No one was very pleased with chemotherapy, but it was one of few options. And eventually, as the first agents were refined, chemotherapy did begin to work against some forms of cancer, especially childhood leukemia. But it wasn't so successful—or its side effects any more tolerable—that doctors like Farber could use it without facing intense opposition from their colleagues. The hostility surrounding Farber's use of chemotherapy was so severe, in fact, that it led to all-out warfare between him and Dr. Louis Diamond, the influential chief of hematology at Children's Hospital. Diamond "absolutely could not stand Farber," W. French Anderson says. "So every time a kid came in with leukemia it was an interesting situation: Who would take care of the patient? Obviously, Farber was the expert, but Lou Diamond was so personally offended that Farber was, in many ways, ostracized. So he went across the street."

In 1952, Farber began a fund-raising organization, the Jimmy Fund (named for a young cancer victim he called Jimmy), and started a children's cancer research institution of his own. "Farber was deeply criticized for his vision," observes Dr. Fred Rosen, a pathologist and immunologist who was a key player overseeing research activities at Children's. Diamond, the chief critic, was a clinician, and his sympathies lay with the patient in front of him. Farber was not insensitive to the suffering of individuals; he himself had had colorectal cancer and would have to use a colostomy bag for the rest of his life.

But he was by nature a man who saw beyond the current day. Rosen recalls that when the Variety Club of New England, a wealthy charitable organization, sent a delegation to see Diamond about doing something to help children with leukemia, "Diamond's answer was, 'Well, I need a new microscope.' They walked out, saying, 'This man just doesn't get the picture.' They went to Farber, who of course had the vision that we needed a cancer center for children."

By the time Alan Davis came up to Boston almost two decades later, Farber was the head of a major cancer research foundation and chemotherapy was a mainstream treatment (by the 1980s, more than 80 percent of children stricken with leukemia would survive because of what he started). Meanwhile, with his energy and savvy, Farber had climbed to the top ranks of the American Cancer Society. He was about to serve a term as its president, and in the wake of the displeasure with Pat McGrady he was asked to oversee the annual press seminar. Farber knew as well as anyone how important an event it was and how it had come to influence the nation's perceptions about cancer as well as the society's ability to raise money for the war against the disease. And so when Davis came to him for ideas about who to recruit for the 1969 press seminar, Farber thought immediately of Judah Folkman.

As busy as he had been with the Jimmy Fund and steering the Variety Club's Children's Cancer Research Foundation, Farber had kept a hand in administration at Children's Hospital, and so he knew Folkman, the thirty-five-year-old star who had recently been named surgeon-in-chief. Folkman had eagerly talked about his angiogenesis theory with Farber, who found the idea enormously interesting and thought it was something that reporters covering cancer ought to hear about. There was a tinge of irony in this suggestion: In the eyes of some people, Folkman's work might have qualified as the kind of half-baked research that Farber's ACS oversight committee was supposed to weed out. But Farber himself was something of an iconoclast, and he had no reservations about putting Folkman up on the ACS podium.

Davis headed for Folkman's lab with the mild anxiety that usually accompanied a visit to a researcher he hadn't met. By nature, most serious doctors and scientists tended to be publicity-shy and not infrequently dismissive of the motives and abilities of reporters and press agents, as public relations people were then called. Indeed, within medicine and science there was a long tradition of branding anyone who spoke too much with the popular press as a blatant publicity seeker to be viewed with suspicion, even if his work was solid. A case in point was the astronomer Carl Sagan, whose public visibility was so disliked by scientists that he was ultimately blackballed from membership in the National Academy of Sciences. (Rejected in 1992, he was later given a public service award and honorary membership.) Even if it was a scientist's human impulse to want attention paid to his work, the correct way was to be published in important refereed journals or to win major prizes, not to be quoted by the Associated Press or *The New York Times*.

So Davis often had to engage in an awkward little dance to gain the trust of doctors and scientists he hoped to present to the public. "You're in their lab, on their turf," he says, "trying to explain why you're there." He would say that his goal was to disseminate information about scientific research in a reliable, responsible way and hope that the recipient of his pitch was not only willing but able to discuss his work without getting hopelessly bogged down in technical jargon. Sometimes it worked, sometimes not. But when trying to recruit speakers for the cancer society's press seminar, Davis had an important advantage: Most researchers were well aware that one of the American Cancer Society's fundamental roles was to supply substantial amounts of scarce research money.

When Davis arrived at Folkman's old, ramshackle laboratory at Boston City Hospital—it was still 1968, before the move to Children's Hospital—he was pleased to find Folkman was an exceedingly friendly man who was only too glad to discuss his work with anyone from the American Cancer Society. "He took me by the hand, almost, and said, 'Okay, let's start talking,' " Davis recalls. "And when you're talking with him he has this twinkle in his eye and he sort of smiles. So there was no problem at all getting into a conversation with Judah Folkman." The hard part was shutting him up.

Folkman carefully outlined his work to Davis: his ideas about cancer and angiogenesis and his belief that the key was in finding the factor that made blood vessels grow toward tumors. He proudly displayed the thyroid perfusion experiments, then walked Davis over to another tissue-growth system, this one filled with little black melanoma tumors growing in perfused slabs of puppy intestine. Davis asked Folkman the goal of his experiments, and Folkman told him he was exploring the question of why tumors triggered the growth of *new* blood vessels rather than calling in those already inside the tissue. "I thought that was absolutely fascinating," Davis remembers.

A few months later, Folkman was standing at the lectern at the 1969 American Cancer Society Press Seminar in New Orleans, explaining his theory of angiogenesis and the substance he was then calling tumor endothelial message. But the message did not get through. His talk was too esoteric and remote from the clinic—he later said he felt like a professor lecturing on vascular biology—and it was overshadowed by a presentation by Dr. Phil Gold, a researcher from Montreal's McGill University who had recently identified a chemical marker, a molecule called CEA (for carcinoembryonic antigen) that seemed to exist on the surface of cancer cells but not on normal cells. CEA might serve as a highly specific target at which to aim the poisons of chemotherapy. The idea that this marker might offer a new and better way to attack cancer cells was the big story of the week. Folkman's report raised hardly a ripple. Davis thanked him for coming and wished him luck with his work. But when Davis went home to New York, he made a mental note to keep track of the young surgeon from Children's Hospital.

DAVIS DID CHECK IN again with Folkman in the fall of 1971. How was he doing? Was he making progress with angiogenesis? Folkman filled him in on the rabbit eye experiments and on his continued search for the elusive growth factor, which he had since renamed TAF. He also told him about a film he had made through his microscope—microcinematography, it was called—showing highly magnified capillaries with blood cells being pumped through them. The film was a tour de force in movie technology, a new and exciting view of live activity that was likely to fire the enthusiasm of science reporters. Davis was sure the short film would be a hit, and he asked Folkman to make a return appearance at the society's press seminar.

This time, Folkman was unenthusiastic. He was in a different frame of mind than when they'd first met in 1968. Despite some exciting successes in the lab, Folkman was feeling the cold shoulder from his peers. His recent talk at Beth Israel and its subsequent publication in *The New England Journal of Medicine* had given him no reason to think his ideas were interesting to many people outside his own lab. The reviewers were dismissive, not to mention that pathologist in Chicago who said he was "purifying dirt." And he remembered the impact he'd had the last time he'd presented his work to the press: none. He wasn't in the mood to try again. But Davis pressed. He thought Folkman had made some significant progress toward seeing and understanding blood vessel growth in the last couple of years and that it would make a fine presentation. Folkman, who felt obligated by the twenty-thousand-dollar cancer society grant that was currently helping support his work, finally agreed to speak at the 1972 seminar in Clearwater, Florida.

Folkman might not have sensed it immediately, but from the moment he arrived at the waterfront Clearwater Hilton, there was a buzz around him. Davis had told Pat McGrady how far Folkman seemed to have come since his talk in New Orleans and about the film he had made. And McGrady, who was overseeing his last press seminar before retiring, was intrigued enough to call Folkman himself. When he did, he realized Folkman's idea seemed more and more likely, and he suspected that a treatment for cancer might be an eventual result. Folkman showed his film, and the showman in McGrady was sold. The master medical press agent decided that for his last press seminar—his swan song—he would promote Judah Folkman and angiogenesis as a major story.

McGrady gave Folkman a prime slot—Monday morning—and billed his talk as "a fitting sequel to the outstanding report he made at the 1969 science writers' seminar." The billing gave the impression that the topic had some history and substance, even if few of the journalists remembered it. All McGrady needed was the cooperation of the sixty reporters in attendance. He made sure they knew all about Folkman before he arrived in Clearwater. Recalls Joanne Rodgers, a medical writer from Baltimore then working for the Hearst chain of newspapers: "Pat McGrady briefed us on it a full day before the meeting actually started. We all sat in this cavernous room, just dying to go out to the beach. Pat said this was important, and everybody got excited, because here was clearly a really interesting and novel idea."

On Monday morning, March 27, Folkman made his way to the microphone as the reporters sat before him, notebooks and pens in hand. "Recent work in our laboratory," he said, "has disclosed a critical point in the early life of a solid neoplasm where a new therapeutic approach may be decisive in preventing a tumor from expressing its malignant potential." It was a carefully crafted and explosive sentence—a preamble to a much more tantalizing report than the one he had delivered in New Orleans three years before. In 1969, he had explained his theory that tumors could be held dormant without access to a fresh supply of blood from new vessels, and that this process was triggered by an unknown substance. Now, to a rapt audience, he announced that he and his colleagues at Harvard thought they had isolated, though not purified or identified, such a chemical signal.

Folkman talked about the still-undefined substance he was calling tumor angiogenesis factor and described the experiments that had led him to conclude that it was a ribonucleic acid (RNA), complexed with a protein (the RNA theory later turned out to be untrue). The semantics of *isolating* versus *identifying* the factor was not an issue any of the reporters in the audience bothered to raise. They were hooked. Folkman showed his film of the moving blood cells, a visual aid that many of them found as compelling as Pat McGrady had. It gave Folkman an extra measure of credibility as a visionary researcher and made his audience pay even closer attention when he offered his theory of antiangiogenesis. If one kind of substance triggered the growth of blood vessels that tumors needed to thrive, he speculated, then perhaps there were others that inhibited it and would cause tumors to be both malnourished from lack of blood and poisoned by their own wastes. "Our work has shown that there is a crossroad early in the life cycle of a solid tumor at which it may be sidetracked into a state of permanent dormancy, while still no larger than a millet seed," he said, a reference to the observation first made in his navy work with Fred Becker a decade earlier, that tumors always stopped growing at a tiny size unless they could draw in a blood supply.

In the audience, a wave of astonishment washed over the reporters. Among those most gripped by the idea was Jane Brody of *The New York Times*. "It was seemingly a breakthrough about the mechanism of cancer," she recalled years later. "It offered a potential to attack tumors that was completely new. We hadn't seen anything like it. Nobody had seen anything like it. It absolutely fired the imagination." Eyeing Folkman, Brody thought he had the manner and the medical credentials of someone to be taken seriously. "He was a very sober scientist," she said, "and he didn't present this as pie in the sky." She decided she would push the story hard when she talked to her editor in New York.

Ron Kotulak, from the *Chicago Tribune*, was similarly struck. "I thought it was really exciting, a brand-new strategy," he said later, a breath of fresh air at a time when there seemed to be a lull in invigorating cancer research. He was also impressed by Folkman's deportment: "He had that very nice disposition. He was polite and explained it very clearly."

But if the reporters were excited about a good story, the scientists who had come to the meeting to give their own presentations were, not surprisingly, somewhat less impressed. Folkman had been speculating, and unlike many other speakers he had not come armed with peer-reviewed publications to back up his assertions. Worse, he was just a surgeon who seemed to be dabbling outside his field of expertise. "The other docs were polite, but nobody recognized it as either fundamental, insightful, or important," recalls Carl Cobb, who was covering the seminar for *The Boston Globe*. "It was kind of 'Let's wait and see if it has any clinical relevance.' "

That was the number one question on the minds of many of the reporters: What would this mean for the treatment of cancer?

After the talk, Brody asked Folkman to come back to the journalists' writing room, where several dozen reporters were feverishly hammering away on typewriter keys, preparing their stories on Folkman for the next morning's papers. Brody was a short, slim, effervescent woman who would soon be one of the nation's leading medical reporters. She questioned Folkman closely, sorting out the details and making sure she understood him. "This is the first time to our knowledge that it has been possible to deliberately hold a carcinoma in the dormant state in an animal," he said, referring to the experiments with the rabbit eyes, as Brody took down his words. Then Brody asked the ultimate question: What were the chances that these discoveries would lead to actual treatments against cancer? Folkman told her that the trick would be to find a way to counteract TAF, either by stopping tumors from producing it or by blocking it from triggering new capillary growth. How long might that take? Perhaps two to five years, Folkman guessed in what proved to be a burst of naive enthusiasm.

The next day, Tuesday, March 28, 1972, page 1 of *The New York Times* was, as always, full of all the news that was fit to print. The Senate finance committee had voted to increase Social Security benefits to $200 a month; American investments in South Africa were being attacked and defended; and New York's mayor, John Lindsay, was thinking of running for president. And squeezed into the bottom right column of the front page were the first two paragraphs of a story out of the American Cancer Society's annual press seminar:

Tests Hint Protein Is Vital to Cancers

By Jane E. Brody

CLEARWATER BEACH, Fla., March 27—A Harvard surgeon said today that his research team had demonstrated in animal and test tube experiments that the growth of most cancerous tumors was dependent on a protein substance without which the tumors reverted to a dormant, harmless state.

The surgeon, Dr. M. Judah Folk-

man, said the discovery could open
an entirely new approach to cancer
therapy—the possibility of forcing
tumors into indefinite hibernation by
depriving them of this substance.

The story jumped to page 34, where the *Times* ran a photograph of a half-smiling Folkman, along with a drawing illustrating the tumor growth process as an interaction with the growth of blood vessels. T.A.F. AND CANCER was the headline over the illustration. Meanwhile, all across the country that morning, dozens of other newspapers reported Folkman's findings. Ron Kotulak's story ran prominently in the *Chicago Tribune,* Carl Cobb's story was on the front page of *The Boston Globe*—helped by the local-guy angle—and scores of smaller papers picked up stories from the Associated Press and United Press International. Suddenly the theory of angiogenesis was out in public view, and Judah Folkman was something of an instant, if accidental, scientific celebrity. As he was to find out, the publicity would be both a blessing to his career and a real curse.

From the outset, it was an odd sort of validation. The public notice seemed to Folkman a recognition that the idea he had been working on for ten years was credible and promising to objective minds. But a crowd of reporters writing news stories on deadline hardly constituted professional peer review. As a succession of colleagues soon let Folkman know, he had just taken his penchant for openness and optimism to hazardous new heights. It was premature, for instance, for him to be blabbing in public about curing cancer. Although he hadn't actually claimed a cure was in sight—the word he used was "treatment"—that was how his message was interpreted, and why his talk had gotten so much play. In the weeks following the newspaper stories, Folkman took more than a few phone calls from people with cancer wanting to know when his treatment would be available. One even showed up at his door. Even Sidney Farber, a big fan of Folkman's and the man whose suggestion a few years earlier had led to those momentous few hours in Clearwater Beach, seemed to have second thoughts. He later told Folkman that it was never good to lead people to believe, even unintentionally, that a new treatment was just around the corner when in fact it might never make it out of the lab.

Farber was not the only one who thought Folkman had said too much. Folkman's colleagues and friends were not shy about telling him he had been too openly optimistic about his pursuit of TAF. Folkman recalls, "A lot of people called up and said, 'You are jumping too fast. You said you might [identify] one of these factors in five years, but it might be ten years or twenty years. It might be never.' In fact, they were right." His colleagues would have been justified if they had pointed out that Folkman had been less than precise, even less than honest, in saying he had "isolated" the angiogenesis trigger. Calling it a ribonucleic acid–protein complex might have sounded impressive to the average newspaper reader, but scientists knew it was shorthand for a mess of genetic material that hadn't been completely purified. That didn't count as isolating the substance.

The public attention also renewed the carping among some members of Folkman's surgical staff at Children's Hospital. To them, a surgeon's job was surgery—even more so for the surgeon-in-chief, who was on call for the most extreme and difficult cases. Folkman reminded them that his department was named Surgical Research. They replied that his research wasn't really about surgery; it was about cell biology, something they didn't see much use for. Remembers Dr. David Nathan, then the hospital's chief of medicine: "They wanted him in his underwear"—dressed in his surgical gown—"not monkeying around up there on the tenth floor." "I don't think he really had their loyalty," observes the hematologist Fred Rosen, Folkman's colleague at the medical school. "They were bad-mouthing him."

Folkman was wounded by the disrespect of his colleagues. He couldn't understand why some of them seemed to regard his research as so trivial that they didn't even bother trying to understand it. Still, their attitude hardly compared to the offense taken by scientists in "the cancer establishment," who were essentially in competition with Folkman. These were cancer researchers who were certain that tumor cells themselves were the best targets for therapy and who were resentful that a surgeon had burst onto the scene with what they regarded as a half-baked notion, threatening to distract attention from what they considered more legitimate (and more grant-worthy) avenues of research. Especially within the populous Boston biomedical community, word began to get around that Folkman, with little hard science in his background, was playing with biology and biochemistry and making claims he couldn't support. Among the expert life scientists at Harvard and the other nearby institutions, Folkman was treated as a pretender, a man ill-equipped to play among the big boys who dug into the very nature of cancer and explored the core of the problem in the cancer cells themselves.

A good bit of the skepticism was based on how and where Folkman had presented his thesis—not in peer-reviewed scholarly journals such as *Nature* and *Science,* with their technical argot and requisite charts and graphs. Instead Folkman's work showed up in surgical journals—seldom read by "real" scientists—and even in newspapers, which almost all scientists distrusted because they explained the work in simple statements and crudely drawn illustrations. The establishment believed no true scientist would tell his results to journalists first. How could anyone assess his data? It wasn't by choice, of course, that Folkman had managed to publish only a couple of peer-reviewed papers on his angiogenesis work to this point. But the fact remained that he was vulnerable to criticism from the other side of the Charles River, the Mason-Dixon Line of the Boston medical science community.

The river was a natural dividing line symbolizing the long-standing antagonism between clinical researchers and laboratory scientists—the battle between M.D.'s and Ph.D.'s. The river isn't very wide as it flows between Boston and Cambridge, but it represents a gulf between medicine and science that can be as broad as an ocean. On the south side, in Boston, are most of New England's large and prestigious medical schools, major hospitals, and specialized medical institutions. On the Cambridge side are the ivy-covered brick buildings that turn out men and women of hard science, the Ph.D.'s of Harvard, MIT, and, some miles farther north, Tufts University. For most of the twentieth century, the two communities seemed to dance at arm's length to the beat of different rhythms. Those dedicated to lab work often viewed M.D.'s doing research as amateurs who were unqualified to sort out all the complexities of what they saw in patients. And clinicians were often wary of lab researchers, believing they did not look beyond the tiny snippets of tissue they saw under their microscopes, barely aware of the connection between disease and a living person.

Of course, there have always been those who swam to the other side of the river—doctors who trained first in one of the basic science departments at Harvard; biologists, biochemists, and biophysicists who migrated to research jobs in the labs at Mass General—but the animosity between Ph.D.'s and M.D.'s has been a constant. As Fred Rosen put it later, "There is still this antagonism. It will never go away." In the case of Judah Folkman—a surgeon, no less, performing basic research—the enmity might be traced to an even more difficult clash of cultures. From the very beginning, the cancer research community could not fathom someone so adventurous, so big-thinking, so willing to outrun his headlights, as Folkman. Lab researchers, says Fred Rosen, "are extremely committed to the truth of their details. Whereas someone like Judah says, 'You know, we'll deal with the details later.' "

All the talk in the months following the press seminar was sub rosa. There were no real broadsides, no public confrontations, no rebukes in print. Instead, circulating among the Harvard postdoctoral fellows, lecturers, and some professors was a murmuring disapproval of Folkman's style, with only a facile familiarity with his actual work. A common view, recalls Fred Rosen, was: "It's all hype. There's nothing there. It's all glitz." Even those who were willing to reserve judgment were baffled and unsure what to think about work that had been presented in such an unconventional way. "Most people were wondering," Rosen says, "if it was just a show—or was it real?"

FOLKMAN WAS FRUSTRATED by the doubts of his peers, but only to a point. Unlike Sidney Farber, who was combative by nature and found himself in a protracted battle that turned on moral judgments and the lives of real people, Folkman was involved in what was, for now, a much more abstract, academic conflict. He knew on some level that his critics were right about one thing: He hadn't proved his case. Not yet. So rather than stubbornly arguing that he had, he did his best to tune out the bad-mouthing and simply returned to his lab to do more work. Instead of debating, he would accumulate more data, arm himself with new facts, look for more convincing ways to show he knew what he was talking about and prove this wasn't just a show.

As the dust settled from the Clearwater press seminar, Folkman and his team focused on the fundamental missing piece that the critics demanded: an absolutely clear way to demonstrate that blood vessel growth was controlled by growth factors. Many people outside the lab harbored stubborn doubts that TAF even existed. In their eyes, Folkman could not prove that blood vessels growing toward tumors weren't the result of inflammation, for instance. And the results Folkman reported in living animal systems—the eyes of live rabbits, the backs of rats, the fertilized eggs of chickens—were still open to too much interpretation and too riddled with ambiguity to be accepted as solid evidence. They showed that blood vessels grew toward tumors, but not why.

There was a paradox in this: Folkman had earlier been roundly criticized for always working in vitro—in lab containers, outside the natural environment of living bodies. But now it seemed that in vitro was exactly where he needed to be. To be convinced of the existence of a tumor growth factor, experts wanted clear data that demonstrated how much TAF was necessary for angiogenesis, how quickly the cells responded, how long the response lasted, and what percentage of cells survived. They wanted to see hard numbers, and they wanted to be able to repeat the experiments with the same results. But the only way Folkman and his team could answer those questions was to create a reliable culture system for endothelial cells. They needed a way to make blood vessel cells grow in a dish, in specific directions, in direct response to purified growth factors. If they could do that, they might learn what actually controlled the growth. And *then* they could test the growth factor in animals. So the first step was to figure out how to do something that had never been done: grow endothelial cells in culture. Although a few scientists had tried to do it through the years, their failures had led to the firm conclusion that it was impossible. Research by a Japanese team in the mid-1960s had already indicated that endothelial cells would not live and divide in culture dishes. After struggling to isolate the cells from human umbilical cords, the Japanese scientists found that the cultured cells quickly converted themselves into fibroblasts—ordinary connective tissue cells—suggesting that endothelial cells didn't like to grow outside the body. As a result, it had since become gospel among cell biologists that endothelium could not grow in vitro. Subject closed. "That issue was nonnegotiable, and the challenge was on," recalls Ramzi Cotran, the Harvard pathologist who was one of the first established scientists to begin collaborating in some of Folkman's endothelial cell experiments.

Cotran, Folkman, and Michael Gimbrone had actually been trying to do this on and off for several years, ever since they were working in Folkman's lab at Boston City Hospital in 1968. But they had made little progress: They could keep the endothelial cells alive in the lining of intact blood vessels, but they couldn't keep them alive as a pure culture in a petri dish. And so they had moved on to other things. Now, four years later, the problem took on a new urgency and an even greater sense of difficulty.

"We tried and tried and tried to get endothelial cells to grow, and they wouldn't grow," Folkman recalls. It didn't matter what animal the endothelial cells came from—mice, rats, humans—they still would not grow in culture. "The pathologists said they cannot be grown. They thought it was ridiculous, like, 'You're trying to invent a way to walk on water.' It was considered an absolute law. Many people had tried, and it had turned out to be fibroblasts, just a contaminant."

But Folkman had little choice but to keep trying. "If we couldn't grow them, then the field [of angiogenesis] would have been dead," he says. "I could not see how we'd get out of that bind. It was sort of checkmate." Cotran and Gimbrone agreed that they were at a crossroads. If they—or someone—could not devise a tissue culture system for endothelial cells, it would take far longer to prove Folkman's fundamental idea that tumors called in their own private blood supply, if it could be proved at all. So they pressed on, Gimbrone in particular, even though his time in Folkman's lab was about to end. As he neared the end of his second one-year stint before going on to residency, he was drafted for military service, and he would soon be off to the National Institutes of Health.

Gimbrone's friends had advised him to forget about trying to culture endothelium—the Japanese study showed it's a waste of time, they told him—but he knew how important it was to Folkman and decided to make one last stab. He was encouraged by a few hints that it might be possible after all. Word was that over at Boston University, vascular biologist David Shepro had managed to cut some endothelial cells out of cow and pig aortas and keep them alive in culture, although they hadn't grown. And soon Gimbrone learned that a research team on the West Coast—biologist Denis Gaspodarowicz, microbiologist Bruce Zetter, and others at the University of California, San Francisco—was also having success inducing endothelial cells from cows' aortas to grow in culture dishes. Oddly enough, endothelial cells were not the original target of the research being done in California. Instead, Gaspodarowicz and his team were intent on finding growth factors—agents that make cells start dividing—and it was serendipitous that the crude factor they were studying could induce cells from the cow aorta to grow. So their focus was on inducing growth, with little interest in endothelial cells specifically. As Zetter later explained the use of cow aortas, "These arteries are so big you can just scrape [the endothelial cells] off, put them on a plate, and hope they grow. People started with these because they could get them from the butcher. And serendipitously, cow and pig turned out to be very easy endothelial cells to grow. No one knows to this day why some species are easy and some are hard."

Human cells were hard—very hard. But Folkman's determination to tackle daunting problems had rubbed off on Gimbrone. In his last two months in the lab in 1972, he made a pitched effort to try to culture isolated endothelial cells. No one had ever cultured human endothelia, and nobody had ever studied their biochemistry. But he was fascinated. "I began to think about blood vessels as not just little conduits, but as a functional part of the different organs of the body," he said.

Gimbrone started with aortas taken from rats, rather than from cows or pigs, simply because they already had a perfusion system up and running for rat-size vessels. Working in a small, dimly lit alcove in Folkman's lab, he pumped a nutrient-rich fluid through the aortas day and night. Looking through an old microscope, Gimbrone saw that the fluid was keeping them alive. They were in the right place, inside the blood vessel, and they looked normal—they weren't fibroblasts. It wasn't the same as actually growing individual endothelial cells in a laboratory dish, but it did show that the culture medium pouring through the tubes was the right stuff. It was not killing the cells.

The next task was to see if he could take the cells out of the aorta and get them to grow in a dish. But there was a problem: Only about ten intact cells could be harvested from each rat aorta, not nearly enough for a culturing experiment. So Gimbrone considered the Japanese idea: What about trying with human umbilical cords? Folkman liked that. He and Gimbrone headed over to the Boston Lying-In Hospital, and asked the head of pathology if they could have some umbilical cords left over from births. Soon Gimbrone was walking over to the hospital for regular collections of fresh umbilical cords that would otherwise be discarded. "I became the perennial expectant father," he recalls. "I'd be in the waiting room and there'd be these people looking at me, saying, 'You're back today? I thought you had the kid yesterday.'"

Back in the lab, Gimbrone and Cotran filled up sections of umbilical vein with collagenase, an enzyme that dissolved the supporting structure around the cells. At first, they had no idea how long to let it steep, so every fifteen minutes they'd drain off one of the sections and see if any endothelial cells had been liberated. They learned that thirty minutes seemed to do it. When they flushed the vein with culture fluid, thousands of endothelial cells came washing out. But would these liberated cells grow? When Gimbrone plunked the endothelium into the bottom of a dish, the answer was clearly no. The cells just sat in the plastic petri dish, alive but not responding.

This was no surprise to Folkman. It merely indicated the cells needed stimulation by some growth factor. But there were no growth factors available to play with, so he and Gimbrone decided to see what would happen if they manipulated the culture medium. The culture fluid normally contained between 5 and 10 percent fetal calf serum, a commercial laboratory product widely used in tissue culture because it contains a rich variety of growth factors, which act as a fertilizer to make cells grow, although no one knew exactly why. Little by little, they increased the concentration of serum in the fluid. From 15 percent to 20, from 25 percent to 30. Finally, in a corner of the image, Gimbrone saw what he thought were new endothelial cells. The next day, he thought he saw a few more. Excitedly, he showed Folkman. "This is growing," Gimbrone told him. "I think we've got them!"

Folkman thought he might be right and that it might offer a point of entry to the all-important problem of endothelial cell growth. They prepared the cells for a bigger test: viewing them through Ramzi Cotran's electron microscope. Cotran was the first to see that it was true: The cells in the petri dish contained telltale tiny granules found only in endothelial tissue. They looked just like cells seen in normal tissue. It was handshakes and elation in the lab—"You can't imagine how exciting that was," Cotran later said—for they'd scaled a formidable barrier. The Folkman team had done what the conventional wisdom said wasn't possible: They'd coaxed *human* endothelial cells to grow in a petri dish. And they had invented a system in which human blood vessel growth could be turned on and off at will, either by adding or withholding serum. This opened the way to future experiments in the search for other agents that would make human endothelial cells grow or stop growing. So thrilled were they that for the moment they even looked beyond their immediate goal of testing angiogenic substances. Maybe, they mused, a way could be found someday to attach these blood vessel cells to surfaces, like the inside of an artificial heart or the plastic patches used to repair aneurysms. Using endothelial cells as a natural lining for these devices might help solve the dangerous clotting problems encountered when artificial organs are used.

The achievement wasn't ready for publication—Folkman wanted to repeat the experiments and double-check everything—but he did note the tissue culture results in the process of applying for research grants. More than a few of the reviewers, Folkman heard, refused to believe it. Pathologists at leading universities and at NIH itself were heard to say that these could not be endothelial cells because, as everyone knew, it was impossible to grow endothelial cells. They were sure Folkman's lab was looking at something else—perhaps fibroblasts, as the Japanese researchers had warned—before anyone actually tried to duplicate the work. But Gimbrone, who had spent his early research time as a Harvard medical student examining endothelial cells through the electron microscope, eventually found an answer for the critics. He concluded that what he was seeing and what the Japanese had reported seeing years earlier were not quite the same. Because the Japanese team was limited to using an ordinary light microscope, Gimbrone thought they had misidentified some of the cells in their samples.

The spindly things the Japanese called fibroblasts were actually pericytes, cells that mature into the smooth muscle cells that surround blood vessels. In the Japanese experiment, a few smooth muscle cells had apparently come out of the umbilical veins along with the endothelial cells. Gimbrone suspected that the growth factors in the culture medium that the Japanese were using caused these pericyte cells to grow wildly, eventually taking over the culture. "These smooth muscle cells were like crabgrass in the lawn," Gimbrone explained years later, after he had become a leading authority on blood vessel structure. "They overgrew the endothelial cells, and they looked like fibroblasts. They said, 'Well, one kind of cell transformed into the other.' But that was wrong."

Folkman's lab wasn't the only place where progress was being made in endothelial cell growth research. New thinking and better tools led researchers to believe that each type of tissue in the body had specific, potent growth factors to which it responded. The quest to discover these growth factors was becoming a hot area of research, and a number of research groups, like Folkman's, were trying to develop ways to test various biochemical substances for their growth-spurring abilities. Factors that triggered the growth of nerves and skin had recently been discovered, and the search was on for more. So Folkman found himself in an unaccustomed position. Though he was the only one hunting for a tumor growth factor, he was no longer alone in the woods. In New York, Eric Jaffe, a hematologist at the Cornell Medical Center, had become interested in the purported factors that could spur the growth of endothelial cells and had also joined the quest to grow endothelium in culture. Unbeknownst to Folkman, Jaffe had also found a way to strip cells from large veins found in human umbilical cords and was getting them to grow in culture. But Jaffe and his group also met with stiff resistance from peer reviewers, who were convinced that both research groups were wrong. Meanwhile, out on the West Coast, similar research was moving apace, though not with human cells. On the San Francisco campus of the University of California, biologist Denis Gaspodarowicz and his postdoc microbiologist, Bruce Zetter, had recently discovered a hormonelike growth factor that Folkman and Gimbrone noted with great interest.

Gaspodarowicz's search led him to grind up pituitary glands from cows. The pituitary had long been considered the body's master gland, a likely place to look if one is trying to understand hormones and similar growth factors, where they come from and how they act. And it was a choice that went to the heart of why the field was suddenly so hot: Scientists realized that if they could decipher the growth control systems for different kinds of tissue, they might then be able to better understand how different organs developed. And although it was just a gleam in the eye, down the road the use of potent growth factors might give scientists control of organ growth, perhaps even a way to grow new organs to replace old ones.

In their San Francisco research, which was performed in 1973 and 1974 and published a year later in *The Journal of Biological Chemistry*, Gaspodarowicz and his colleagues had found that the pituitary contained a substance that seemed to be a potent agent for cell growth. It made cells grow in culture dishes. He hadn't isolated or identified the factor but found first that it could induce growth in ordinary fibroblast cells, those found in the connective tissue that is widely distributed throughout the body. So he named his mysterious agent fibroblast growth factor, or FGF. But then Gaspodarowicz began testing it on every kind of cell available, and he found that despite its name, FGF worked best on the bovine version of Folkman's favorite, endothelial cells.

Only a handful of researchers paid much attention to the discovery of FGF at the time, but it would turn out to be a big step in a landmark development for medicine. The new growth factor was one of the first among dozens of hormonelike substances biomedical researchers discovered beginning in the mid-seventies. These natural agents seemed to have extraordinary powers, finally giving researchers—and also doctors—the ability to spur growth in specific tissues. That would become especially important as researchers learned how to selectively augment the growth of specific kinds of white and red blood cells to overcome some of the damage done to bone marrow by chemotherapy. It also became important in the neurosciences, where experimenters began to control the growth of nerve cells in culture dishes and also in living tissues. The discovery of whole families of growth factors opened up a new world of possibilities for research and medical progress. Their emergence gave biologists and biochemists glimpses of an entirely uncharted realm of discovery.

In fact, scientists would in time find a huge variety of tissue-specific growth factors that seemed to do almost magical things within the body. By the 1970s, it was already well known that hormones regulate much of what happens in the body. There was the "fight or flight" hormone called adrenaline, which is an emergency response system. There was insulin from beta cells on the pancreas, which is the critical player in balancing blood glucose and is the hormone that is given daily to control diabetes. There was human growth hormone, which, when in short supply, leads to stunted growth and dwarfism. And there were the sex hormones—estrogen and testosterone—which control secondary sex characteristics such as body hair, breast growth, and voice development. The modern study of hormones and growth factors was also full of surprises. For many years the pituitary was considered the body's master gland, since it secretes a host of hormones that control what other glands are doing. It later turned out, however, that the real master gland is the hypothalamus, which is controlled by the brain.

The identification of all these hormones still would not prepare scientists and doctors for the discovery of a flood of tissue-specific, growth-triggering "factors." In response to a wound, for example, EGF (epidermal growth factor) would be released to speed the repair of torn skin. Damage to peripheral nerves would stimulate the release of NGF (nerve growth factor) to spur the rebuilding process. And the bone marrow has a whole suite of stimulatory factors that can drive the production of specific cell types. Erythropoietin is a potent stimulator of red blood cell production, while GM-CSF (granulocyte-monocyte colony-stimulating factor) causes bone marrow to start making extra disease-fighting white blood cells, which in turn secrete other factors called cytokines. As the research continued, whole families of factors called interleukins would be found, some made by disease-fighting T cells, others by monocytes and macrophages, fibroblasts, bone marrow cells, thymus cells, endothelial cells, and alveolar cells in the lungs. In time, it would become clear that the body is constantly being fine-tuned by the flow of invisible factors, some stimulating cells to grow, others turning off such growth. It is yin-yang in the extreme.

The first successes coaxing endothelial cells to grow in culture were so exciting to a small group of scientists that they formed an informal association dubbed the Blood Vessel Club. An inaugural meeting was held in Atlantic City on the Sunday before the huge annual meeting of the Federation of American Societies for Experimental Biology in 1973. It was at that meeting that the two leading groups working with human endothelial cell growth—Folkman's and Jaffe's—gave their first reports of success. "It was electric," recalls Cotran, who chaired the session. "Jaffe gave the talk, and Gimbrone gave a blitz" (a five-minute presentation, almost an abstract, usually given by graduate students or postdocs who are not yet senior scientists). The results got a warm reception from the Blood Vessel Club, but nonmembers, especially the pathologists on grant committees, continued their skepticism, because only the two teams headed by Folkman and Jaffe had reported success at growing human endothelial cells. But they were the only two who had tried; only a small number of people were even remotely interested in the subject of blood vessel growth. With the available literature telling the world that blood vessel cells would not grow in laboratory dishes, few budget-strapped academics were going to commit to such an unpromising pursuit or be able to find graduate students who would sign on for an assignment that seemed more likely to stall their careers than build them. So the old dogma that no one could grow human endothelium continued to hold sway.

Now the race was on. The two teams became friendly competitors, each hoping to be the first to dispatch the doubts and announce, in a peer-reviewed publication, that it had done the supposedly impossible. Folkman's team had a handicap: Gimbrone had by then reported for duty at NIH, meaning he had to commute to Boston to tie up loose ends. Jaffe's group won the race by about three months, publishing in late 1973 in *The Journal of Clinical Investigation*. The Harvard paper came out in spring 1974, in *The Journal of Cell Biology*. But Folkman didn't fret much about losing the credit competition—he was much more excited about the milestone both teams had reached. Finally getting endothelial cells growing in petri dishes meant they could now get on with the pursuit of TAF. Even now, though, many researchers outside the Folkman laboratory maintained their skepticism about growing human endothelial cells and the existence of TAF.

For this first try, Folkman took tumor-conditioned medium—the fluid that tumor cells from rats had been growing in—and added it to the growing endothelial cell culture. It was a moment he had anticipated for years; he expected to see a burst of growth from the cells, a clear signal of the potency of the fluid containing the elusive TAF. But the results were crushing, almost worth tears. Nothing happened. There was no burst of growth. Not even an extra wiggle. The cultured cells just sat in the bottom of the dish, ignoring the bath of stimulating chemicals washing over them. Folkman had convinced himself that the factor hidden in the fluid would jump-start the growth of the endothelial cells. It worked in live animals—on the rat's back and in the rabbit's eye—so why not in cultured cells?

Were the cultured cells just dead-end kids, duds incapable of growing vigorously even if they were stimulated by the correct growth factor? Or worse, was the growth factor, TAF, a dud? Folkman figured there were three possibilities. First, maybe conditions in the dish were too cramped. Once they'd filled the bottom of the dish, perhaps growth was halted by the phenomenon called contact inhibition, in which cells in close contact stop growing. The second possibility was that something else, another kind of cell, perhaps, needed to be present to help the endothelial cells respond and grow. Third, maybe Folkman's team was working with the wrong kind of cell. Was it possible that there was more than one type of endothelial cell, a diversity that no one had imagined?

This last possibility seemed unlikely. Everyone in the business was convinced that since the body's entire network of arteries and veins is interconnected, it was only logical that all blood vessels are lined with the same kind of cells. This logic was simple, elegant, and—as it would later turn out—dead wrong. The future would bring new lessons about blood vessel physiology, lessons that no one could have anticipated.

EVEN IF HE FIGURED OUT what was wrong with his endothelial cells, Folkman still had to face the other puzzle that had bogged him down: purifying TAF. He was up in the lab fractionating the fluid from rat tumors, and he was stuck. He had managed to get human endothelial cells to grow in a dish but had been unable to use them to show the powers of his long-sought fluid, TAF. To go further, he needed to discover a way to purify his tumor soup down to the one little molecule that specifically triggered blood vessel growth, without being inflammatory. And that's why he asked the National Cancer Institute to give him another hundred thousand dollars.

Folkman needed so much money because he was becoming ever more dependent on help from technicians and postdoctoral fellows, and he had to make sure they were supported. Folkman was still spending the first half of every day in surgery, was still teaching classes at the medical school, and was still bearing all of the administrative duties of being chief of surgery. He also had a young family to raise, which involved being constantly on guard because of Laura's susceptibility to infection. What all this meant was that Folkman was stretched very thin, and a good, solid grant from the NCI would allow angiogenesis research to continue even though he couldn't be in the laboratory full-time.

In 1974 Folkman's big grant application went in, and a site-review committee was sent out. A half-dozen reviewers, all highly accomplished researchers, arrived at the John Enders Building to inspect Folkman's new facilities, talk to the staff, assess the quality of the work, and hear from the principal investigator, Judah Folkman, why he thought the United States government should quintuple the amount of money it was giving him to support his angiogenesis research. Folkman made his pitch and fielded questions.

Then he heard the visitors say things like "I don't think you can do it" and "This is not feasible." And then they left.

Back in Bethesda, the visitors and bureaucrats studied Folkman's written proposal and saw a vital flaw in his efforts. What this project was really about, they realized, was biochemistry, the science that deals with organic chemicals found in living systems, their origins and interactions. On his team Folkman had only the help of a junior biochemist on loan from Fred Rosen's lab working part-time. What he needed was a deeply experienced biochemist who had the time and knowledge to make a big difference. At first Folkman only modified his proposal, essentially ignoring the study section's urging that he hire more high-powered help. But when the proposal came back with the same criticism, he realized he probably wouldn't get his money if he didn't bring in someone special.

Harvard, of course, had no shortage of able, experienced biochemists. But Folkman knew he needed a great one, someone who would be particularly well suited for the work he was pursuing. After some inquiries, he decided the man to approach was Dr. Bert L. Vallee, a professor of biochemistry whose work was so focused on medical research with direct clinical applications that his spacious lab was located in a research hospital—the one next door to Children's, Peter Bent Brigham Hospital.

Bespectacled and bow-tied, a native of Luxembourg, Vallee was a serious man with an international reputation for doing rigorous, painstaking research. He was so thorough that he would always repeat his experiments at least three times before reporting his results. He was most noted as an expert in the metabolism of zinc—one associate liked to refer to Vallee as "Dr. Zinc"—but he was also studying the biochemistry of alcoholism and was an authority on enzyme chemistry.

Vallee's interest in fundamental biochemistry and biology grew out of a half-century-long fascination with the problem of organ development, a process called organ generation, or organogenesis. He later explained to *Harvard Magazine* that his interest had first been piqued by a book he'd read when he was eighteen: Hans Spemann's *Embryonic Development and Induction*, which became his cherished scientific bible. Spemann's experiments with salamanders had ignited Vallee's interest in the intricate natural process of initiating and building living organs in the body. Blood vessels—in fact, the whole vascular tree—could be considered a single functioning organ that must develop accurately step-by-step during embryonic life. So Folkman had no doubt Vallee was the right man to ask. What he doubted was Vallee's interest. "I thought he would be terrific," Folkman recalls, "but I didn't think he would work with us. He was already a member of the National Academy of Sciences, he had both M.D. and Ph.D. degrees, he had a very big laboratory. And I was only a surgeon."

Folkman went to see Vallee, told him about the site visit from the cancer agency, and asked if he might be interested in collaborating. Vallee asked around on the medical campus and heard enough good things about Folkman—and found his research intriguing enough—to lead him to agree. He had only one condition. He wanted to set up blind tests on both sides of the collaboration, each side testing and retesting coded samples they were exchanging. The idea was to objectively compare their results, double-checking to make sure they weren't fooling themselves. It was sure to be an odd mix of personalities and approaches, but potentially a good match: Folkman, a fervent man who liked looking at the big picture, and Vallee, a cautious and meticulous researcher who had no trouble with taking years on a piece of work. Folkman and Vallee were awarded enough NIH money to begin supporting the TAF work in both labs.

To begin their collaboration, Folkman's small team grew the rat cancer cells, popped them open in the pressure chambers, and separated the proteins as far as they could. Then they sent their active fractions over to Vallee's lab for finer, much more sophisticated biochemistry. Vallee assigned a researcher to squeeze out what he could from Folkman's fluids, then send it back for Folkman's team to test on the chicken eggs and the rabbit eyes. But it was clear very quickly that this wasn't advancing the work. Vallee's lab couldn't get much closer to isolating TAF than Folkman's lab had. Vallee's first major contribution was to drive home to Folkman why this was so and what they needed to do about it.

The problem was in the numbers. Folkman had initially assumed that TAF was a relatively prominent part of the tumor soup, its molecules perhaps as numerous as one part per thousand, or even one in a hundred. (The recently discovered nerve growth factor, Folkman knew, was present in fluids at one part in twenty.) But Vallee suspected that TAF was probably so minuscule a part of the tumor fluid that any given amount of juice might contain perhaps one part TAF to a trillion parts everything else. If Vallee was right, TAF had to be extraordinarily powerful: Great effects were coming from a minuscule amount of the substance. But it also meant that TAF was too small to isolate in the amounts of tumor fluid they were working with. It was worse than the proverbial needle in a haystack—it was more like trying to find one person on a planet whose population was 250 times that of the Earth, with neither an address nor a map.

To Vallee, the only way to attack this problem—and to make the collaboration anything but futile—was to drastically increase the scale. Vallee thought it probable that TAF was present in tumor fluids only in vanishingly small amounts. Folkman had originally suspected that large amounts of TAF—maybe a few milligrams—might be found in every liter of tumor-conditioned medium, but their experiments indicated far smaller concentrations, micrograms if not nanograms per liter. And to extract even a small amount of TAF from the fluids at such low concentrations would require huge amounts of the tumor-conditioned medium.

"We need a huge scale-up of cell cultures," Vallee told Folkman. Until now, Folkman had been trying to isolate TAF from two or three liters of tumor cells at a time, taken from half a dozen rats. Vallee told him that wasn't anywhere near enough; they would need *hundreds* of liters. And Vallee was ready with an idea for how to get it.

Vallee had a connection with a major American chemical corporation that might have the wherewithal and interest to produce prodigious amounts of culture material. The idea of hooking up with a large industrial company would have made many academic scientists wary, but Folkman perceived it as more of an opportunity than a hazard, for it might mean the difference between actually isolating TAF and failing forever. It would turn out to be an odd but an entirely sensible partnership. Big money was not headed his way from the government, and now Folkman had a chance to partner with a man who viewed himself as "an expensive person," in the view of one medical school administrator. Bert Vallee required, and commanded, solid financial support for anything he got involved in.

Chapter Nine

———

THE WARNING SIGNS from the Middle East were all too clear. With Arab nations and their allies poised to gain control of the world's oil, the giant American chemical company Monsanto had little choice but to look beyond the petrochemical business. For Monsanto, much of the immediate threat came from Saudi Arabia, which was gearing up to refine and process its own crude oil and come barging full force into the global market for oil-based chemicals.

It was 1972, and St. Louis–based Monsanto, then America's thirty-eighth largest company, had to confront the reality that serious competition for sales of chemical feedstocks and products like ethylene and propylene was looming. And few at the company were more acutely aware of the threat than Monte C. Throdahl, Monsanto's vice president for research. He realized that for the company to remain strong, it would have to reinvent itself. And he knew that he was one of the people who had to figure out how to do it.

Throdahl was already a veteran of industrial-strength pressures. Trained as a chemical engineer at the University of Iowa, he had graduated in 1941 and almost immediately hired on at Monsanto, just a few months before the Japanese attack on Pearl Harbor forced the United States into World War II. The expanding global conflict soon touched off a dire need for a substitute for the natural rubber no longer coming in from Asia. Throdahl's task was to help solve that problem, and he did. Discoveries from the research labs at Monsanto and other companies led to new petroleum-based chemical products that became tires, gaskets, and other plastic goods that mimicked the performance of natural rubber. After the war, this new business expanded dramatically as synthetic materials made from petroleum became more and more common. And by the time the global energy crisis arrived in the early seventies, Throdahl had climbed to the upper reaches of the Monsanto corporate ladder. He was in charge of the entire technical program. From that lofty perch, he was keenly alert to fields of research that might lead to innovative new products for Monsanto, which might even mean survival for the company. The most promising area seemed to be what was called "the new biology."

Continuing advances in the then-obscure fields of molecular biology and genetics were yielding fundamental new information about how life works at the molecular level. The first complete gene had been isolated by Jonathan Beckwith and his colleagues at the Harvard Medical School, and a few genes' nucleotide sequences—their chemical spelling—were on the way to being deciphered. Enzymes that snip genes apart and stitch them back together had been discovered and were used in pioneering gene-splicing experiments. The first efforts to rearrange genes in "unnatural" combinations were on the near horizon. The world of biology was in enormous ferment. A whole new arena of science and experimentation was beckoning, and it seemed likely that new biochemical products would soon be emerging from this strange new field of genetic engineering, especially for agriculture, which was an area of special interest for Monsanto.

The company was among the first of the large multinational corporations not only to become interested in primary biotech research, but to put its money where its mouth was. As the company's point man, Throdahl first tried to induce a few biologists to hire on at Monsanto, but he quickly found that the best of them had zero interest in joining industry. Many regarded taking a job in the private sector as a sign of failure, an admission that they couldn't compete in the rigorous research environment of academia. But if Throdahl could not lure the country's most promising young scientists to Monsanto— even at salaries that universities couldn't match—he, like executives at other companies, did have some success persuading scientists in various fields to sign on as consultants, arrangements in which the academics advised companies on specific technical projects for brief periods of time. In the back of his mind, he wondered if this haphazard, arm's-length relationship might somehow lead to a more formal affiliation between Monsanto and a major university. If scientists wouldn't come to Monsanto, maybe Monsanto could come to them.

In the meantime, the existing consulting arrangements gave Throdahl regular contact with scientists. At meetings and lunches and in informal chats he made it a point to steer the conversation toward the future. "I was looking for things to do once we couldn't do what we were doing," Throdahl later explained. He also wanted to use these connections for vital in-house education. He hoped to get the top executives at Monsanto—even the nonscientists—interested and familiar, quickly, with the emerging biology research.

One day late in 1972, Throdahl heard something especially interesting from a biochemist who had a consulting arrangement with Monsanto: Harvard professor Bert L. Vallee. He was an expert on enzymes, the natural chemical molecules that help speed up chemistry's reactions without getting consumed themselves. Monsanto, like other chemical conglomerates, was developing ways to use enzymes for consumer products, such as laundry detergents. Now Vallee had something else on his mind. He told Throdahl that he had recently agreed to work with a young Harvard surgeon who was researching an exciting but elusive idea about cancer. He explained Judah Folkman's angiogenesis thesis and the problem he was facing. Folkman had evidence that tumor cells oozed a chemical substance that signaled nearby blood vessels to begin growing toward the cancer. But purifying that substance, TAF, had proven difficult. Some critics didn't even think it existed. If TAF was real, they argued, where the hell was it? With good laboratory practices, it should have been found after ten years of vigorous search. But Vallee and Folkman knew that few other researchers were even seeking molecules like TAF, so it wasn't surprising that it hadn't been identified. So what he and Folkman needed, Vallee told Throdahl, was a way to grow great numbers of tumor cells. Did Monsanto want to help?

Throdahl had recently read up in technical journals about the newest research in biology, so he was ripe for Vallee's overture. In fact, it was exactly the entrée Throdahl had been trying to find for Monsanto. "It was clear that we'd found two guys"—two *Harvard* guys—"who were eminent scientists in their own right, and that we might have a lot to offer each other," he said later. What Throdahl sought for Monsanto out of this, primarily, was an entry into the burgeoning new world of genetic manipulation. Education—meaning the education of Monsanto executives and other staff—in the fundamentals of biology was needed in order to explore the promising new field. There was, of course, also the promise of new products—something to put in a bottle and sell—that might emerge from such collaborations.

For his part, Folkman was enthusiastic about a partnership with Monsanto, given his own needs. He was comfortable with the idea primarily because of Throdahl. He thought the Monsanto executive was imaginative and forward-looking, and he liked what appeared to be Throdahl's interest in the public good—his desire for Monsanto to have a beneficial impact on humanity in ways it had not before—even if he took this position because it made good long-term business sense.

Folkman had been growing his cultures of rat tumor cells in "shaker bottles," jugs that were constantly agitated to keep the fluid moving so that nutrients were well distributed in the liquid growth medium. Vallee presumed that Monsanto had the resources to figure out a way to scale up production. The company's scientists and technicians had never done something like this before, but Throdahl was confident they could learn.

Throdahl suggested a two- or three-year agreement, but Vallee thought that would be too short for such a large and complex project. He thought much bigger than that—maybe ten or twelve years, the time he suspected it could take to isolate TAF, since it seemed to be present in such small amounts. And he was also thinking of a major commitment of money. Fortunately, Throdahl was willing to seriously explore the proposal. He knew how much time and effort Folkman and Vallee were spending to maintain the flow of federal research money. They constantly worked on grant requirements just to keep their laboratories open. He liked the idea of Monsanto being the one to liberate them from this burden and let them devote their talents to pursuing their research, which might lead to unanticipated advances, perhaps even the same way chemists at rival DuPont had stumbled on to useful plastics through laboratory errors and failed experiments. Certainly, big projects were nothing new to Monsanto, which had created a pre-emergence weed killer that had cost millions of dollars and taken years to perfect.

But such a long-term arrangement, involving millions of dollars, would be fundamentally different from the ordinary consulting agreements companies like Monsanto had with scientists like Vallee. This would be a partnership between Monsanto and the institution of Harvard—an unprecedented and potentially touchy arrangement that Vallee and Folkman knew might get a cool reception from the people above them, whose enthusiasm they would need. The general proposal went up the line. Vallee took it to Henry Meadow, the associate dean of the medical school, who took it to Robert Ebert, the dean, and then Ebert and Meadow brought it to the president of Harvard, Derek Bok.

Bok knew that even to go forward with discussions would be a momentous move on his part. Ebert and Meadow were not only talking about accepting millions of dollars from a multinational corporation, but about a host of complicated issues that would come with the money: questions of academic freedom, the ethics of profit, even the very process of science. At the proposal's

core there was a true clash of cultures. Though it had some reservations about
the details, Monsanto's top management embraced the basic idea enthusiastically. An arrangement with as prestigious an institution as Harvard would be
a coup—more than a foot in the door of the new biology. At Harvard, though,
an alliance with a profit-driven corporation was politically more of a mixed
blessing. It would end the university's long-standing policy barring direct
commercial ties, much to the chagrin of many in the university's scholarly
community. Complex issues were involved that could influence the school in
fundamental ways for decades to come.

Whatever his reputation among grant reviewers or some Harvard colleagues, Folkman still had enough support from the top leadership at the
medical school to make his ideas about angiogenesis the basis for one of the
boldest moves in the university's history. The pieces were in place for a block-
buster deal, thanks to a powerful man at Harvard with no philosophical objec-
tion to shaking hands with corporate America and the power to make it
happen. As associate dean, Henry Meadow was responsible for the financial
affairs of the Harvard Medical School, but for all practical purposes, he actually ran the school on a day-to-day basis. White-haired and distinguished,
Meadow was regarded as one of the last great lions of Harvard, a scion of Old
Money New England and a man very much entrenched in the school's culture. Even so, he was not nervous about breaking new ground. In 1946 he had
been instrumental in getting the Office of Naval Research to start sponsoring
research at universities, a move that contributed greatly to the explosion of
postwar federally supported primary research. He also traveled in august circles, counting among his friends Elliott Richardson, whose resignation as
President Nixon's attorney general later that year would be part of the notorious "Saturday Night Massacre," and top executives at the major pharmaceutical companies. One of his newest acquaintances in business was, in fact,
one Monte Throdahl, vice president of the Monsanto Corporation.

On a practical level, the largest stumbling block to a deal was the question
of patents. Throdahl insisted that under the agreement Harvard had to patent
any devices or treatments the two scientists came up with during the term
of the contract and to give Monsanto the first opportunity to license those
patents to develop products. Throdahl considered this an eminently reasonable proposal, but Harvard's bylaws expressly barred either the institution or
its faculty from retaining ownership of discoveries that came from research at
the university. The policy, adopted decades before, was that inventions had to
remain in the public domain. The notion that the university should own

patents and then license the rights to a specific corporation was new and unsettling; it was simply not done at Harvard. The idea was so far off the map, Throdahl was amazed to learn, that the university had no patent attorney even to discuss the proposal with.

There was a piece of irony in this, given that Folkman and one of his navy colleagues, David Long, had already encountered Harvard's ingrown reluctance to play with patents. A decade before, the two drafted doctors had serendipitously invented a drug-delivery system by discovering that certain small, oil-soluble molecules could slowly leak through the walls of plastic containers. The navy recognized the potential value and quickly patented the discovery. But it lost interest a few years later and turned the patent over to Folkman and Long after they left the service. The two men, though offered good sums of money for the patent rights, instead tried to pass them on to Harvard. But the university had no interest in profiting from the discoveries of its faculty and declined the offer. Folkman and Long retained the patent and in 1968 gave a royalty-free license to the Population Council, a nonprofit group in New York City. Folkman and Long's "leaky plastic," as they referred to it, was eventually developed into Norplant, the slim, implantable capsules that would become one of the world's most widely used forms of birth control. Neither of the researchers nor Harvard University would reap a dime of profit from the discovery. It was hardly the first case of its kind. Harvard researchers had in years past developed a drug to cure a condition called pernicious anemia and built the first iron lung, among other devices and treatments. The tradition was firm: Harvard held no patents on therapeutic or health agents.

With Folkman and Vallee playing the role of very interested bystanders, continuing their research as best they could on a limited scale, Meadow spent nearly two years with Monsanto executives, trying to hammer out an acceptable compact. The talks broke off several times, but somehow the duration of the prepared contract kept getting longer and the numbers kept getting bigger. Eventually Meadow prepared a thirty-five-page contract covering all the vital issues, a groundbreaking agreement that, by Harvard's lights, would do more to ensure the advance of science than the growth of corporate profits. "The two cultures wanted their own things," Folkman recalls. "Monsanto needed the new knowledge to be kept secret, and the university needed the new knowledge *not* to be kept secret." The contract drawn up by the university stipulated that any new knowledge that came out of any professors' heads could immediately be published. There would be no secrecy. And Harvard was not obliged to guard any of Monsanto's trade secrets: If Monsanto had information it didn't want disclosed, it should withhold it from Folkman's lab.

Nor would Monsanto's commercial interests compromise the timing of publications. The contract specified that the university would only be required to send the team's research papers off to Monsanto at the same time they were submitted to journals. "That meant that they couldn't hold a paper up," Folkman remembers. "You could write a paper and not have to sit around while it went through tiers of lawyers." It would be Monsanto's job to survey the scientific papers quickly and decide whether the work ought to be patented. Another key part of the complex agreement made it clear that the research agenda would be determined by the scientists, as would the pace of the work. "That meant that whatever was decided should be done would be decided by us," Folkman said. "They would be partners. They could suggest things, and we might say that's a great idea. But we didn't want any takeovers." And Harvard said clearly that all of the funding for the research had federal money mixed in, so if Monsanto didn't want to work with the government, it shouldn't make the deal.

By the end of 1974, after many rounds of negotiation, Throdahl and the Monsanto people had agreed to virtually all of Meadow's proposals. Now it was for Bok, Harvard's president, to sign off on the deal. What he had before him was a quid pro quo whose simplicity was overshadowed by its sheer heft. Harvard would be given an enormous grant: twenty-three million dollars over twelve years— enough to pay for one new endowed professorship in Folkman's lab and two more in Vallee's, salaries for them and their staffs, and equipment to fill up more laboratory space in the John Enders Research Building. Monsanto would be given a chance to profit from anything that emerged from the research. For Bok, the issue boiled down to this: What was all this going to cost Harvard? Would the relationship with Monsanto affect the university's "distanced objectivity"—its collective credibility and precious prestige? Would the world still look to Harvard for honest answers? Or would it wonder if those answers were colored by the interests of some deep-pocketed company? Bok decided that Meadow had done a good job of protecting Harvard's integrity. Not without some trepidation, he approved the deal.

Bok was right to worry about where the deal might lead. The landmark arrangment would mark a sea change in American life-science research. In the very short term, though, the effects would be seen primarily in the two labs run by Folkman and Vallee. They were instantly a well-heeled research team.

Besides the new endowed chairs, each lab received $200,000 a year for operating expenses, and Folkman's team would get important new equipment, including an $80,000 electron microscope, high-speed centrifuges, and other cutting-edge gear. With the promise of new tools and remarkable financial stability, they could dig deeper into their search for the elusive TAF. Everything was wonderful—until Loretta McLaughlin found out about the deal.

In the nearly two years since the negotiations had begun, the proposed alliance had been kept virtually secret, both at Harvard and Monsanto. Along with Folkman and Vallee and a very few people in their labs, only the highest officials at the university and the company were privy to a deal everyone knew would be controversial. One decision they hadn't gotten around to was how, when, or even whether to announce the partnership. But that question became moot on the morning of Thursday, February 6, 1975. HARVARD MEDICAL, MONSANTO JOIN IN HISTORIC PROJECT ON CANCER, screamed the *Boston Herald American* from the top of page 1.

As the *Herald American*'s medical editor and reporter, Loretta McLaughlin was closely tuned in to the goings-on at Harvard Medical School and its hospitals. One day late in 1974 she was chatting with Herb Shaw, the medical school's longtime public relations man, when Shaw matter-of-factly mentioned that Harvard had made a research agreement with the Monsanto Corporation. McLaughlin used an old reporter's trick: She pretended she already knew about the deal and bluffed Shaw into supplying a few more details. When she told Shaw she wanted to break the story, he realized he'd made a big mistake. "I've *got* to have this story," McLaughlin said. The thought of scooping the more powerful *Boston Globe*, which had four medical writers, on an important story about the Harvard Medical School was as exciting to McLaughlin as it was embarrassing to Shaw. He didn't want to alienate the *Globe;* he didn't want the story to get out at all until the school could decide how to let it out. But Shaw was cornered. McLaughlin said she was ready to run the story immediately, even with some of the details missing. Shaw went to Robert Ebert, the dean of the medical school. "Loretta's gotten wind of this," he said, "and she wants it exclusively. She's threatening to go with what she's got."

Ebert thought it would be better to help her get the story right and also avoid suspicion that Harvard was trying to keep the deal secret. He consulted with his colleagues, then called Shaw back. "Show it to her," he said.

McLaughlin went over to Shaw's office. "He slipped me a copy of the contract," she recalled. Then she went to the medical center library, sat down,

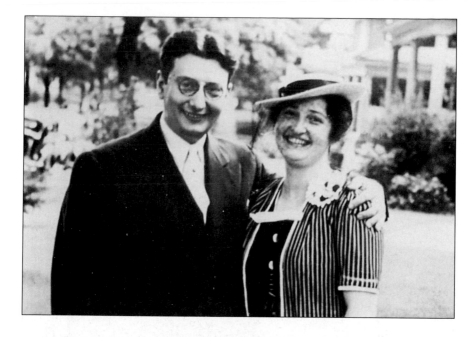

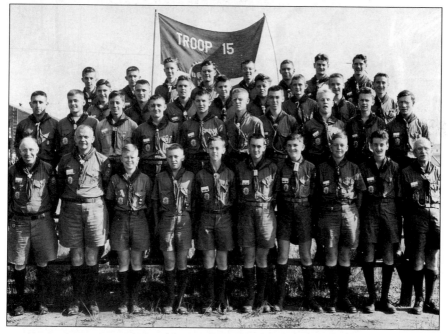

TOP: In the early 1930s Rabbi Jerome Folkman and his young wife, Bessie, were just settling into married life. *(Courtesy of Judah Folkman)*

Boy Scout Troop 15 from Grand Rapids, Michigan. Judah Folkman is in the first row, second from the end on the right. *(Courtesy of Judah Folkman)*

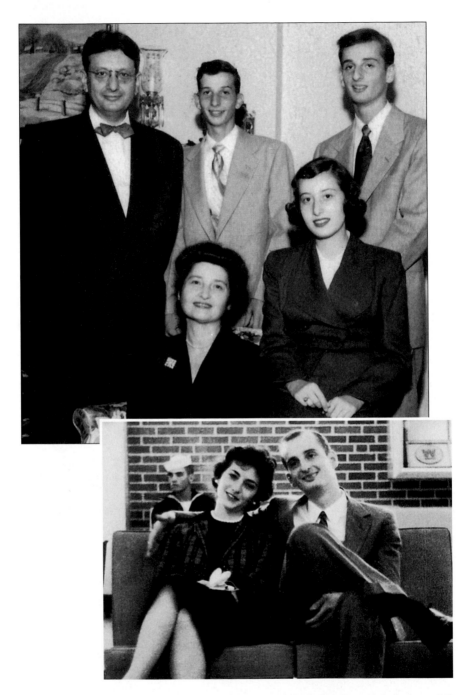

TOP: The Folkman family: Rabbi Jerome Folkman; his wife, Bessie; and their three children, David (standing center), Judah, and Joy. *(Courtesy of Judah Folkman)*

Judah Folkman, then assistant resident at Mass General in Boston, and his bride-to-be, Paula Prial. *(Courtesy of Judah and Paula Folkman)*

As a medical student at Harvard working with pediatric surgeon Robert Gross, Judah Folkman devised a way to insert a small sheet of plastic in the wall separating the chambers of the heart. Before the invention of the heart pump, it offered a potential way to save infants born with leaky heart chambers. *(Harvard Medical School)*

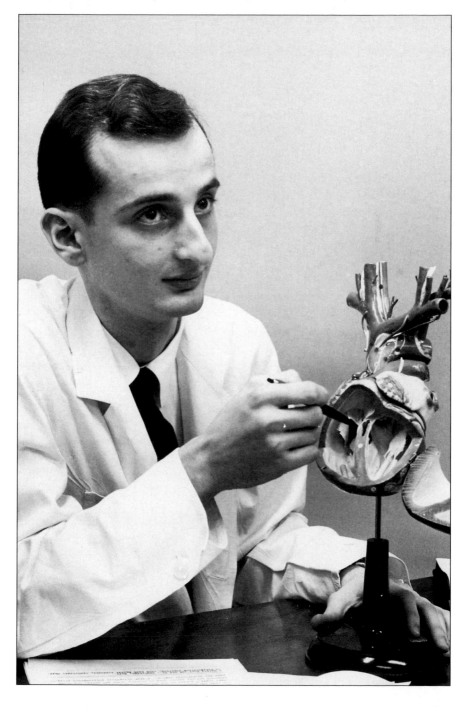

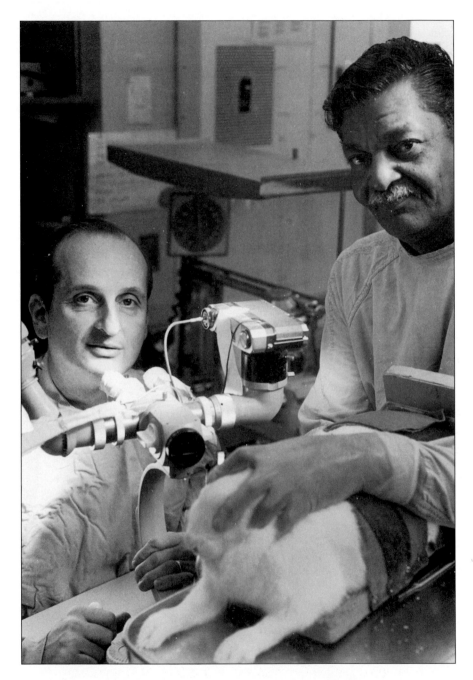

Judah Folkman discovered a way to test substances that might spur blood vessel growth by watching new blood vessels grow toward a tumor sample in a rabbit's eye. Here Folkman's longtime technician, Paul Wesley, calms the rabbit as Folkman prepares to photograph the growth pattern. *(Harvard Medical School)*

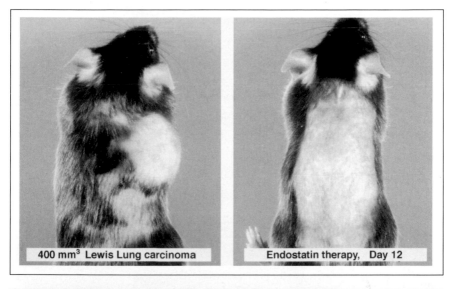

400 mm³ Lewis Lung carcinoma   Endostatin therapy,   Day 12

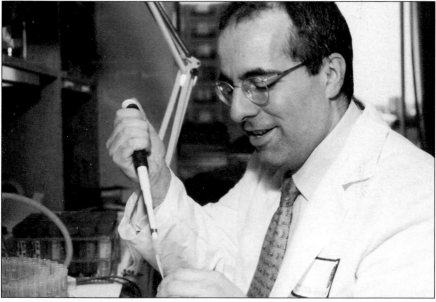

TOP: After just twelve days of endostatin injections, this mouse's tumor had shrunk dramatically. The tumor grew back after the first treatment was stopped, but after being "cycled"—growing and shrinking in response to endostatin—the tumor never came back. *(Harvard Medical School)*

Dr. Michael O'Reilly spent several years collecting and analyzing urine samples from mice, an onerous but worthwhile task. It led directly to the discovery of the potent antiangiogenic agents angiostatin and endostatin, each capable of shrinking large tumors, rendering them dormant. Both agents went into clinical trials within a few years. *(Lori DeSantis/Children's Hospital)*

RIGHT: Ophthalmologist Dr. Robert D'Amato was the first to propose that thalidomide—a drug that causes terrible birth defects—inhibited blood vessel growth in the fetus. This led to trials of thalidomide as an anticancer agent and as a drug to slow or stop the progress of macular degeneration, the leading cause of blindness in the elderly.
(Lori DeSantis/Children's Hospital)

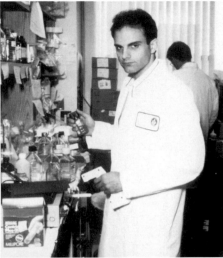

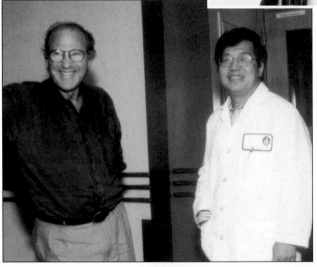

Biochemists Michael Klagsbrun and Yuen Shing were the first to purify basic fibroblast growth factor, a potent natural agent that makes endothelial cells grow in culture. It was a landmark discovery on the way to controlling blood vessel growth.
(Lori DeSantis/Children's Hospital)

Biologist Bruce Zetter played a central role in making endothelial cells grow in culture. His discovery, that interferon-alpha could stop endothelial cell movements, led to treatments for tumor-like hemangiomas.
(Lori DeSantis/ Children's Hospital)

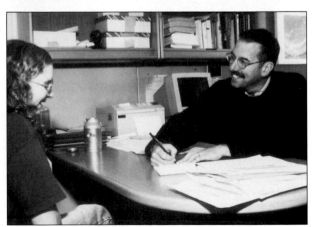

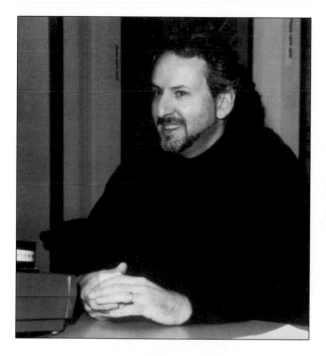

Donald Ingber is credited with the discovery of TNP-470, the first drug to have potent angiogenesis-inhibiting properties. In combination with chemotherapeutic agents, it has shown encouraging signs of effectiveness against tumors. *(Lori DeSantis/Children's Hospital)*

Ophthalmologist Anthony Adamis and his coworkers ran experiments showing that the angiogenesis stimulator VEGF causes tiny blood vessels to grow in the eye, gradually destroying vision in diabetics. *(Lori DeSantis/Children's Hospital)*

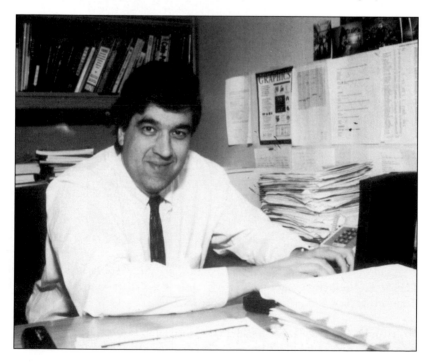

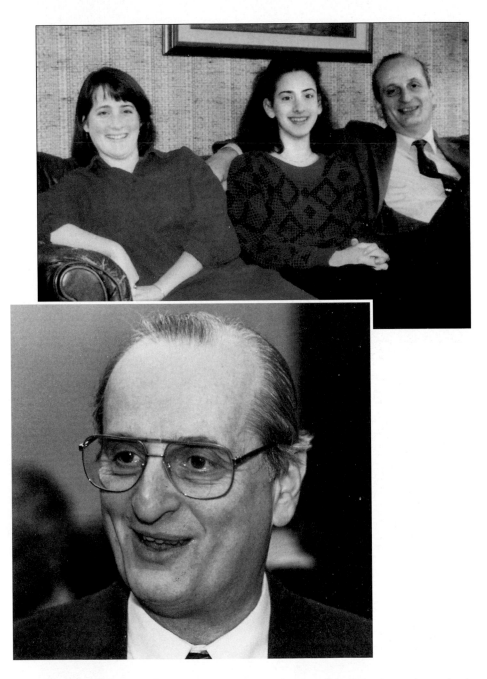

TOP: Dr. Folkman and his daughters, Laura (left) and Marjorie. Laura is a school-teacher in Northern California and Marjorie is a dancer with the Mark Morris Company in New York. *(Judah and Paula Folkman)*

BOTTOM: Dr. Judah Folkman at Children's Hospital in Boston in 1994, soon after the discovery of angiostatin in his laboratory. *(Barbara Steiner/Harvard Medical School)*

and raced through the pages, taking notes. The document Shaw shared with McLaughlin didn't include all the particulars—such as exactly who was paying what to whom—but she knew it all added up to twenty-three million dollars and that it was the first collaboration of its kind. That made it a huge story. Medical news rarely made page 1, but this was going to lead the paper. The next morning, McLaughlin's story, copyrighted and branded EXCLUSIVE, announced the biggest research agreement ever made between a university and a company—and declared that the two Harvard researchers at the center of it were considered by the science community to be "on the threshold of a breakthrough" in cancer. In that respect, of course, McLaughlin was not fully informed. Within the science community, few who knew about it thought Folkman's theory would actually pan out, and some were dubious about the man himself. But once again, to his dismay, Folkman found himself staring at his own half-smiling face in the press, this time on the front page, alongside that of his new partner, the stern Bert Vallee. Vallee was even more unhappy than he appeared in the newspaper photo. A man who insisted on absolute secrecy within his lab, he was furious when McLaughlin broke the story and even angrier when he felt the repercussions.

The news was picked up by the wire services and spread worldwide, unleashing a ferocious and enduring backlash against the deal, the deal makers, and the scientists at its core. The agreement was branded an unnatural union, and it sparked fierce debate at Harvard, along with amazement at other universities, and even inner turmoil at Monsanto, where Throdahl said some middle managers and in-house scientists wondered why the company was giving outsiders all that money. Of course, most of the clamor was heard at Harvard and in the Boston research establishment, a community with an extraordinarily high aptitude for indignation. As Folkman recalls vividly, "Everybody was upset. They said, 'You are selling the university's soul.' " Some directed their remarks personally at Folkman.

Folkman was honestly mystified at all the fuss. Naively, he did not realize that the Monsanto "grant" would be seen as a threat to academic freedom. The aim of medical research was to make treatments available as soon as possible, and to him this was what the agreement was designed to accomplish. He actually agreed with Monsanto's insistence that Harvard reverse its patent policy. He thought it was high time universities started getting legal protection for discoveries—not to make them rich, but to ensure that the inventions found their way to the public and weren't seized upon, patented, and privately exploited by someone else.

The outcry over the Monsanto deal was, of course, entirely predictable. Harvard's leaders had always been so wary of outside money that even government funds had once been considered suspect: Years earlier, Fred Rosen had been ordered to return half of a twenty-five-thousand-dollar career development grant to the National Institutes of Health because it was thought that he didn't need that much money. Not that Harvard was afraid of money. It avidly solicited big gifts from alumni, and tycoons were welcome to endow professorial chairs and pay handsomely for the privilege of having their names chiseled into the facades of campus buildings. But to accept corporate money and guarantee the corporation the exclusive rights to patented research results was almost inconceivable.

Making matters worse, a deep distrust of big business had surfaced in the later years of the war in Vietnam. Corporate recruiters, especially from big chemical companies, were no longer so welcome at some American universities, including Harvard. Protests routinely erupted around military-corporate connections, such as Monsanto's manufacture of the defoliant Agent Orange, which the United States had used liberally in Vietnam and which was beginning to be blamed for a variety of health problems among veterans. Across town, MIT was being driven by student discontent to divorce itself from the famed Draper Laboratory, where much military-industrial research was being done. Now there was the image of Monsanto sneaking into Harvard's medical laboratories through the back door, cash in hand. Throdahl tried to convince the Harvard community that the company's motives were benign, telling the *Harvard Crimson,* "We don't want to direct their research. We're not competent to judge—we were very impressed by the work going on here, and we decided to give them the grant."

To try to deal with the uproar, the medical school called a special faculty meeting, with Bok and Ebert presiding, in one of its white, marble-clad buildings on the Quad. It turned into a raucous and emotional clash of wills, an academic brawl. Folkman was there, and he was stunned by the accusations and fears in the air: Bok and Ebert had sold the university's soul; there would be secrecy in the academic halls; students wouldn't come to Harvard because they'd be exposed to ruthless big business. "Every kind of thing you could think of was said against Vallee and me," Folkman later recalled. Some used the word "prostitution." Others accused the two of "feathering their own nests."

The deal's proponents pointed out that precedents existed around the country. The University of Wisconsin had earned substantial amounts from patented vitamins over the years. Faculty members at MIT and Caltech, the nation's leading technological universities, were encouraged to develop patentable devices and to cooperate with the chemical, electronics, and aircraft industries. A chemist at Caltech, Arnold Beckman, had even started a major technological company, Beckman Instruments, on the basis of his invention of a pH meter in his university laboratory. The Harvard faculty members weren't impressed: "That's them," they replied, "not us." And when someone stood up and said, "Excuse me, but some of us"—including Bert Vallee—"are already taking corporate money; we're consultants to the chemical industry," the reply was "Yes, but that's not the institution."

The hue and cry failed to derail the deal with Monsanto. Later in 1975, the university issued a policy document explaining how business connections would be handled in the future. It officially ended Harvard's cherished old "no patents" policy.

In the aftermath, Folkman could never quite forget that many of their colleagues would always hold that he and Vallee had gone to bed with the devil. Over and over the two were invited to give seminars, first locally and then nationally, on the pitfalls of working with industry. Folkman accepted many more invitations than Vallee and used these occasions to defend the great good of the deal. He found that many university people were naive about what it took to get a good idea out of the laboratory and into the hands of the public. If this helped the battle against cancer, and everybody stuck to the provisions of the deal, then why not?

Still, Folkman did harbor some ambivalence. He was a little bit embarrassed by the immensity of the checks being written. Whereas Bert Vallee reveled in being treated well, Folkman was modest when it came to money. "Bert Vallee, for whom I've negotiated contracts, always sat in the front of the airplane and stayed in very nice hotels, and never understood the logic of being thrifty. It was sort of, 'What are you talking about?'" says Stephen Atkinson, whose job as director of the medical school's Office of Technology Licensing and Sponsored Research was created after the Monsanto deal was struck. But with Folkman "it was almost a Marie Curie syndrome: 'I can save the world from this little shack out back.'" Folkman's frugality started at home: He lived in an unassuming house near the hospital, drove an unremarkable, well-broken-in car, and generally did nothing to make himself a wealthier man. Just as he had declined to exploit such achievements as the invention that led to Norplant, he later turned down lucrative consulting offers and gave his honorarium payments away.

Though he spoke freely and frankly at professional meetings, Folkman resolved to talk as little as possible to the general public about the Monsanto deal or the research it supported. This self-imposed policy had actually started in the wake of the 1972 ACS press seminar, when he'd begun to decline requests for interviews. Folkman liked talking to reporters but was learning that his enthusiasm for the implications of his work needed to be tempered by an awareness of the media's natural tendency to play up exciting prospects and play down the uncertainty of the scientific process.

Folkman became so serious about staying out of trouble that he hired Carl Cobb, the former medical reporter from the *Globe,* ostensibly to help write reports, grant proposals, and research papers but also to fend off the press. Henry Meadow made Cobb's salary part of the grant package. But even this move to keep a low profile seemed to backfire. Some of Folkman's colleagues regarded his hiring of a personal public relations man—no matter the reason—as an unseemly move. "I've always felt that his relationship with the press was very unwise," says one high-ranking colleague, speaking about the span of Folkman's career. "I think he's terribly eager to see press, much too accessible. Having a press agent was an enormous mistake, I think, for a scientist. I think his reasoning was 'If I get enough notoriety I can get enough funds to continue this.' " Of course, Folkman hadn't initiated his appearance at the ACS press seminar, nor did he have a hand in how it was promoted or reported. He wanted Cobb to keep him *out* of the news—the opposite of what a press agent was generally supposed to do. "We never put out a single press release in that whole time," Folkman recalls, and reporters who called for interviews found they almost never got past Cobb, their former colleague. But it was also true that anyone looking on from the outside could easily imagine cause and effect: Press attention. Monsanto grant.

NEITHER THE HARVARD ADMINISTRATION'S stance, nor any defenses by Folkman, silenced the chorus of dismay about the Monsanto deal. Many of Harvard's senior faculty were members of university and medical school boards and committees, and they took full advantage of their positions to speak their minds. The violation of Harvard's sacred trust was a common theme, as was betrayal, surrender, and selling out. "There was no question that the green-eyed monster—greed, envy, and jealousy—was alive and running well," Throdahl recalls.

The Monsanto deal opened a gate, and over the next few years a huge stampede of fortune-seeking biologists would eagerly dash through it. Soon, observed Folkman, "everybody had a company." In a research field accustomed to bowing and groveling for funding from government agencies, foundations, and rich donors, the new industrial money—big money—began pouring in almost immediately from venture capitalists who saw the Harvard-Monsanto deal as a blessing from the gods.

Suddenly it wasn't just Harvard that was facing the prospect of intense commercialization of basic biomedical research. The issue of patenting had come up only rarely at American universities and generally only in the area of devices or products, such as vitamins. University biology departments had been largely immune to such commercialization, primarily because there really hadn't been very much to sell. Until now. Soon after the news broke about Harvard's Monsanto deal, Folkman got a call from MIT's president, Jerome Weisner, who had served as White House science adviser for President John F. Kennedy. "Welcome to the twentieth century," Weisner told Folkman.

At the time, MIT was forging strong ties to industry, especially in engineering and electronics. For twenty-five thousand dollars, companies could join the institute's Industrial Liaison Program and get an inside look at MIT's research activities. But such an idea ran counter to the culture of biomedicine; it might seem like exploiting the sick. So academic medicine and biomedical research had long been insulated from business, for better or worse. "There was no money in biology; it was like taking a vow of poverty," Folkman observes. "Before the Monsanto agreement, there was nothing except for twenty-five-thousand-dollar grants where you test a brand of penicillin."

Now, rather than turning their noses up and dismissing it as prostitution, leaders of many universities wondered how they might grab a piece of the action. Cornell University, for instance, almost immediately created a new biotechnology institute involving the university and several major companies as research partners. Within the American chemical industry, executives were beginning to view Monsanto's collaboration with Harvard as big, bold, and daring—perhaps something to be emulated. Monsanto, in fact, went on to sign deals with other research universities, especially Washington University in St. Louis, the company's hometown.

Now, with the extraordinary advances taking place in the life sciences, opportunity was knocking with a loud bang. And venture capitalists in the Boston and San Francisco areas, who had honed their skills in the burgeoning computer industry, were looking for new fields to conquer. The birth of biotechnology and the store of knowledge in the universities offered them a big one. Suddenly every biology professor seemed to have an idea that was ripe for development. Molecular biologists at research centers such as MIT, Harvard, Caltech, and Stanford had begun to see real possibilities in what came to be called "gene-splicing," moving genes around from one creature to another. At first, it was performed almost solely in bacteria, but biologists could already see promise in the idea of genetically engineering these microscopic organisms to make new products. One of the first to come to mind was human insulin, for which there was a great need and a big market. Some diabetics were allergic to the insulin derived from pigs; making a human version by artificial means in factory vats offered a way to solve that problem.

At the time, in the mid to late seventies, there seemed no end to the possibilities, and the growing list of opportunities included cancer research. The new tools developed in molecular biology—especially the so-called restriction enzymes, which allowed genes to be snipped out of their natural settings—gave cancer researchers a new way to explore the genes in cancer viruses and test genes one by one to assess their importance. So the excitement in cancer research was beginning to focus strongly on genes. In comparison to all these major developments, Folkman seemed like a quiet little church mouse, working away at angiogenesis.

With all this new science—and its commercial potential—it wasn't just Harvard that was facing practical and ethical questions about partnering with industry. Most universities had few if any rules governing how this money-spinning activity should or shouldn't be done, and inevitably turned to Henry Meadow's thirty-five-page contract as a model. The agreement was so detailed and thorough that it became the gold standard for industry-university relationships. Copies were soon in great demand, and Meadow's office spent a lot of time explaining its intricacies. In a dash of irony, Harvard's Derek Bok disagreed publicly with Stanford University's president, Donald Kennedy, over the issue of how closely universities should be allied with industry. Kennedy thought collaborations should be pursued aggressively; Bok, whose university had broken down the walls, favored caution. But the fact that they were engaging in such a discussion was a testament to the power of the Monsanto deal.

Within four years, new firms bearing names like Genentech, Amgen, Cetus, Biogen, Genetics Institute, and Collaborative Genetics would spring forth from this newly cultivated ground, taking root especially in the Boston and San Francisco areas, where biological research was most frenetic. Harvard's Nobel laureate Walter Gilbert helped found Biogen. Biologists Mark Ptashne and Tom Maniatis caused a fuss when they proposed creating Genetics Institute as a Harvard-owned business. Eventually Bok said no, and Genetics Institute was formed as an independent company, with Ptashne and Maniatis involved as advisers while keeping their faculty positions. Down Memorial Drive in Cambridge, at MIT, new companies with "Inc." attached to their names began sprouting like mushrooms as researchers such as David Housman and David Baltimore cashed in on their expertise. Many of these professors chose to keep their hard-won faculty positions but were still able to accept appointments to the boards of directors, or perhaps to the scientific advisory boards, of companies large and small. Many of them set up shop virtually across the street from universities and lured away the best grad students with offers of good salaries and stock options that could make them millionaires when the companies went public. From coast to coast it became an academic-industrial free-for-all, with scientist-businessmen giving up tenured positions to jump into the new industry, hand in hand with venture capitalists. People were getting rich, very rich, fast.

The gold rush raised immediate and serious questions concerning ethics, ownership of ideas, and fairness. Who, for example, could sell an idea that came from a group? Who owned research materials such as genetically engineered cells? Were bacteria and animals patentable? Should lifesaving drugs and devices be held back, awaiting the patent process? Was peer review a thing of the past? Were these business deals cast in concrete? Would graduate students, the academic slaves doing grunt work in laboratories, be exploited by their professors' companies? And what about the professors? To whom should they owe first loyalty—their universities and their students, or the aggressive new biotechnology company setting up shop nearby?

The questions seemed endless, and each university struggled to find its own way through the maze. Within a decade, a valuable sense of community evaporated at some universities. Once open and communicative biology departments began to take on a secretive, competitive atmosphere. Graduate students and postdoctoral fellows were less likely to casually exchange hints, ideas, and results with their peers in neighboring laboratories. Experts began to hold back some of their expertise, fearful of giving away company secrets. Some researchers began spending more time in company labs and less at the university. At the University of California, San Francisco, a researcher snuck back into his old lab, took some cloned cells, and brought them to his new employer, Genentech, Inc. (Years later, Genentech, though denying it had used the materials for commercial purposes, paid a two-hundred-million-dollar judgment to the university.)

Of course, there had always been jealousies and conflicts—academia's reputation for intellectual assassination is well earned—but adding wads of money to the mix made everything more volatile. In a way, the commercialization of academia mimicked what had happened a decade or so earlier with the birth of the computer industry, which in the beginning also grew largely around universities in the Boston and San Francisco areas. With the Harvard-Monsanto agreement leading the way, the biotechnology revolution spawned a brand of academic capitalism that was destined to continue. Indeed, even though the support for biomedical research from government agencies accelerated during the late 1970s and through the 1980s, increasingly large parts of the work were supported by the new biotech companies. And some, like Genentech and Biogen, were doing a lot of the new research in-house rather than spending their money on university professors. Thus the small biotech companies began to become a major force on the research scene, and they were soon being gobbled up by major pharmaceutical firms that began seeing promise in genetics.

But at Harvard, where it first burst into prominence, there was to be lingering hostility. The money was a lightning rod, both for people who resented what the Monsanto deal had unleashed and for those who felt the money had been dropped in the lap of an unworthy recipient. Already under attack as an intellectual maverick, a researcher with alternative ideas and questionable methods, Judah Folkman now carried the added burden of outrageous good fortune.

Chapter Ten

———

HERETICAL IDEAS SELDOM GO DOWN well, and those who espouse them often get burned, one way or another. The early Christian church did it openly and barbarically, pursuing God's kingdom by broiling any dissenters who dared speak up. The Puritans were hardly more subtle, resorting to the stocks, the dunking chair, or, for those accused of witchcraft, crushing the culprit to death beneath a load of stones. Modern academia has evolved its own approaches to heresy, with the result being a somewhat milder form of death. Those who drift too far afield can be denied tenure; their research proposals may go unfunded; and their work may be denied publication by anonymous reviewers. It is a rare person who can withstand sustained scorn and resistance and defiantly continue down a path that, according to everyone else, offers a long journey to nowhere. As many have learned, the problem with being a visionary is that people suspect you're seeing things.

In modern science, a world in which fact is supposed to trump faith, there is a fine line between persistence and obstinacy, and it's often hard to tell the difference. Revolutionaries and critics can be equally blind in defending or opposing a cherished theory—both sides having invested precious time and effort in supporting their own positions. Objectivity helps, but often only with the benefit of time can the cranks, the misguided, and the simply wrong be distinguished from the geniuses. Through the ages any number of prophetic thinkers saw their ideas dismissed at first as nonsense.

One such visionary, early in the twentieth century, was Alfred Lothar Wegener. Born in Germany in 1880, the geophysicist and astronomer—a brilliant teacher, scientist, and lecturer—came up with the notion that the rock-solid continents occupying the Earth's surface were once joined in one supercontinent he called Pangaea. Wegener theorized that this huge mass of land broke into large fragments about two hundred million years ago and that these blocks gradually drifted thousands of miles apart to reach their present positions. Telling evidence for him was the look of some of the larger coastlines of the western hemisphere: South America and Africa would fit together nicely. The thesis was dismissed as absurd, the product of bad judgment, flawed thinking, and a willful neglect of obvious facts. It was clear to leaders in the field that the continents were too stiff, solid, and unyielding to move. Wegener was essentially drummed out of his profession, a pariah among geologists.

Nonetheless he persisted. Though Wegener died on an expedition to Greenland in 1930 and never saw vindication, his far-out ideas eventually led to a major revolution in the science of geology. Because of Wegener's ability to see what others refused to imagine, geologists finally resolved major puzzles, such as why earthquakes occur and why they strike where they do. Wegener's thesis, now called plate tectonics, even helps explain how so many different animal species evolved distinctly different forms—animals became isolated and evolved separately as the major landmasses slowly drifted away from one another. In fact, so much evidence has now accumulated in favor of continental drift and seafloor spreading that Wegener's once-ludicrous heresy has evolved into orthodoxy, and anyone who seriously challenges his scenario faces the same treatment Wegener once faced.

In medicine, too, there have been those whose ideas cost them dearly, such as the Hungarian physician Ignaz Philips Semmelweis, who lived from 1818 to 1865. Like Folkman, Semmelweis made a fundamentally important observation that collided head-on with the conventional wisdom of his time. Semmelweis infuriated legions of hardworking, dedicated doctors with the simple but unsettling idea that they should wash their hands. As sane as that seems today, Semmelweis's suggestion did not go down well with most of his peers in 1847; in fact it was widely taken as a slur on the medical profession. Semmelweis was in effect accusing his fellow physicians of doing harm to their own patients, even killing them. And the charge came out of nowhere: France's biomedical genius, Louis Pasteur, hadn't yet come up with the germ theory of disease.

The idea arose in the course of Semmelweis's work at the Vienna Lying-In Hospital. It had been noticed that the young mothers being cared for by doctors in one of the birthing wards were perishing in alarming numbers, victims of infections called puerperal fever (or childbed fever). The source was not known, but the onset of disease was rapid, and the symptoms included high fever, rapid pulse, bloated abdomen, and intense pain. About 10 percent of the infected women died. What was especially puzzling was that in another ward, where new mothers were instead being tended by midwives, there was a significantly lower incidence of the disease and many fewer deaths.

Semmelweis thought he understood the cause after a friend and colleague of his fell victim to a massive, fatal infection that erupted soon after he'd cut himself while performing an autopsy. Semmelweis noticed that his friend's symptoms followed exactly the same course seen in the young mothers stricken with childbed fever. That was a vital clue. He realized that the midwives had but one job: taking care of the mothers and babies. But the physicians and their medical students were on double duty, sometimes working in the birthing ward and other times in the autopsy chamber, dissecting corpses. At Semmelweis's suggestion, the doctors and medical students doing the dissections were ordered to wash their hands in a disinfecting solution before examining women in the birthing ward. It worked. Within a year the death rate in the doctors' ward dropped dramatically; the women there began doing even better than those tended by the midwives.

Such an important discovery would seem to be a cause for celebration, with many and grateful thanks to Semmelweis. But while a few prominent physicians supported him, many more took offense, despite the logic of his position and the seeming inarguability of his data. The controversy became so intense that Semmelweis was soon forced to leave his post in Vienna and return home to Budapest, where he found a new position at St. Rochus Hospital. The idea of hand-washing traveled with him, of course, and he was allowed to introduce the requirement in his new setting. Success was once again immediate and obvious, but because of what one historian called "reverse gullibility"—an unwillingness to change despite overwhelming evidence—animosity and controversy continued to dog Semmelweis's trail. The Hungarian physicians were hardly more flexible in their attitudes about the need for hand-washing than were the Viennese. Semmelweis's professional life became increasingly difficult, and eventually, after the deaths of two of his children added further burdens to his life, he entered an insane asylum in 1865, where he died of blood poisoning. It wasn't until 1883, at the Boston Lying-In Hospital in the United States, that the basic ideas of cleanliness finally took firm hold. In the meantime, many young mothers, along with other patients and some doctors, paid with their lives for the arrogance that prevented a good and simple idea from getting widespread use.

———

IF ONLY THE WORLD COULD WASH its hands of cancer. A century after Ignaz Semmelweis tried to sell his simple idea to the great unwashed, Judah Folkman was laboring to prove a much less obvious notion about a disease that had long seemed unconquerable. However promising Folkman's work, among the cancer specialists and researchers at Massachusetts General Hospital, Beth Israel Hospital, and the other major units of the Harvard teaching system—as well as the anonymous peer reviewers of grant committees and science journals—his ideas about blood vessels gained little traction. Everyone was focused on cancer cells themselves. In the cancer establishment of the 1970s, angiogenesis was a decidedly fringe idea, and Folkman was the Don Quixote of the Charles River.

The state of understanding and treating cancer remained dismal. There were still few clues about what caused cancer—environmental factors such as tobacco smoke obviously could be central, but how and why were as much a mystery as ever. The number of new cancer cases and the resulting deaths had remained stubbornly high, and even gotten worse, throughout the twentieth century. The success with combination chemotherapy against childhood leukemia was amazing, but the overall number of these cases was too small to have any real impact on national cancer statistics. The lack of progress was disappointing, given the billions of dollars, francs, marks, lira, pounds, and yen that had been poured into cancer research for decades.

One of the most obvious problems was that there remained a wide gulf between the laboratory and the clinic. Pathologists and biologists could detect cellular damage, such as the oddly rearranged chromosomes seen inside some kinds of leukemia cells, but they could not reverse it. Even later, when central players in the cancer drama—the so-called oncogenes and antioncogenes—were uncovered beginning in the mid-1980s, the impact on treatment remained small. Testing for mutant versions of such genes could help diagnose cancer, but the results did not offer a way it could be successfully treated.

Because of ignorance about cancer and its causes, medical scientists in the early 1970s were left to pursue a shotgun approach in the search for therapeutic drugs. Among the largest efforts was a chemical-screening program supported by the National Cancer Institute, which set out in 1966 to systematically test the thousands and thousands of known chemicals that might have some beneficial effect on cancer. In this decades-long program, the chemicals that showed hints of promise by killing cancer cells growing in laboratory dishes were then tested in animals, and if they continued to show promise without overwhelmingly bad side effects, they might advance toward phase I clinical trials, testing for toxicity in humans. As a result of screening, and from efforts to develop drugs in other anticancer programs, an armamentarium of anticancer drugs was eventually created that included methotrexate, cyclophosphamide, cisplatin, vincristine, fluorouracil, doxorubicin, Taxol, and many others. Each of these was useful for some kinds of cancer, and they were frequently given in combinations to multiply their power. But as promising as these drugs were in their ability to drive tumors into remission, their continued use often led to a deadly problem known in the trade as MDR—multidrug resistance. Even if a drug was potent and very effective, the actively mutating tumor cells soon evolved resistance and could no longer be poisoned by it. Worse, the mutant tumors became so adept at avoiding poisons that they could withstand one drug after another, until nothing worked and the patient died. Cancer researchers understood the problem, and even knew how it worked at the molecular level. But it didn't mean they could overcome it.

The most basic thing that wasn't known when Folkman began his angiogenesis research was what turned a normal cell into a cancer cell. It was also not yet clear why some tumors remained safely benign while others became ruthlessly and inexorably metastatic, killing their hosts. And at the time there was no simple way to identify genes, or even to know whether these inherited, fundamental control elements in biology played a central role in the various kinds of cancer. It was clear that cancer cells could be killed by surgery, by poisoning them with chemicals, and by burning them with radiation, but next to nothing was known about *why* that worked: how the cancer cells responded, why they became drug-resistant, and why some seemed almost impervious to beams of X rays or gamma rays. At the time Folkman entered the picture, and throughout his career, most of the fundamentals were missing; cancer remained a stubborn enigma. The Nobel laureate James Watson famously described cancer as "a black box that we're trying to influence with magic."

By the time Watson spoke those words in the late twentieth century, the effort to find some magic that would slow or stop cancer was already ages old. Cancer was familiar in antiquity: In 460 B.C. Hippocrates used the Greek word *karcinos*—"the crab"—as its label. Three centuries later, the Greek physician Galen considered cancer a form of inflammation, and he, like Hippocrates, warned of the futility of trying to treat deep cancers, which could be seen as massive abdominal bulges or knots on limbs. Still, through much of history cancer was relatively less prominent than other diseases that plagued humanity. Even in the mid–nineteenth century, infectious diseases took such a heavy toll that great numbers of people died before they could get cancer, which is primarily a disease of the elderly.

Because they had little understanding of anatomy or physiology, physicians in past centuries proposed any number of theories about the origins of cancer. Some suggested that a special fluid, called "blastema," carried nutrients and "generative substances" throughout the body and was responsible for cancer. The lymphatic system, which had been identified through years of dissections, was also occasionally blamed as the seat of cancer, since swollen lymph nodes were often associated with the spread of metastasizing tumors. And there were also thought to be "cancer personalities," people destined to get the disease because of their personal mannerisms and habits of behavior.

An important step toward understanding cancer—indeed, toward understanding life itself—was naturalist Robert Hooke's discovery in 1665 that living individuals consist of tiny building blocks he called cells. Hooke, in England, could see under crude magnification that a thin slice of cork consisted of tiny empty chambers, but the significance of his discovery—that he was seeing the basic unit of all life on this planet—didn't immediately sink in. It wasn't until 1838 that German botanist Matthias Schleiden proposed that the cell is the fundamental structure for life. Three decades later, in 1867, a German physician, Wilhelm Waldeyer, became the first to suggest that cancer arose from normal cells going bad. Based on the tumor tissue he saw through the better lenses then being built into microscopes, he theorized that tumors expanded through the ordinary process of cell division.

As doctors struggled to understand cancer in the absence of sound knowledge of physiology, they found that the most useful weapon against it was epidemiology. By examining, tracking, and analyzing who got what kinds of diseases, at what ages, in what areas, and how they fared, it was possible to gather impressions, if not firm clues, about the causes of disease. For example, the first strong hint that substances encountered in the environment could cause cancer came in 1775 from Percival Pott, a British surgeon. He made the startling discovery that England's chimney sweeps were far more at risk for cancer of the scrotum than other men. The culprit seemed to be a residue of soot that remained caught in creases in scrotal skin. Pinning the blame for lung cancer on tobacco took far longer. It wasn't until 1951 that the renowned Medical Research Council, in England, paid two doctors—Austin Bradford Hill and Richard Doll—to look for possible causes of lung cancer. After studying cancer patients in twenty English hospitals, they identified smoking tobacco as a likely suspect.

That cancer is so much more prominent in older people than in children and young adults also spawned several sketchy ideas about causation. During the cancer-conscious era inaugurated by the American Cancer Society, doctors and scientists asked, for example, whether it took chronic or even lifelong exposure to various chemicals, or sunshine, or something else, to start cancer. Or was it caused by infection? Equally puzzling, why was cancer more common in some families than in others? Was cancer inherited? Or caused by diet? Were all of these factors involved? Or none of them? Or was there a mixture of causes?

Likewise, from the beginning scientists argued another familial theme: Was cancer a family of different diseases with different causes, or a single disease that comes in different forms? How could they make sense, for example, of skin cancers? Some tumors could be black as ebony, or white, or blood red. Leukemia could be fulminant, killing within weeks of diagnosis, or a relatively benign chronic disease that took years to progress. And some inherited forms of cancer would strike family members all in the same organs, such as breast, ovary, or colon, while in other families any organ or multiple organs seemed to be vulnerable. Why? How could one disease manifest itself in so many ways, strike so many different organs, and respond so differently to treatments?

No one knew, and until about 1975 the research tools didn't exist to find out. Only when molecular biologists began dissecting the internal structure of cancer cells and revealing their biochemical machinery did the mystery begin to clear up, if slowly. Only years later, as the century ended, was it finally clear that cancer is a result of genetic instability. When cells lose control of their genetic integrity, cancer grows. It could be that gene-repair mechanisms fail to correct the errors that normally occur during the gene-copying process in cell division or that mutations arise from exposure to chemicals and radiation. But when errors accumulate, and control of growth is lost, cancer erupts.

Answers to the enigma came so slowly because of the complexity that results from this genetic instability. The different forms of cancer behave very differently, seldom look alike, and grow at different rates. Some tumors metastasize rapidly and some don't. Some tumors may sit for years, seemingly dormant, while others grow explosively and kill in a matter of weeks, or months. But toward the end of the twentieth century, molecular biologists gained a toehold toward understanding and manipulating DNA, the stuff genes are made of, and biochemists discovered, altered, and created chemicals that seemed to be active against tumors, at least temporarily. Much of the work was purely scientific—science for science's sake—but a few physicians would occasionally try exotic substances on the chance something might work. As early as 1947, for example, Sidney Farber had experimented with a derivative of folic acid—a natural chemical found in plants—and showed that it tended to inhibit acute leukemia in children. It was the first so-called antimetabolite drug that could be used to interfere with the cell's internal processes. His work led to a new category of drugs that work because they share structural similarities with compounds the cell needs for its normal activity.

Meanwhile, because of a massive amount of nuclear research done during and immediately after World War II, nuclear medicine—meaning potent beams of X rays, protons, neutrons, and gamma rays—was being tailored for use against cancer. This was an increasingly sophisticated use of an old idea: Experiments in 1903 had shown that the radioactive metal radium, which had been isolated by Marie and Pierre Curie in 1898, was effective to some degree against tumors. So progress existed, but it didn't produce much of a dip in the cancer statistics. The types of cancer that responded best to new treatments—childhood leukemia to multidrug treatment; the type of lymphoma called Hodgkin's disease to radiation and chemotherapy; and testicular cancer to surgery, drugs, and radiation—afflicted only a small percentage of victims. In general, the American Cancer Society's annually updated graph showing cancer incidence in the United States was almost flat, essentially unchanged since 1900. The only startling exception was a huge upsurge in lung cancer among men, followed decades later by a similar upsurge of lung cancer among women. Liberation—"You've come a long way, baby"—wasn't an unmixed blessing.

By the 1960s and 1970s, doctors focused their efforts on cutting tumors out surgically, poisoning them with chemicals, or cooking them with radiation, all the while hoping their patients could stand the treatments. The cancer death rates remained stubbornly high. Clearly, something new and different was needed. Maybe it was time to seek answers elsewhere—to look for a cause of cancer inside the cell, at the molecular level. For biochemists and molecular biologists, this meant looking into the genes, and into the things that can change genes.

They focused first on viruses. These tiny invisible agents, so small that some of them could infect microscopic bacteria, had long been suspected as a cause of cancer, ever since Peyton Rous, in 1911, discovered a strange virus, later named the Rous sarcoma virus, that caused cancer in chickens. Viruses were already an enigma because biologists had always struggled to define whether they were actually alive or not. Unlike a living cell or a bacterium, a virus has no internal cellular machinery of its own. It cannot reproduce on its own, and never needs to eat or dispose of wastes. Instead, viruses are the ultimate parasites, utterly dependent on their ability to infect living cells. In general, once a virus has invaded a cell it commandeers its host's control system—a microscopic coup d'etat—and orders the cell to begin making multiple new copies of the virus. After enough new viruses have been made, either the cell bursts, liberating the new virus particles to attack other cells, or individual viruses "bud" themselves off the surface of the infected cells, then infect others.

What virologists eventually learned about the Rous sarcoma virus and its kin—a family called the C-type viruses—was a surprise that overturned one of the central dogmas of biology. Scientists had carefully worked out the premise that biological information flowed in only one direction: away from the gene, which is comprised of DNA, the double-stranded, twisted, and coiled molecule that serves as the central carrier of inheritance, making up the chemical codes that are passed from one generation to the next. The DNA produces an exact but single-strand copy of itself called RNA, and then the RNA molecule slips out of the cell's nucleus to tell the cell what kind of protein to make. Virologists knew that a virus consisted only of a DNA message wrapped inside a coat of protein. In an infection, the virus hooked itself to the cell's membrane, and then squirted its small chunk of DNA into the cell's interior. The virus's DNA soon worked its way in among the cell's existing set of genes, and began to issue orders and gain command of the cell.

The puzzle posed by the C-type viruses was important because it upset this scenario. The Rous sarcoma virus and its C-type brethren arrived at the cell surface carrying no DNA of their own. Instead, all that was wrapped inside the virus's spiky coat—resembling a floating sea mine—was a small length of RNA, the messenger molecule. So instead of full-strength genes, C-type viruses did their dirty work with mere shadows of genes, the fragile messenger molecule, RNA. How could this work? Everyone who worked on viruses knew that genetic information flowed in only one direction, from DNA to RNA to protein. C-type viruses seemed to break that rule. And because Peyton Rous and later others had found C-type viruses so closely associated with cancer, they seemed certain to offer important clues—if only they could be deciphered.

As it happened, the 1975 Nobel Prize in Physiology or Medicine went to Howard Temin at the University of Wisconsin and David Baltimore at the Massachusetts Institute of Technology for their discovery five years earlier of an obscure enzyme called reverse transcriptase, which was the tool a C-type virus used to capture the genetic machinery of a cell and make genetic information flow backward, from RNA to DNA. It opened a new world of exploration in biology, quickly focusing scientists' attention on this family of strange viruses that did things backward and managed to cause cancer in the process. Thus there was great excitement in science that cancer could, in some instances, be an infectious disease. Indeed, a few viruses were firmly linked to certain cancers, such as the Epstein-Barr virus as a cause of Burkitt's lymphoma, and the hepatitis B virus as a cause of liver cancer. Researchers, especially those working with hepatitis and herpes viruses, naturally thought that if cancer was sometimes a virally transmitted disease, then maybe it was possible to come up with vaccines that might protect against it. After Baruch Blumberg, at the Institute for Cancer Research, near Philadelphia, won the 1976 Nobel Prize for Physiology or Medicine for pioneering work with the hepatitis B virus, for example, vaccines did become available that promised to reduce the incidence of infection, and later liver cancer, especially in Asia, where hepatitis B was endemic. Also, because viruses were genetically as simple as it got, studying cancer-causing viruses seemed a good way to learn what goes wrong genetically to turn a normal cell into a cancer cell.

This exciting new work with viruses, especially the C-type viruses, helped introduce cancer researchers to the very important concept of oncogenes—mutant or misplaced normal genes that spur the growth of tumor cells—developed in 1969 by Robert Huebner and George Todaro, then at the National Institutes of Health. One theory held that since viruses insert themselves among the cell's normal genes, they can sometimes extract an extra, growth-promoting oncogene and pass it on to the next host cell. If this new growth-promoting gene is inserted into the next set of genes incorrectly or has been damaged, it might spur abnormal growth—cancer. That was one way that a virus infection might set off the cancer process.

Proving it was difficult, and not until the mid-1980s would molecular biologists Robert Weinberg, at the Massachusetts Institute of Technology, and Michael Wigler, at the Cold Spring Harbor Laboratory, identify the first one, an oncogene given the unassuming name *ras*. Their discovery, and the development of ever-more-powerful techniques for finding genes, soon led to the discovery of dozens of oncogenes, as well as their opposite number, antioncogenes. Roughly described, oncogenes such as *ras* act like a car's accelerator pedal; when activated they cause accelerated growth. Antioncogenes serve as the brakes; they are there as a safety mechanism to keep growth under control. So either mechanism, the accelerator or the brakes, can fail and lead to the accident called cancer. When viruses insert themselves into a cell's DNA, they can damage either an oncogene or an antioncogene, touching off the uncontrolled process of cell division that can lead to cancer.

These developments in virology and molecular biology, along with the increasing success doctors were having treating cancer with combination chemotherapy, more sophisticated anticancer drugs such as cisplatin and doxorubicin, and more precisely controlled radiation treatments, amplified the enthusiasm for cancer research and encouraged the political action to make the money available to pay for it. Pushed by advocates and pressure groups, in 1971 Congress approved and President Richard M. Nixon signed legislation kick-starting the so-called War on Cancer, an initial outlay of five hundred million dollars that would eventually stretch into the billions of dollars.

The War on Cancer set off an explosion of fundamental biological research. For the first time, huge amounts of money began pouring into genetics, molecular biology, and biochemistry. The money allowed scientists to develop powerful new tools to learn what goes haywire inside a cell to turn it cancerous. And that's where the world of cancer research was going—into the tremendous excitement of gene discoveries, understanding the cell's growth cycle, and getting at the roots of cancer. And then there was Judah Folkman, this *surgeon,* arguing for an utterly different approach, one that was literally and figuratively at the periphery. Here were the mainstream scientists, finding the dangerous genes, sorting out the rules and regulations of cell growth and life itself, collecting their Nobel prizes, while Folkman was poking his nose in with these strange ideas about blood vessels. He was more interested in figuring out how those misbehaving cancer cells sustained themselves and how their sustenance might be blocked, but to most in the field these ideas were barely worth noticing. He was in the loneliest of positions. No matter how many dollars he got from Monsanto or anyone else, the only way to change that would be to generate some real results.

FREED AT LAST BY THE MONSANTO DEAL from short-term financial pressures, Folkman set out to turn his collaboration with Bert Vallee and Monsanto into a triumph: the isolation of the magical tumor angiogenesis factor—TAF. His first obstacle was his working arrangement itself—not the one between Monsanto and Harvard that everyone else was worried about, but the one within Harvard. For the collaboration between Folkman and Bert Vallee was not a marriage made in heaven. Their work began at a distance and proceeded to gradually grow farther apart, not least because the two men were so different in personality and style. The environments of their labs were also poles apart, and the effort to blend them was like trying to merge two distinct civilizations built on fundamentally different principles. Vallee's participation was vital, and he would contribute important work, but the notion that he and Folkman would forge a close bond, isolate TAF, and then conquer cancer together turned out to be wishful thinking.

In the first place, Vallee already had major research projects of his own under way. He was, at the moment, focused on sorting out the role zinc played in both the structure and activities of enzymes. It was becoming ever more clear that metal atoms were extremely important parts of biological molecules. Iron was the best known of the essential metals because its vital role in the structure and function of hemoglobin had long been understood, and now zinc was increasingly seen as important in cell metabolism. It was a subject of fundamental importance in Vallee's world, so he could devote only small resources to the TAF project. Nor, for that matter, was Folkman spending anywhere near all his time on angiogenesis. He still spent most mornings and many nights in surgery, and still had to administer the department of surgery. It was important to perform well in all these tasks. Surgery was his livelihood and first love. Being chief of surgery gave him clout, which lessened the danger that his research and office space would be squeezed away. But the competing demands on his time were relentless. He knew very well he was on to something big and important in angiogenesis, that it would eventually have lasting value, and he was counting on Vallee to make a crucial difference.

Vallee was the embodiment of the Old World scientist. He ran a disciplined, regimented laboratory. Everyone had a specific piece of research to do, carefully planned and mapped out step-by-step, without much room for deviation. Vallee was directly in charge, and insisted on reliable, top-quality work at every step in a way that tended to quash whatever creative, risk-taking impulses his researchers might harbor. He could not abide what he saw as sloppiness, and he had little use for people whose results weren't rock solid. His attitude was described as almost Prussian: absolute dedication to a single-minded goal. Still, Vallee's rigorous and unyielding standards did not mean he was unkind. He endowed a foundation to support visits by outside researchers. Nor was he humorless. He was known for his deep, rumbling belly laugh.

Folkman's humor was more a part of his everyday personality, and his laboratory was, in contrast to his collaborator's, almost familylike, with a flexible, easygoing atmosphere—the kind almost guaranteed to make Vallee uncomfortable. Folkman never stopped being a teacher. His weekly lab meetings were a friendly free-for-all, the atmosphere bubbling over with ideas and enthusiasm. Some postdocs showed slides and graphs summarizing their results, then asked for any advice their colleagues might have for improving separation techniques: What tools might be available to buy or borrow? What biological or chemical tests might be done to push the research on cell growth and tumor-conditioned medium? For the students looking to finish their research, publish, and move on in their careers, Folkman acted as a facilitator, making suggestions, asking questions, and soliciting opinions from the other participants: What do you think that means? Why aren't the cultures growing? Is the temperature right? What about acidity? Did you get these cells from a reliable source? Maybe they came with contaminants. Maybe someone else ought to test them. Did you try a different test? Can anyone else here help on this? Oh, that's interesting; it looks like something new; maybe you're opening a new area! Bravo!

Scribbled on the board behind him in the conference room was a long list of "burning questions" that Folkman felt the laboratory needed to answer about angiogenesis. Some questions got erased after just a few weeks, others remained on the board for years. Each question offered a possible research project for anyone who cared or dared to take it on. The choice was voluntary, but the need to address these questions was clear, and they were among the first things encountered by the handful of postdoctoral fellows who joined Folkman's team each July, replacing the ones who had moved on after the completion of their two- or three-year stints. Some were surgical fellows who came in expecting to hone their skills under Folkman's tutelage, working in the operating room under intense pressure and finding research projects to work on during their off hours. But others were young physicians who joined Folkman primarily to take part in the angiogenesis work in his laboratory, hoping to get their feet wet in research, establish their credentials, and move on to medical centers to carry on their careers as physician-researchers. Their decisions about research projects were important, and Folkman tried to make sure they made good choices. He assumed responsibility for helping the young people build their self-confidence and making them willing to tackle important, even audacious problems.

Folkman's researchers also tended to share ideas and materials without much territoriality. He was remarkably open about the work: The blinds were rarely closed in the conference room next to his laboratory. He wanted no one even to suspect something secret was going on. His laboratory meetings, usually held at nine A.M. on Fridays if he was in town, were open to just about anyone. Some colleagues even worried that Folkman was *too* open and that some outsider might steal his ideas. He was amused by the suggestion. "If it's a really new idea," he'd reply knowingly, "you can't even give it away."

Vallee, meanwhile, almost never discussed results until all was complete. "His philosophy is that everything done in his lab has to be kept very quiet," observes Michael Klagsbrun, a biochemist who had come to Folkman's laboratory as a postdoctoral fellow in 1973, a year before the Monsanto agreement was signed. "Nobody was allowed to give seminars on it; no publications until the whole project was over, which took many years. He would not let anything out of his laboratory, including information. He would not allow people to attend conferences." Folkman not only allowed people in to observe the work in progress; he went out into the world and gave talks about it. "Folkman is the creative and imaginative type," remarks Klagsbrun, a muscular man with a soft-spoken intensity. "So you could talk about things that might not necessarily have been fully accurate yet, or totally nailed down. But he would be out there talking with sort of an optimistic outlook, while Vallee was definitely from the old school. So there was quite a lot of friction between these two." There was, before long, a certain arm's-length aloofness. It was a polite but distant relationship that did not get better with time. There were some small tiffs about experiments, responsibilities, schedules, and materials.

IN THE EARLY DAYS OF THE TAF PROJECT, Folkman worked closely with Monsanto's Joe Fedder to figure out how to scale up the production of tumor fluid from rats in order to have a better chance of isolating TAF. Culturing animal tissue was something new for the chemical company's research people, though they did have some expertise in growing plant cells in culture. At first, Folkman personally brought the tumor cells to the company headquarters in St. Louis, carrying them aboard a plane in a quart jar filled with fluid, sometimes accompanied by Vallee and Meadow, the medical school's associate dean. Folkman taught Fedder the arcane craft of cell culture, and Fedder and his team got to work on the problem of scaling up. When designing a system, they had to pay close attention to all the things that could mess up a culture and on a grand scale—temperature, acidity of the fluids, balance of nutrients, flow patterns, and, of course, sterility. Bacteria, viruses, and fungi were all capable of ruining a batch of cultured cells, so the vats, pipes, and pumps required constant monitoring and cleaning with ultrahot steam. Any loss of control could kill the growing cells. The pipes feeding a stainless-steel tank were first made with right-angle turns, creating small pockets where contaminating viruses would hide. Fedder substituted curved pipes that could easily be swept clean by blasts of steam.

Once the tumor cells began growing in huge amounts, regular shipments of frozen tissue samples placed in big boxes of dry ice began to arrive in Folkman's lab, where the cells would be thawed and broken open to liberate the tumor soup. Now Folkman had batches of tumor fluids containing TAF big enough to measure in grams, rather than the milligrams or micrograms he had before. Once the tumor fluids were released, the supply was split between the Folkman and Vallee laboratories. Both teams were working on fractionation techniques—removing solids from the fluids, changing the acidity or the salt concentration of the liquid—to isolate the small amount of TAF hidden within the complex soup of tumor broth. The work was difficult, time-consuming, and, for a long time, not very productive. This struggle was to continue for almost a decade.

In the meantime, Folkman pursued other aspects of the angiogenesis question. The set of notions at the core of angiogenesis was simple, but these ideas were bound by many disparate threads—observations, hunches, impressions, guesses, impulses—all of them, he suspected, vital to understanding what drove or stopped cell division, and to yielding better ways of testing the premises. One of the threads he now found sticking out from the rest, demanding attention, was this physiological curiosity: There were apparently only two places in the body where blood vessels were not normally found. One was the cornea, for good and obvious reasons. The other was cartilage. Why? Was there something inside this dense, gray-white tissue material that obstructed the growth of capillaries? Might it be that cartilage contained some sort of angiogenesis-inhibiting molecule, an agent that actively kept blood vessels out? And if that were the case, could that substance be recruited as a tumor fighter?

If Folkman was on the periphery before, now he was—to some people like Harvard hematologist Fred Rosen, who liked to laugh at Folkman's ideas and ridiculed the notion that cartilage had anything to do with cancer—off in outer space. Here was blatant speculation, ideas reached without supporting evidence, an obvious waste of time, money, and research energy. Anyone who cared to look could see plainly that cartilage was inert, a plasticlike tissue that grew in place, did its job, and didn't get involved in anything else. Cartilage had no blood vessels because it didn't need them.

Still, Folkman convinced a few students and postdocs working in his lab that cartilage could be a fruitful avenue for research. Embryologists had shown that very early in fetal life, blood vessels help cartilage grow, but before birth the vessels shrink back and then disappear completely. Something causes them to go away. And there was this: Many aggressive tumors seemed incapable of penetrating cartilage, even if they surrounded it. Folkman had first realized this years earlier, while performing an autopsy at Boston City Hospital on a woman whose breast cancer had metastasized to her spine. Her cancer had been so overwhelming that every vertebral bone had been invaded by tumors, and every part of the tumor was fed by blood vessels. But the vertebral discs, the plasticlike cushions made of cartilage that sit between each segment of backbone, remained white and tumor-free. Folkman filed the observation away.

One clue came from researcher Steven Brem, whom Folkman had brought in as a postdoctoral fellow to study tumors three years earlier. Brem, whose younger brothers Henry and Harold would also work in Folkman's lab later, looked at dozens of tumors from pathology labs, counted the capillaries he saw in each, and ranked them. At the top of the list, those most thoroughly vascularized, were brain tumors. And at the bottom were chondrosarcomas, tumors of cartilage. These tumors, which were rare to begin with, were the least well served by a blood supply. Folkman found still more evidence in the recent literature. While ordinary, healthy cartilage avoided being invaded by new blood vessels, one research team in Chicago had found that new capillaries did arrive after they killed cartilage with chemicals. This was crucial: It meant that something chemical, not just a physical roadblock, was keeping blood vessels out of cartilage.

Folkman found it hard to contain his enthusiasm for this new line of inquiry. One day, he ran into Fred Rosen on the street and asked, "Do you know the tissue that grows fastest?" Rosen said he had no clue; he'd never really thought about it. "Antlers. A deer, a moose, whatever. It's the fastest-growing tissue in all of biology," Folkman answered. He'd done some zoology reading and found that antlers are an outgrowth of cartilage, which, once formed, do very nicely without blood vessels. What was interesting was how antlers change. Early in life, they're surrounded by a soft, velvety tissue richly populated with blood vessels. But when the antlers grow to full size, the soft outer layer begins to disintegrate and peel away. They become hard and barren, totally devoid of arteries and veins. Did cartilage have a built-in property that made this happen? "Everything needs oxygen and a blood supply or else it can't exist," Folkman said to Rosen. "So what is this?"

To explore the properties of cartilage, Folkman and Henry Brem went back to the rabbit's eye. As Michael Gimbrone had done earlier, they inserted a small chunk of tumor into the cornea, close enough to the iris so that it would begin drawing in blood vessels. But then they altered the experiment by inserting a sliver of fresh rabbit cartilage between the chunk of tumor and the edge of the cornea, right in the path the blood vessels would most likely follow. Then they watched to see what happened. A month went by, and the tumor was unable to draw in a blood supply; the tiny capillaries would not grow through, over, or around the little barrier of cartilage. Then, in a contrasting experiment, an identical piece of cartilage was boiled, killing its cells. Then it was inserted into a rabbit's eye, again between the tumor and the cornea's edge. Soon tiny blood vessels began growing in, driving right past the cartilage barrier and rapidly engulfing the tumor. Even though it still presented a physical barrier, the sliver of dead cartilage couldn't block the arrival of new capillaries.

The implication, of course, was that live cartilage contained, produced, or excreted some kind of chemical that kept blood vessels at bay. And that suggested to Folkman that a potential inhibiting molecule actually did exist, and that it was a natural substance present in the body. It was an exciting finding, the first evidence that there might actually be a way to block or slow down blood vessel growth toward tumors. Nearly three decades later, elegant drawings of the experiment would remain hanging in the hallway of his lab.

But Folkman knew it was a long leap between observing a result and figuring out how it happened—and how it could be applied to the ultimate problem at hand. The cartilage question was just one of several puzzles that were accumulating in Folkman's lab. He needed to attract as many first-rate minds as he could. Given his unsettled reputation, this was no easy task.

FOR A LONG TIME, THERE HAD BEEN a doctrine at play in the world of scientific research, especially along the banks of the Charles River in Boston: Real scientists don't work on applied problems. Among some of those who were submerged in "pure" research there was open contempt for colleagues who thought too much about how their work might be used outside their laboratories. Oddly, it was an attitude reflected at times even in the arena of medical research. It was no accident, for instance, that the cancer research program at MIT had no direct connection to any hospital. This was pure biology; patients were not in the loop.

But things were going to change. As the twentieth century entered its last quarter, the divide among researchers would begin to crumble. It would be the age of biotechnology, and the discoveries being made in pure-research settings were becoming almost immediately useful. Hormones, growth factors, enzymes, and antibodies isolated and produced in research labs would quickly become treatments for real diseases. Human insulin would be made—by the ton—in factories. And, spurred in part by Harvard's collaboration with Monsanto, talent would flow toward young biotech companies whose reason for being was to discover things that sell. So many scientists would see that pure and applied research—and even science and commerce—would effectively merge. Science for the sake of science would be an increasingly quaint notion.

Among the many researchers responsible for this union would be chemical engineer Robert Langer of the Massachusetts Institute of Technology. A headline in the MIT alumni magazine, *Technology Review,* offered a pithy assessment of Langer's career: THEY USED TO CALL HIM CRAZY. NOW THEY CALL HIM SMART. By the time the article appeared in 1998, Langer was MIT's Kenneth J. Germeshausen Professor of Chemical and Biomedical Engineering. His name was on more than 330 patents and scores of scholarly papers; in addition to countless rewards, he also received, in 1998, a check for half a million dollars from MIT itself, the honorarium from the Lemelson Award, an annual prize given to an American for invention and innovation. Langer had the further distinction of being the only active member of all three of America's major national academies—the National Academy of Sciences, the National Academy of Engineering, and the National Institute of Medicine. He is a living rejoinder to the haughty credo that true scientists don't work on applied problems.

In the spring of 1974, Langer was a freshly minted graduate of MIT, trying to decide what to do with his new doctoral degree in chemical engineering. The decision marked the culmination of a long road for the young researcher, a short, slightly built man with dark wavy hair and an engagingly crooked smile slanting slightly down to the right. As a boy growing up in Albany, New York, he had been given a Gilbert chemistry set, a microscope, and many words of encouragement by his mother and father. Langer gravitated toward engineering after enrolling at Cornell University. He didn't really know what being an engineer entailed but thought it seemed a logical choice. His performance was less than brilliant in his first semester away from home, however, and his grades, adequate but disappointing, stirred him to reorganize his life. He studied almost obsessively the rest of the way. He settled on chemical engineering because that's where his best grades were, graduated with honors, and headed for MIT. There, he completed the tough chemical engineering curriculum in just four years and produced a doctoral dissertation, "Enzymatic Regeneration of Adenosine Triphosphate."

The newly titled Dr. Langer had no shortage of job opportunities that spring. The worldwide oil crisis was getting under way in earnest, and chemical engineers who might help figure out ways to squeeze more energy out of a barrel of oil were in great demand by the big oil companies. MIT-trained research specialists like Langer were a corporate recruiter's dream. Exxon alone made him four strong offers, with annual salaries exceeding twenty thousand dollars plus bonuses and perks—compensation that far surpassed what he might make in academia. During one interview in Louisiana, a recruiter told him that if he could find a way to improve the yield by .1 percent, it would mean billions of dollars of profit for the company and a sizable bonus for him. Langer's fellow MIT graduates were avidly accepting these lucrative jobs, but he couldn't get excited about spending his life in a refinery or running a corporate laboratory. It didn't seem a useful way to employ his hard-earned skills. He turned down all the Exxon offers, along with almost a dozen more from other companies.

Langer asked his professors at MIT about research possibilities in the chemical engineering laboratories. But that, too, held little allure. The professors were interested in extremely esoteric subjects that had little or no immediate impact on real life, research whose big payoff was to have one's name on a paper that might be read by a handful of people. Some people found this work extremely satisfying, but not Langer; he would rather invent a new clothespin than a new clothespin-shaped chemical molecule that was of no real use to anyone. "I kept asking my advisers: How is this going to do anybody any good?" he recalls. "It was very disillusioning to me." His research thesis—about the biochemical reactions that give cells their energy—was technically interesting, and he was proud of it. But the value of most of the work going on in the labs seemed remote and abstract to him. "I just felt I wanted to do something important," Langer explains. "Some people are drawn to science by enormous curiosity, and love the beauty of it. But that's not me. I think science is an incredibly powerful thing that can change the world. And that's what I wanted to do."

Frustrated with the standard options in chemical engineering, Langer had a thought: What about medical research? Maybe he could apply his experience to work that might actually make a difference. He began writing to hospitals, to little avail. Then a friend, a postdoc in his lab, told him he should write to a man named Judah Folkman. His friend, a physician studying engineering at MIT, told him about the buzz of controversy around Folkman in the Boston medical community because of his unconventional ideas. He told Langer he had a hunch that Folkman might be interested in a chemical engineer looking to segue into medical research. Langer wrote to Folkman and soon got a phone call suggesting a meeting. Folkman was always on the lookout for talent, always open to creative collaborations. He thought the idea of a chemical engineer from MIT coming to work in his lab was positively inspired.

Langer made his way to the Enders Building and rode the elevator to the tenth floor. Folkman welcomed him with his usual friendly manner and warm smile, and filled him in on his lab's work on angiogenesis. Then the conversation took an important turn. When Langer began talking about the techniques he'd learned as a chemical engineer, Folkman heard an entirely different language from the one he and his students spoke. Where biologists look at a living system and try to take it apart, engineers begin with the parts and try to build them up, seeing how they fit and how they work together. Folkman was excited by the prospect of a fresh perspective and by Langer's combination of brains, tenacity, and vision. Here was an ideal person to try bold new approaches to the stubborn problems Folkman was trying to overcome in his angiogenesis research. Folkman told Langer that he had a number of projects that he'd love a top postdoc to tackle, and that though he couldn't pay him what Exxon would—even with Monsanto's money—he'd have the chance to work on something exciting and important. It was music to Langer's ears. The conversation had opened his eyes. He could see all the things that engineers could do in medicine. Here was something that could change the world.

Langer's idealism was genuine. He was a chemical engineer with a social conscience. During graduate school at MIT, he had somehow found time to help start an alternative high school for low-income teenagers in Cambridge, called Group School. Langer taught chemistry at the school, and in his spare time, he did magic tricks for the students.

Langer's gift for magic would turn out to be a kind of metaphor for his performance on the laboratory stage. Years later Folkman would paraphrase physicist Richard Feynman to describe the young engineer's breakthroughs as the work of a "magician genius." As Folkman said to reporter Robin Lloyd in *Natural Science:* "There are all kinds of geniuses in the Harvard area, so we classify them. There are standard geniuses, and you can follow how they got from here to there, once they show it to you. But with a magician genius, you have no idea how he did it. Langer is that kind of genius—like an Einstein or a Feynman."

When Langer accepted Folkman's job offer in 1974, it seemed to almost everyone but them a curious match, a brilliant chemical engineer entering a surgery department.

That so many people outside Folkman's lab found the partnership strange was a reflection of how little they understood the direction of his work. First, there was the matter of cartilage. Some substance in it seemed to block the growth of blood vessels, and it was reasonable to think that a chemical engineer might succeed in discovering what it was, where biologists and biochemists had failed. A superior chemical engineer from MIT might at least conjure up new ideas to try.

Folkman also wondered what Langer might bring to the TAF question. For several years now, the lab had been working with complex soups extracted from living tumor cells, trying to isolate the elusive angiogenesis factor by separating out different parts of the fluid, testing to see if activity remained. Folkman was convinced these fluids contained one or more hormonelike agents that caused blood vessels to sprout new branches and begin growing toward tumors. In pursuit of this, Folkman had a particular area he wanted Langer to work on: leaky plastics.

This arose from the discovery Folkman and David Long had made while they were in the navy nearly fifteen years before—the one whose patent they had given royalty-free to the Population Council when Harvard didn't want it. Now it was on its way to becoming the Norplant contraceptive, but Folkman thought he might be able to exploit the concept himself after all. He had already shown that TAF consisted of large molecules, because it wouldn't fit through some ultrafine filters. So why not try to come up with a plastic material that would allow bigger molecules to seep through slowly and at a precise rate, so that any growth factors they found might be easily tested? That would be another of Langer's assignments.

Arriving for work in Folkman's lab, Langer had to first become acquainted with his new biological world. He had to learn to work with living animals and cells, for one thing. And he had to learn the rudiments of cell science and everyday techniques like culturing tissue. But he and Folkman were anxious to get started on the questions at hand, with cartilage the first order of business. Folkman told Langer about Henry Brem's work showing how cartilage blocked the path of blood vessels in a rabbit's eye, the best indication so far that cartilage was worth looking at as a potential source for an antiangiogenesis agent. The question he posed was: Is this a physical blockage? Or is it—as Folkman thought—a biochemical one? Folkman was asking Langer to isolate the first angiogenesis inhibitor.

Doing serious research on cartilage required, first, a serious amount of cartilage. Henry Brem had used rabbit cartilage, but Langer decided that rabbits simply weren't big enough animals to supply the heaps of cartilage that would be needed for research. He scaled up. He went and got cows—a lot of cows. He visited all the meat markets in South Boston, before settling on an old slaughterhouse called Treligan's, in a run-down part of Cambridge. "It was a real dump," he later recalled, "but I could get cow shoulders."

Langer started making regular trips to the slaughterhouse and loading up his old Plymouth—the seats, the floors, the trunk—with hundreds of pounds of cow bones. He hauled the shoulder bones up to the tenth-floor lab, then cleaned and prepared them for his experiments. Scraping the residue of drying meat off the bones was an arduous chore. "I recruited anyone who walked by," Langer would recall, though he wound up doing much of it himself. Once the bones were clean, Langer cut off the pure white cartilage, chopped it up, and dumped it into a chemical solution until it was partially dissolved, leaving a fluid that could then be put through a series of separation steps in an effort to isolate antiangiogenic activity. Finally, after about a year, he started seeing some results: Using rabbit eyes as the testing chamber, he discovered that a substance drawn from the cartilage seemed to inhibit the growth of new blood vessels.

As the cartilage research started producing data that looked interesting, Folkman agreed to put enough extra money into the project to hire people to help clean and prepare the cow bones. Every afternoon, flocks of local high school students came in and scraped the raw meat off cow bones, so many bones that they had to work in the hallways. "A lot of people laughed at us, and at Dr. Folkman's theory," said Catherine (Kit) Butterfield, a tissue culture specialist who joined Folkman's team after Langer. Fred Rosen, an important research supervisor in the Enders Building, was one of them. He found the commotion amusing, if not downright ridiculous. "That was quite a wild scene," he recalled later, the years having softened his scorn. "They were out in the corridors, breaking the fire laws. They were everywhere." The lab was so crammed with cartilage scrapers that accidents happened. One day a technician accidentally spilled a whole jug of cartilage extract across the floor, and the group had to start over. But that was nothing compared with the scene that came after Langer decided he needed even more cartilage than the slaughterhouse could supply. Sharks, he realized, have more cartilage than bone. He started visiting fish markets and soon came up with a source of sharks. The first shark he bought weighed hundreds of pounds, and Langer and his assistants had to bring it up in chunks. They stored it in a cold room, but that didn't help much. "The stench," remembers Sandy Smith, a technician, "was unbelievable."

Langer was thinking big, and it paid off. After nearly two years of hauling cow and shark meat upstairs and separating the constituents of their cartilage, he and his partners extracted a material that inhibited angiogenesis in the test chambers of rabbit eyes and fertilized chick eggs. The substance wasn't a pure molecule; it consisted of protein mixtures that—as with TAF—couldn't yet be identified. But it was the first real inhibitor, and for Folkman's team it was a major discovery. Langer thought he would have a good chance at publishing the work in a leading journal, and he was right. It was accepted for publication in *Science* in 1976. But while he and Folkman were ecstatic about the discovery, they weren't prepared for what came next.

In their article, Langer and Folkman remarked that sharks had not been known to get cancer, and hinted that maybe it was because they were so full of cartilage. "If Bob had sent this to *The Journal of Biological Chemistry*, no one would have ever paid attention," observed one member of the lab. "But it got published in *Science*." And that's where I. William Lane saw it.

Lane was a biochemist, a nutritionist, and a vice president at W. R. Grace & Co., the large international chemical company, which had facilities in Boston's suburbs. He also had an entrepreneurial bent, and he took Langer and Folkman's report on cartilage—shark cartilage, in particular—as a call to commerce. He had no trouble imagining a market for the stuff as a cancer fighter. It could be manufactured and sold as a food or a food supplement (not as a drug), thus avoiding the scrutiny of the U.S. Food and Drug Administration. Soon after the publication of the paper in *Science,* Lane called Langer, asked him some questions, then began buying huge quantities of shark and rendering the cartilage into a product he called BeneFin, which he began selling through health food stores. Much to the chagrin and consternation of Langer and Folkman, Lane built his sales pitch around them, even using their names and photos in his early promotional materials. A Harvard attorney got that stopped, but he couldn't prevent Lane from prominently citing the researchers in a book he published years later, *Sharks Don't Get Cancer,* as well as in a sequel, *Sharks Still Don't Get Cancer.*

Unfortunately for Lane, sharks do get cancer; it was just that no one (including Langer and Folkman) had taken the time to research it before. And several clinical studies later showed that the oral use of shark cartilage preparations had no discernible anticancer benefit. Langer's original finding that cartilage contains an angiogenesis inhibitor was confirmed but simply eating it was of no use. The active ingredient apparently didn't get through the wall of the human intestine. For Folkman the episode was damaging. Even if he and Langer were innocent victims of Lane's sly publicity, the vague impression remained that they had some connection with yet another unproven cancer theory. Lost in the fuss was their discovery that angiogenesis could be stopped. Folkman and Langer were going in the right direction.

MEANWHILE, LANGER WAS ALSO THINKING hard about his other assignment, leaky plastics.

Folkman's idea was to develop some sort of device that would simulate a tumor—a kind of depot that would release small doses of largish proteins capable of influencing the growth of nearby blood vessels. He wanted Bob Langer to come up with an experimental device that would reliably keep chemicals flowing at a slow, steady rate because—as Michael Gimbrone had shown—that's what tumors do. They pump out a little at a time, all the time, for a long time. Ultimately Folkman wanted to develop a system to test the leaking chemicals for their ability to stimulate or inhibit angiogenesis in assays such as the live rabbit eye or the fertilized chicken egg. So Langer needed to create a plastic akin to Swiss cheese—a material with holes just the right size to let specific kinds of molecules through. There were already plastics that allowed substances made of very small molecules, such as birth control hormones, to pass through. Langer would try to come up with one that allowed bigger molecules—like TAF—to slowly migrate through. But he also needed plastics that did not cause irritation of the nearby tissues, as in rabbit eyes. Folkman did not want to hear once again the dreaded inflammation argument.

Langer was eager to work this out. He had found the cartilage research intriguing and challenging, and he demonstrated his enthusiasm with every load of smelly shark he brought up in the elevator. But it was the plastics project that appealed to him most as a chemical engineer, and, eventually, it was this work that fulfilled his wish to have an impact on the world. Using heat or solvents, he molded the contenders—various kinds of plastic he had bought as beads or sheets—into tiny tube-shaped chambers. Then he put various large-molecule substances inside the chambers and had bacteria growing in culture on the outside, and watched what happened. If the lawn of bacteria changed in appearance, it meant the plastic was allowing the substances inside to leak out.

"Langer attacked it with a chemical engineering approach, which is called working the problem," Folkman recalls. "That's fundamentally different from biology, where you discover phenomena, and you don't have many organizing principles. We have Darwin and the double helix. But in chemical engineering you have hundreds of principles and laws. So when you work a problem you pick out the best principle, and then it will explain everything." Langer, for example, did not take a solid material and then poke holes in it or try to alter it mechanically. Instead, he began by listing what properties he wanted in a plastic—pliability, a certain minimum porosity, chemical reactivity—and then set out to use materials with these properties to build into his new product.

Langer tried silicone rubber first, but it wasn't porous. The fluid wouldn't come out. He tried vinyl acetate, polyvinyl alcohol, every kind of plastic he could find. All but two inflamed the eye. One of the exceptions was a material called Hydron that had been invented by Bausch & Lomb for use in soft contact lenses. The other came from Alza, a pharmaceutical company that owed its existence, in good part, to Folkman and David Long's work in the navy, and on whose scientific advisory board Folkman had once sat. Alza's material, called Occusert, was already in use as a method of delivering drugs via the eye. It resembled a crescent-shaped lens that fit under the lower eyelid and secreted a drug for glaucoma. With those two plastics in hand, Langer began experimenting to see if they could be tailored to allow large-protein molecules to seep out. Neither plastic worked; they were too impermeable.

But then Langer found out that the plastics could be purchased in powder form, and this gave him an idea. He added alcohol to the powder, and it became a gooey fluid, rather like Karo syrup. Once the alcohol evaporated off, the residue was a rubbery polymer, a plastic. But still the big molecules wouldn't seep through. Then he had a very good idea. To the syrup mixture containing alcohol, he added dry, powdered proteins. If the proteins had been wet, the alcohol would have ruined them. But because the protein was dry, the solid granules could be mixed in without harm. Then he evaporated off the alcohol, leaving what looked like a white piece of rubber. The protein grains were locked inside the plastic, sitting cheek by jowl. Then Langer added water, which was soaked up by the millions of protein grains, expanding them and creating interlocking channels, passages within the plastic that made it resemble Swiss cheese on a microscopic scale. And with time, the wet proteins diffused out of the microchannels, in some cases taking months to escape completely, depending on how big the original protein granules were. What was left was a piece of plastic riddled with microscopically small channels. The tumor-conditioned medium, with its TAF, was able to leak through.

It was a momentous discovery that made possible an entire new industry, an achievement that would define the rest of Langer's career. He and many of his colleagues would go on to develop an array of leaky plastic capsules that could be implanted under the skin to deliver medicines and hormones in precisely regulated amounts over very long periods. The benefits would be enormous, both for patients and for MIT's endowment fund, the beneficiary of Langer's 330 patents. But the plaudits were a long time coming. When Langer made the first of these discoveries in Folkman's lab in the mid-1970s, they were not hailed as vital achievements. Langer remembers trying to tell the world—or at least the world's polymer chemists—about his findings, only to see the news land with a dull thud. It was another case of entrenched experts looking askance at the work of a newcomer.

A number of these experts sat alongside Folkman on the scientific advisory board of the Alza Corporation in California. Among them were two Nobel laureates, Stanford University's renowned Paul Flory, a world-class specialist in polymer chemistry and winner of the 1974 Nobel Prize for Chemistry, and Arthur Kornberg, winner of the 1959 Nobel in Physiology or Medicine. Alza was founded specifically to develop medicine-delivery systems based on leaky plastics, so Langer expected his work to immediately attract the company's interest. To test the waters, Folkman brought his eager young postdoctoral fellow along for a West Coast board meeting, where they carefully explained how Langer was succeeding in getting large-protein molecules to ooze reliably from his special plastic capsules. "And they said no. Just forget it,"

Langer recalls. "They said the literature says no." To the experts, there was no chance that large molecules could ever be made to leak out of plastics—even though Langer had the data to show otherwise. No less an authority than Paul Flory said it couldn't be done. Though disappointed, Langer persisted.

As Folkman's early mentor, Robert Gross, had done for him two decades before, he escorted Langer to his first major technical meeting, where he would offer up his findings to a large group of experts. They flew to Midland, Michigan, and Folkman introduced his twenty-seven-year-old protégé to an international gathering of distinguished polymer chemists. Then Langer took the podium and told them that big stuff could leak out of plastics. As Langer remembers the moment: "It was the first talk I ever gave at a national meeting. I had practiced for weeks. So here I am, this young guy, and I'm feeling pretty pleased because I didn't stammer or stutter much. And when I get done, I expect all of these nice guys will want to encourage me, this young guy. But all they say is 'This is impossible. We don't believe anything you've said!' It was very shocking to me. I hadn't realized how hard it would be."

It really didn't matter that Langer's data was solid. His findings did not mesh with the conventional wisdom, and there were enough small gaps in his work—a few relatively minor questions he couldn't answer immediately—to allow technical quibbling. "We didn't understand everything, but then you never do in science," Langer says. "But I think this idea just went so much against the grain of everyone's thinking that they thought you can't do it. It was met with a lot of skepticism which, of course, is kind of damaging to your career."

In this, of course, Langer didn't have to look far for commiseration.

Chapter Eleven

———

HARVARD'S MONSANTO DEAL WAS SIGNED late in 1974, but one of its provisions was potentially so thorny that it took two years to carry out. The idea, advanced by Harvard and accepted by Monsanto, was to put together a five-member advisory committee to ensure that each side—but mostly Monsanto—honored the agreement. The committee would monitor the relationship and make sure the company respected Folkman and Vallee's academic freedom—their right to publish, for instance—and responsibly developed any products that emerged.

The oversight committee idea had come from Hale Champion, an executive dean at Harvard's Kennedy School of Government who had been involved in the original negotiations as an adviser. He thought a board of respected outsiders, formally acting "in the public interest," might allay some of the fears he accurately predicted would erupt among the faculty after the deal was disclosed. But selecting the members turned out to be as complicated as the agreement itself. It was like picking a jury. Monsanto didn't want anyone who might harbor antibusiness attitudes, Harvard didn't want anyone who lacked an appreciation for the academic culture, and each side had the right to reject the other's suggestions. So it wasn't until early 1977 that Monsanto issued a press release finally announcing the appointment of five distinguished men, two with long experience in public affairs and three with eminent careers in science. Frank Stanton, the former vice chairman of CBS who was now president of the American Red Cross, would be its chairman. The other members would be William Ruckelshaus, the former administrator of the Environmental Protection Agency; Stanford's Nobel laureate in chemistry, Paul Flory; biochemist Alton Meister from Cornell University; and hematologist Maxwell Weintrobe, from the University of Utah. The latter three were members of the National Academy of Sciences.

But the announcement, long after the controversy about the deal had simmered down to a background rumble at Harvard, had an unintended effect. It stirred things up again, triggering a new round of indignation and hand-wringing, especially in the wake of a long and skeptical article in *Science,* one of the world's most respected sources of science news. For the uninitiated, the author of the article, Barbara Culliton, took the opportunity to review the events that had led to the appointment of the committee: Folkman's angiogenesis theory and the search for TAF, his collaboration with biochemist Bert Vallee, the negotiations that culminated with a deal between America's leading educational institution and one of its largest corporations—an arrangement, Culliton noted, that was "unprecedented in the annals of academic-business affairs."

Among the things that Culliton found most notable was the secrecy that still surrounded the deal. Both Monsanto's Monte Throdahl and Harvard's Henry Meadow tried to avoid giving interviews—Throdahl said he didn't want to do anything to disturb the agreement, "a fragile flower just ready to bloom"—and Folkman and Vallee didn't want to talk either, particularly about the research. (Folkman told Culliton that he had not given an interview in four years, ever since the 1972 American Cancer Society press seminar. "I really do not want to talk about the work until we have something new to say," he told her over the phone.) Throdahl and Meadow eventually did speak, but they refused to divulge financial details of the contract. That concealment, along with nagging concerns at Harvard that the twenty-three-million-dollar grant had not gone through the normal peer-review system and that the research agenda was being dictated by commercial interests, prompted some to wonder if the oversight committee was not so much a precaution as a sign of trouble. "If everything is on the up-and-up," one faculty member told Culliton, "why do we need a committee for civic virtue?"

The article reopened all the half-healed sores from two years earlier. It quoted unnamed sources who were still questioning the ethics of the agreement and even the value of Folkman's angiogenesis research. Introducing Folkman's elusive tumor-produced growth factor at the top of her story, Culliton noted: "TAF may or may not exist." She had no trouble finding people willing to gripe anonymously that Folkman's work seemed to have a lot of financial support but little scientific merit. One grant reviewer told Culliton: "I believe that anyone who has a 'factor,' which means they don't know what it is, has five or six years to prove it. After that, I stop reading about it."

Such comments were an accurate reflection of how Folkman's work was being perceived everywhere except in his own laboratory and at Monsanto. Despite the corporate windfall—or because of it—Folkman had continued to apply for grants from the government. In this, he was looking not so much for money as for assessment: He felt it was important to put his work through the normal NIH peer-review process. But in a few instances this backfired: Among some grant referees, the Monsanto deal seemed reason enough to reject him. One committee actually turned him down on grounds that he didn't need the money, though an oversight committee later ruled that the decision was unfair. But some reviewers were against the grants because they had doubts about the work. A friend on a review committee told Folkman that one of the other members had said, "Haven't we supported Folkman long enough on this hopeless search?"

Sometimes, the disrespect took the form of people walking out of sessions when it came Folkman's turn to talk at conferences. At one meeting, Folkman came into a room to give a twenty-minute talk and found only three people waiting for him. At another large gathering of experimental biologists, he watched a hundred people get up and leave as he came to the podium to give a brief lecture.

Folkman also ran into resistance when he tried to recruit top people to work in his lab. He heard from many promising postdoctoral students who were initially interested in his work, but who were warned by their professors that accepting a position in Folkman's lab would be a dead end—he would turn them into mere technicians. When Donald Ingber, a physician and cell biologist from Yale, was considering moving to Folkman's lab, he asked his closest professors what they thought. "Well, I've never met the guy," one replied. "But I'm worried. I've heard from a lot of people that he's a charlatan." Ingber did hear some good comments—"Judah? He's a good man," George Palade, a Nobel laureate, told him—but when he decided to accept the position, many others were less than impressed. The attitude was: Oh, that's junk. You're wasting your time. We're never going to see a cure for cancer in our lifetime.

"These were hard times," remembers Carl Cobb, the former medical reporter who became an aide to Folkman. "His grants were getting 'special' reviews. I remember one had gotten a low rank and had been turned down, and then the team was sent up here. One of the members of that team, a pathologist, made it blatantly and absolutely clear he thought that Folkman didn't know what he was talking about. He said Folkman had it backward, that it was well known and well documented that blood vessels actually came from the tumors. He said Folkman's work was nonsense and that something so far out should not be supported. People were saying, 'You don't understand the biology, and you're a surgeon, not a biologist'—they never let you forget that he was just a surgeon, not a scientist—and that bright, reputable people shouldn't be spending time in his laboratory. So there were years of swimming against the tide. Of not being in prestigious journals. Of struggling to get grants. Of being, in many ways, bad-mouthed by his peers."

The bad-mouthing was severe enough and became so widespread that twenty-five years later the Nobel-winning biologist Harold Varmus, speaking as the director of the National Institutes of Health, would introduce Folkman with the remark: "The first time I ever heard of Judah Folkman, he was described as this guy in a hair shirt working on an island in Boston Harbor." In those years, Varmus was a cancer researcher at the University of California, San Francisco, and it was his impression that Folkman—despite his gargantuan grant from Monsanto, which, in the eyes of some, further eroded his credibility—was an isolated, obsessed man, a kind of misguided martyr.

"Judah was thought of as sort of a renegade scientist, trained as a surgeon, pursuing a phenomenon that most of us thought of as peripheral to the central issues of cancer," Varmus recalls. "He was definitely out of the mainstream, not known for a high level of rigor. There was institutional skepticism about what he was doing. We didn't see his work in the major journals. We were going to tumor meetings, talking about cancer genes, while he was over on the periphery, working on the vasculature, asking what growth factors make the difference."

It was the 1977 *Science* article that again brought Folkman's sagging reputation to the attention of the top administration at Children's Hospital, where his role as surgeon-in-chief made him very visible—and vulnerable. The griping had generally been confined to colleagues whispering in hallways or to meetings of grant review committees. But now it was out in the open, for everyone to see. It was *national*. With its critical, almost cynical tone, the *Science* article was an embarrassment, and it turned the hospital's board of trustees against him. "You're making a mockery of research here," Folkman recalls being told by one person. The heat was being turned up. Colleagues began insisting that Folkman be subjected to an official, external review of his work.

Under normal circumstances, such reviews were not all that uncommon. The medical school and hospital made a practice of asking independent experts to evaluate two of the twenty laboratories every year, a process in which the lead researcher spent an entire day essentially justifying his lab's existence. When it was over, the visitors reported on whether they thought the research was worthy. The process was grueling, sometimes traumatic, and aimed at clearing out dead wood. Being identified as dead wood could be a career-ending event, sparking immediate and intense debate over the definition of dead wood. All that was under normal circumstances. These were extraordinary circumstances. As everyone knew, the Harvard Medical School had staked a good piece of its reputation—and Monsanto's money—on a man Children's Hospital was now considering kicking out.

Even apart from the outside committee, Folkman knew he was in a precarious position. The people at Children's who made decisions about space allocations for the Enders Research Building weren't convinced that Folkman's project even belonged there. "It wasn't their kind of science," Folkman recalls; the only reason he had been able to hang on to his big space was that he happened to be the chief of surgery. But that kind of clout would have little effect on the committee of outsiders, which was headed by a renowned pathologist, Henry Harris, from Oxford University in England.

On the appointed day, Folkman showed the visiting scientists around and described his efforts to purify TAF and his experiments with such systems as rabbit eyes. The scientists were unimpressed. "They just blew up," remembers Dr. David Nathan, then the hospital's chief of medicine. "I can still remember [Henry Harris] saying, 'I've got about two hundred reagents in my laboratory that will give me pinkeye if I put them in my eye.' He said, 'This is ridiculous work.' " To no one's surprise, Harris's committee issued a scathing report. It said that Folkman was working on "nonspecific inflammation" and that his project was unlikely to be of great relevance.

Stunned, Folkman found little support among his surgical colleagues. Though he had the firm loyalty of some younger members of the staff, who considered him a mentor, many of his peers agreed with Harris. "[They thought] this was a lot of rubbish, with bad assays chasing ridiculous agents," Nathan says. "Nobody understood what the hell was going on. People thought [Folkman] was out to lunch." Many of Folkman's colleagues thought his two main systems of observing angiogenesis in action—the eyes and the eggs—made it impossible to see what was actually going on. Folkman was well aware of the shortcomings of his research thus far but found the intensity of the resistance puzzling. There was little sympathy for his contention that it was still early in the game and that there was still much to be learned about blood vessel growth, especially as it related to cancer.

The devastating reviews opened the door to more and even louder grumbling about Folkman's priorities. There had long been complaints that he was always off in his lab when he should have been in the OR, gowned up and operating on sick children. Now, despite the support of the medical school and Monsanto, the critics claimed he was disregarding surgery for something unworthy. That was how the decision was framed when the controversy reached its inevitable climax. Something had to be done. And William Wolbach, president of the hospital's board of trustees, had to decide, finally, what to do about Folkman.

His research aside, Folkman saw no reason to be ashamed of his performance over a decade as surgeon-in-chief. He performed some of the most difficult surgical procedures daily. He was always on call for major emergencies. And he oversaw a team of outstanding surgeons who went on to brilliant careers of their own even as he continued to teach at the medical school. Folkman also pointed out to his detractors that he had reformed the surgical service during his tenure, to the benefit of the patients and the hospital. When he got there in 1969, the department was being run almost like a private practice; he instituted weekly meetings to thrash out what had been done correctly and incorrectly in the operating room. He also insisted that every patient, rich or poor, be visited regularly, day and night. Some veteran surgeons resisted this rule, but over time he prevailed as new people came in. "We began to get the best residents in the world," Folkman later reflected, and he was able to get them involved in leading-edge medical research. An organ transplant team was set up, and with the arrival of Dr. Joseph Murray as head of plastic surgery, Children's Hospital put together the best cranial-facial reconstruction program in the world.

Folkman also brought up his predecessor and mentor, Robert Gross, as an argument that the surgeon-in-chief could do both surgery and research. But there was a difference. Folkman, David Nathan notes, "was a classic case of somebody trying to be chief of surgery in a very busy surgical service, and not being in the OR that much, whereas his predecessor was one of the great inventors of operations, and lived in the OR."

Wolbach was a businessman—he ran the Boston Safe Deposit and Trust Company—and he didn't find the call a particularly difficult one. He didn't want to hear any more complaints. He wasn't convinced Folkman's blood vessel research would ever pay off, and, in Nathan's words, "he wasn't going to screw up surgery," which was, of course, one of the hospital's main thrusts.

Wolbach called Folkman to his office. You've got your choice, he told him. Either be surgeon-in-chief, a full-time surgeon, or you're getting out. We're kicking you out, and you can go back to your laboratory. And stop giving pink-eye.

To Folkman and those on the staff who supported him, this was less about medicine than about public relations. He was essentially being bounced because of the article in *Science*. "It was terribly damaging because the trustees said, 'Gee, the criticism and ridicule we hear locally from Harvard professors is in fact felt nationally, and we have somebody here who doesn't know what he's doing, and we don't understand it either.' So we were constantly getting this flak from Mr. Wolbach. They only want on their staff people who are solid, fashionable, and noncontroversial." The huge Monsanto grant certainly kept Folkman from being described as noncontroversial. What it did was make him the target of bile—an academic admixture as hard to isolate as TAF, but one in which strains of jealousy were evident.

Folkman was as angry as he had ever been. The stresses were so intense that Paula even suggested that he get out of medicine altogether; at that moment it didn't seem worth the grief. Folkman would never do that, of course. He had other options. He knew there was a way he could still be a chief of surgery and also continue his angiogenesis research: He could accept one of the many offers he was receiving from medical research centers around the country. There was an especially appealing offer from the rapidly growing M. D. Anderson Medical Center in Houston. He could have a department of his own there, as well as a professorship, a huge salary, and ample staff, though the Monsanto money would stay at Harvard.

Folkman didn't want to act rashly; he could not lightly give up a tenured professorship at the Harvard Medical School, the very tip of the top in medicine, a position signifying enormous ability and accomplishment. The Boston area would also be hard to leave. The concentration of research talent and resources kept the level of scientific excitement high. And the Folkmans liked their lifestyle. They had a nice home within walking distance of the hospital. Their two girls, now adolescents, were in good schools. Paula was involved in her music career in one of the most musically rich parts of the country. She later sang with the Boston Symphony Chorus at Tanglewood.

Folkman also felt a deep responsibility for the careers of people he'd brought into Children's Hospital, most of whom supported him through these tough times. One of these surgeons was Dr. Joseph Vacanti, a Nebraskan whom Folkman had encouraged in 1973 to apply for an internship in surgery at Massachusetts General Hospital. Vacanti had succeeded, and he had gone on to become chief resident in surgery at Children's Hospital, and later chief of organ transplantation. "For many of us, through more than one generation, Dr. Folkman was almost the ultimate mentor and teacher," Vacanti later said. "The way he teaches, the way he inspires; he's very charismatic, and he can really ignite the mind." Not everyone felt that way, certainly; there were always colleagues and competitors who didn't put much trust in charisma. "I guess if you're a strong leader or a strong personality, people don't come down on you halfway," Vacanti mused. "They either love you or you're hated. Dr. Folkman once told me that you can tell a leader by counting the number of arrows in his ass."

It was a rise in the status of angiogenesis, perceptible to few other than Folkman, that ultimately led him to stay in Boston. Ironically, considering the seeds of his political problems at the hospital, he felt a sense of progress. Some of his students, like Michael Gimbrone, and collaborators, such as Ramzi Cotran, were pursuing angiogenesis studies on their own. So now the work was no longer solely confined to Folkman's laboratory; other scientists were trying to unlock the mysteries of blood vessel biology and hunting for growth factors, research that seemed destined to explain angiogenesis and its relationship to cancer. "It was like we were working on a big jigsaw puzzle, for which all of the pieces had been handed to us in a bag," Folkman says. "It was at the point where I could begin to see what image was emerging." It wasn't the time to pack up and start over somewhere else.

Folkman agonized over the decision for months but finally agreed to step down in 1979 as chief of surgery at Children's—though he was to stay on until a replacement was named two years later—and resolved to devote himself even more vigorously to angiogenesis. He had a long-standing written agreement with the hospital that allowed him research space, and his problems at the hospital couldn't threaten his tenure at Harvard. To some of his colleagues, this was the right move. Though Wolbach was forcing him out of a field he'd been part of since he was a teenager in Ohio, he was also allowing him the opportunity to focus his energies and his talents fully—for the first time, and at a critical moment—on his true passion, angiogenesis. "Judah must have hated [Wolbach]," Nathan observes, "but it was the break of a lifetime."

———

IN 1972, FOLKMAN AND MICHAEL GIMBRONE had first suc-
ceeded in growing endothelial cells extracted from human umbilical veins,
but they couldn't understand why nothing happened when they dribbled
fractionated tumor fluid on the cells. Folkman was sure there was TAF, the
unpurified tumor angiogenesis factor, in that fluid. So why didn't the blood
vessel growth factor spur the growth of blood vessel cells? Arguably, his entire
theory rested on the answer to that question. He had to prove there was a
growth factor that specifically stimulated blood vessel cells. It was the fundamental property underpinning his ideas, and it wasn't working.

Desperate for an answer, Folkman had in the intervening years taken a
bold and intuitive leap in his imagination. With essentially zero evidence to
back it up, Folkman mused that maybe there was a fundamental difference between the endothelial cells lining the big blood vessels and those in the capillaries, the very tiny blood vessels found throughout the body. He didn't spend
much time worrying about the existing dogma, the firm belief that endothelial tissue is the same everywhere in the body, extending like a uniform layer
of carpeting throughout the circulatory system. Was there a hidden difference? He had kept mulling this possibility until, one day in 1976, it struck
him: Of course, of course—it was so obvious. *Tumors don't recruit large blood
vessels. They recruit capillaries.* Maybe capillary cells were somehow different
from other blood vessel cells—and maybe they responded to different growth
factors.

Pursuing this thought meant breaking new ground. Folkman had learned
how to culture endothelial cells from large blood vessels. Now he needed to
learn how to grow them from capillaries, the tiniest blood vessels. He wrote up
a grant proposal that necessarily included the adventurous, if not heretical,
idea that endothelial cells varied within the body. To his disappointment, but
not surprise, the application was summarily rejected on the ground that it was
nonsense. "It is well known," came the reply from the NIH reviewers, "that
all endothelium is the same."

Folkman persisted anyway, squeezing money from whatever accounts he
could—including Monsanto's—to keep the research going. The first order of
business was to find some way to get a supply of capillaries. Capillaries are
small, fragile, and easily destroyed during dissection. It was extremely difficult to extract them from living tissues. Folkman turned to the literature and
found an abstract from a researcher in Florida who reported isolation of cap-

illaries from rat adrenal glands. It seemed there was a rich and easily accessible capillary bed under the rodent's adrenal gland. Folkman put in an order for rats and assigned tissue culture specialist Kit Butterfield to the laborious task of dissecting the rats to harvest the small amounts of capillary tissue each animal yielded. "You had to do about twenty rats to get enough tissue to even think about going anywhere," Butterfield recalls. Soon Folkman realized that using rats wasn't practical. He thought again of cows: Their adrenals would be considerably bigger. So back they went to the slaughterhouse. Butterfield showed the meat packers what she needed, and she began making regular trips to Cambridge, which yielded an ample supply of capillary endothelial cells.

That solved the supply problem, but not much else. The endothelial cells derived from cow capillaries stubbornly refused to grow in a culture dish. It looked like another dead end, but in a way it was critical: It bolstered Folkman's belief that he was right and the prevailing dogma, about all endothelial cells being the same, was wrong. In the same medium where the umbilical vein was growing, the capillary endothelium was *not* growing. "So they *must* be different," Folkman recalls thinking. "There must be a big damn difference." Still, the grant requests to the National Institutes of Health kept coming back with comments from anonymous reviewers who were not going out of their way to be kind. "Blistering, really murderous" is how Folkman remembers their criticisms.

For two years after the idea about capillaries struck him, Folkman kept trying to get the endothelial cells from cow adrenal glands to grow, but it wouldn't happen. It was in the midst of that failure and frustration that he was invited to a presentation at Dana-Farber Cancer Institute by a young microbiologist visiting from San Francisco. Bruce Zetter had flown in to give a talk about blood vessel biology, but what he really was doing was prospecting for a job. It wasn't the first time Folkman found himself presented with the right person at the right time.

In 1978 Zetter was a microbiologist who had devoted the past few years to the new science of growing endothelial cells. He was a New England guy— anthropology degree from Brandeis, microbiology doctorate from the University of Rhode Island, postdoctoral fellowship at MIT—but he had spent the last few years in California. Now he was ending his second fellowship, a postdoctoral tour of duty at the University of California Medical Center in San Francisco that had felt to him something like indentured servitude. He spent a difficult two years working in the laboratory of biologist Denis Gaspodarowicz, a cantankerous and argumentative man famous for vigorous arguments at scientific meetings. Now Zetter felt the need to find a real job in someone else's research lab. What he wanted most was a tenure-track position that would allow him to pursue the work he'd been doing in California—exploring blood vessel growth—in a more pleasant atmosphere. There wasn't a lot to choose from. Only a few labs were doing research in vascular biology.

Zetter had first joined the Gaspodarowicz laboratory at the Salk Institute, an ultramodern research center in La Jolla, California, about six months before the whole laboratory shifted north to San Francisco. Their overall research subject was the pursuit and study of growth factors, the newly discovered hormonelike agents that cause specific kinds of cells—such as fibroblasts, bone marrow cells, skin cells, and nerve cells—to grow on demand. It was then an exciting new research area; Nobels were to be won, and the competition between laboratories all across the nation was intensifying. Natural substances that spurred the growth of skin and nerve cells had already been discovered; more were on the way. Gaspodarowicz and his team had contributed a factor they named FGF, for fibroblast growth factor, which turned out to be a misnomer. FGF was not best at stimulating fibroblasts (ordinary connective tissue cells). Instead, it was very potent on endothelial cells extracted from the huge blood vessels, or aortas, of cows and dropped into petri dishes. The achievement put the Gaspodarowicz lab at the forefront of research using bovine endothelial cells.

One problem Zetter faced in his job hunt was that the research field of vascular biology was tiny, so opportunities were scarce. Zetter began by calling friends for ideas and leads. One of the first he called was a close research associate named Lan Bo Chen, who had been hired at the Harvard Medical School just a year before and was doing research at Dana-Farber. Chen offered to invite Zetter in as a guest lecturer and try to make sure the right people—the right professors with vacancies to fill—attended.

Now Zetter just had to make sure he gave the best talk of his life. He didn't find that particularly daunting. He had grown up in a house in which public-speaking ability was valued. His mother was an actress in community theater in Rhode Island, and his father, a furrier by trade, went around the country competing in Toastmasters Clubs oratory contests. His older sister became a Broadway actress and later an actors' manager in Hollywood. Zetter himself once briefly considered becoming an actor, but even as a microbiologist he prided himself on the polish of his speeches. For the crucial meeting with the professors in Boston, he carefully tailored his talk to pique the interest of a small number of people: experts in blood vessel biology. He knew there were big names in that very small field at Harvard: Judah Folkman, Ramzi Cotran, and the éminence grise of vascular biology, Professor Morris Karnofsky, a renowned pathologist who had conducted some of the pioneering studies of the circulatory system. Chen invited them all.

Zetter flew in to Boston from California and went straight to Dana-Farber, where he delivered his talk on how endothelial cells interact with blood platelets. He mentioned during his lecture that as part of Gaspodarowicz's team he had experience in growing vast amounts of endothelial cells in culture dishes. That caught the attention of several researchers, including Folkman. He thought the young man from San Francisco might be able to help him solve one of the puzzles he had been stuck on for years.

Folkman hoped Zetter would be an important addition to his lab at a critical time, but he realized the young researcher would have to ignore what he was hearing. "People advised me not to come," Zetter recalls. "Some very famous, very established, Nobel-type scientists. One reason [they gave] was that the science wasn't very good. It was too iffy and too biological. At that point everybody was doing biochemistry, thinking about molecular biology, and he was sticking things into rabbit eyes. That wasn't considered hard science. And the other reason was 'Don't go there, he's in the pocket of industry.' " For what it was worth, Gaspodarowicz, too, advised Zetter against joining Folkman's lab. "He's too controversial," he told him.

Zetter was undaunted—he'd put up with a lot worse while working for Gaspodarowicz. He decided that Folkman's work had unique promise, enough to outweigh the risks to his career. And how valid were the criticisms? Zetter couldn't help but notice that they hadn't stopped Folkman and the people he worked with—Gimbrone, Cotran, and Vallee in particular—from making Boston a mecca for anyone who wanted to be involved in blood vessel research. Besides, whatever nasty things people said about Folkman, Zetter liked him. He found his enthusiasm and determination contagious; it was obvious that the atmosphere in his laboratory was the antithesis of the tense, antagonistic Gaspodarowicz lab. Any attacks came from *outside* the lab.

Arriving in 1978, just as Folkman was being pressured about his duties as surgeon-in-chief at Children's and at the height of the fierce bad-mouthing going around NIH circles, Zetter was quick to realize that Folkman's lab was like a garrison. And yet, more than he'd imagined, Folkman seemed surrounded on all sides by hostility and resistance that seemed to persist no matter what discoveries his lab produced. "Out in the street, if you asked somebody, 'What do you think about angiogenesis?' they'd say, 'Oh, it's just inflammation,'" Zetter recalls. "It was this low-level buzz; it never completely goes away." It made Folkman's optimism and perseverance all the more remarkable. As he got to know his new boss and see him in action, Zetter figured out that Folkman's problem was that he was simply too candid. He presented his ideas lucidly and energetically; his delivery was engaging, laced with the wry humor those close to him knew so well. As always, Folkman didn't go out of his way to be circumspect about the adventure he was on. A teacher of renown at the medical school, Folkman was almost too willing to speculate, to see meanings where others saw only jumbled data, to pull lessons from events that others felt were unremarkable. Of course, this had always been off-putting to scientists who rely on nothing but data and don't trust the imagination, especially the imagination of a surgeon. "There is a type of established scientist who tends to be very, very cautious and never speculates," Zetter says. "But Judah is not like that. His strengths are his vision and his *ability* to speculate. So the more conservative scientists react negatively when they hear Judah give a talk."

There were also the lovely pictures Folkman used in his presentations. He had the services of a very talented medical illustrator named Janis Cirulis, whose full-color drawings of the phenomena observed in Folkman's lab were a staple of Folkman's talks. He had inherited Cirulis from Robert Gross, for whom Cirulis had illustrated surgical procedures. Now, he was drawing gorgeous, detailed illustrations comparing, for instance, how blood vessels grow toward tumors when they are blocked by fresh cartilage and by dead cartilage. "Folkman only had to say, 'Draw me a picture of a tumor with blood vessels,' and it would be a fabulous picture," says Zetter. Other scientists illustrated their lectures with crude, hand-scrawled diagrams shown on overhead projectors, so to them Folkman seemed a little too slick. Some of the crusty, conservative scientists would ask, "Why are you showing these, when you should be showing us data?"

Zetter perceived what many others had before him: Folkman was not only smart, but creatively smart. "Scientists aren't jealous of someone being intelligent," he observes, "but they are jealous if someone is both creative and intelligent. Especially if he has an idea you never thought of yourself, and it's something you've been thinking about for twenty years. That sometimes takes people aback."

Zetter decided to do as Folkman did: ignore the rumble of disparagement and just focus on the work. After all, that was where the real frustration was. In the short term, the problem was what to do about growing capillary endothelial cells. Folkman was in dire need of some fresh ideas, and Zetter was anxious to supply them. He, too, was interested in growing capillaries. It was the next frontier, and he actually agreed with Folkman that endothelial cells might very well be different from one another, behaving differently although they didn't appear to be different even under high magnification. But they still couldn't prove it—until they could grow capillary endothelial cells in culture and show that they responded to different kinds of growth factors. He would later reflect on how that very failure should have made it obvious that the endothelium included different kinds of cells. Why else would it be relatively easy to grow cells from aortas and umbilical veins, and so hard to grow capillary endothelium? It seemed that the differences hadn't been found, in part, simply because very few people had even bothered to look. Everyone knew all endothelial cells were the same, so why spend time or money trying to show otherwise?

Zetter and Folkman tried to approach the problem together but from slightly different perspectives. Folkman came up with a process he called "weeding and feeding," in which he used a small, curved glass instrument to remove, one by one, any pericytes (the smooth muscle precursor cells) that he saw contaminating the capillary endothelial cell sample under the microscope. He didn't want to repeat the mistake made earlier in Japan, letting the pericytes grow and overtake the entire culture. So, like a homeowner yanking weeds from a lawn, Folkman would wait a few days, then see if any more pericytes had grown among the endothelial cells. If there were any, these were weeded out with the little glass tool. "Only a surgeon would have thought of this, weeding and feeding," Zetter remarks. "He was very good with his hands. He could go in and cut out or squish the cells he didn't like." It was an extremely slow and painstaking task; the microscope, the sample, and Folkman's hands all had to be enclosed within a glass-fronted cabinet called a fume hood, for the sake of sterility. Still, even when they were purified by this technique, the capillary cells stubbornly refused to divide.

Zetter took a different tack. He considered the possibility that capillary endothelial cells had built-in, genetically controlled preferences or requirements for their local surroundings. Feeding them and keeping them wet and warm obviously weren't sufficient; maybe they needed something else. Like many microbiologists, Zetter tended to think in terms of the needs of the cells, trying to be aware of what it took to keep them "happy." In the case of capillary endothelial cells, he wondered if the problem was that they didn't like the unnatural taste or feel of the plastic petri dish into which they were

deposited. During his time in San Francisco, he and his colleagues had experimented with different coatings on the petri dishes they were using to culture
cells, trying to come up with surfaces that more closely resembled the cells'
natural home. Under normal circumstances, cells live within a complex fluid-
like structure called extracellular matrix, a good part of which is collagen, a
gelatinlike substance. (In fact, gelatin is actually just denatured collagen extracted by boiling cows' hooves, horns, hides, and all kinds of other tissues.
Zetter's advice is to never, ever take a tour of a Jell-O factory.) So one coating
Zetter and his colleagues had come up with was a dilute form of pure gelatin.
They had covered the floor of petri dishes with the gelatin, let them dry, put
the culture media in, and then added the endothelial cells. It seemed to help
endothelial cells from large blood vessels grow. Maybe the same trick would
work with capillary endothelial cells.

The results were immediate. The cells adapted readily to the gelatin-
covered floor of the petri dish; they grew slowly but perfectly. They finally had
capillary endothelium alive and thriving in tissue culture, long enough for
them to run the experiments Folkman had waited six years to conduct.

Carefully, almost holding his breath, Zetter picked up the small flask containing tumor-conditioned medium, tipped it gently, and began dribbling a
tiny amount of the substance onto the thin layer of cells. As the crucial test
began, Zetter could see the clear fluid spreading across the bottom of the
plate, engulfing the waiting endothelial cells whose response would be their
way of saying whether TAF was real and whether Folkman was right. Would
it actually stimulate speedy growth?

Bingo. Small clumps of capillary endothelial cells began growing on the
floor of the dish. Zetter and Folkman were ecstatic, bowled over. "The cultures really took off," Zetter recalls. "They kept going and going and going."
The clumps of cells kept expanding in size, showing the exact behavior Folkman had predicted. For both Zetter and Folkman it was a true peak experience. Finally, after all those years, after all the experiments, the days, the
nights, the endless disappointments—they grew! The achievement documented the wisdom of a sign Folkman kept hanging in his lab: INNOVATION IS
A SERIES OF REPETITIVE FAILURES.

Now they began trying to document the triumph. "We must have taken a
thousand pictures of these colonies," Zetter says. "No one had ever seen
colonies [of endothelial cells] growing that big!" It opened the door to finally
being able to test TAF and any other agents that might have the stimulatory or
inhibitory properties Folkman was seeking.

Folkman and Zetter wrote up the findings in a paper, which was published in 1979 in the *Proceedings of the National Academy of Sciences.* It was a hit. They had proved, for the first time and irrefutably, that endothelial cells in large vessels are fundamentally different from those lining capillaries. Now researchers could investigate what those differences were, what they meant, and how they governed the properties of blood vessels. Requests for reprints of the paper poured in, and scientists from around the world began streaming into Folkman's lab, excited to learn a brand-new technique that promised to open new research avenues. They came from all across the United States, from Europe, from the Soviet Union. They came from university laboratories and from major pharmaceutical companies. Each visiting scientist had to commit a week to the training, mainly to become adept at Folkman's weed-and-feed method of removing contaminating pericyte cells from among the capillary endothelial cells. In a sense, of course, he was training the competition. But Folkman had an unusually altruistic view of the role competition played in medical science. Keeping everyone's creative juices flowing was a good thing, he felt, and he was disappointed when some researchers did not reciprocate—when those who had received materials from Folkman, or who had sent people to Boston for training, would refuse to send materials of their own to the Folkman lab, fearing competition. Others, for the sake of protecting patentable information, declined to share data that might help Folkman move ahead.

While his peers learned about growing cells, Zetter turned his attention to the next critical question: Might these tiny capillary endothelial cells have the ability to migrate, to creep or drag themselves across the floor of the dish, going from one point to another? It seemed to Zetter that blood vessel cells had to do more than just divide and make more copies of themselves to reach a growing tumor. They had to actually move and work their way through living tissues, and then form into tiny tubes that would become blood vessels. Within the body, movements were facilitated by special enzymes that open holes in surrounding tissue, allowing the migrating endothelial cells to creep through. The cells move by changing shape and oozing through small gaps. In tissue culture, the cells would not need to creep through small holes but would instead migrate across the floor of the dish. One ruffled edge spread out forward and then the rest of the cells gathered themselves up to follow along. Zetter suspected that this phenomenon, cell migration, was a key to the process of angiogenesis. The growing cells had to have the ability to creep through tissues, heading directly toward a source of TAF, if they were going to build new vessels fast enough to supply a growing tumor with blood.

To test his ideas, Zetter exploited a newly discovered technique called the phagokinetic assay. This was a test system in which a thin layer of very tiny gold particles is placed on the petri dish's floor to track the migration of cells. As the clear, translucent cells crawl along the dish floor, they engulf the gold dust and take it inside their cell membranes, leaving a thin, cleared trail that could be easily measured, showing where they have been and how far they have moved. The speed of migration could also be measured by noting how far the cells traveled in a given amount of time.

Zetter put a group of capillary endothelial cells on a gold-covered floor, where they did not move, naturally enough. But then he added some TAF to the dish, and the cells began to move very rapidly. Oh, my God! Zetter thought. The tumor really was producing something vital to its existence: The TAF made blood vessel cells migrate. Endothelial cells did have all the properties and abilities that Folkman had been postulating for a decade.

The results were thrilling, and Zetter wrote them up for publication. In the process he also ran a small test to see if he really wanted to stay in Boston and build his career in Folkman's department at Children's Hospital. After he wrote the paper, he put a cover page on it with the title and his name alone. Then he gave the paper to Folkman and asked for his thoughts. What Zetter wanted to see was whether Folkman was, like many well-known professors, the kind of boss who insisted on being in charge of everything and having his name on every research paper published through his department. "I realized very early that I had to be doing things that would build my own, independent career, and this work on cell migration was all my own work," Zetter recalls. "If he said, 'Go ahead and publish it,' then that was great. That would mean he was the kind of person I wanted to stay with because he was interested in my career, and in being fair. But if he said, 'This is great. Please put my name on it,' then I would know that he wanted what we call the old Germanic Herr Professor system, that he was going to continue to be part of everything."

Folkman quickly read Zetter's paper, handed it back, and said: "This is great. This is your work. Go publish it."

Zetter sent his paper to *Nature* in 1978. The report, when published later, would turn out to be the first and last paper in which he had sole authorship; it marked a prominent entry into the field of blood vessel and cell migration research, and it cemented his decision to stay with Folkman and pursue his research and teaching career at Harvard. With that question resolved, Zetter soon dug into another experiment with endothelial cells, one that would have major unanticipated consequences.

Zetter was working at that time with a visiting cancer scientist from France, Danielle Brouty-Boye from the Institut de Recherche Scientifique du Cancer, near Paris. Brouty-Boye had access to interferon, a natural substance that some laboratories, mostly in Europe, were coaxing out of living cells in huge culture systems. Interferon's discovery had set off a huge burst of enthusiasm among cancer researchers, who thought it might have strong—if undefined—antitumor properties. Though its natural role in the body seemed to be to guard against viral infections, interferon was being widely trumpeted as a potential cure for cancer because early tissue culture studies suggested it might be capable of slowing or even stopping the growth of tumors, especially if the cancer was caused by viral infection. The first human tests with interferon alpha, which began in 1978, yielded inconclusive results, but still the news media began touting interferon as a great hope for the future.

In the late 1970s, interferon was still so new and hard to come by that it hadn't been studied very much. But Brouty-Boye had some interferon to play with, so she and Zetter decided to put a few doses into the petri dishes where endothelial cells that had been stimulated by TAF were crawling around on their golden pastures. When hit by interferon, the cells suddenly stopped migrating. Folkman realized that this was a major moment. Could this be the kind of *anti*angiogenesis factor he had dreamed about? Folkman knew, though, that much work had to be done. Even though these results hinted that antiangiogenesis might be a possibility, interferon was extremely scarce and expensive, little understood and hardly studied. Folkman and Zetter were far from even doing animal experiments, much less getting the idea of angiogenesis inhibition into the clinic. That would have to wait—for years.

Zetter and Brouty-Boye hurried to write up their results, and they submitted their manuscript to *Science,* where it was accepted quickly. By coincidence, the publication of Zetter's earlier paper on cell migration had been delayed, and it was finally published in *Nature* the same week in 1980 that the interferon paper was published in *Science.* With two important papers published simultaneously in leading journals, Zetter made a big splash. And the real payoff from the work was yet to be seen. Although interferon soon became widely available, it turned into one of those heralded cancer treatments that failed to live up to its early promise. Yet it was not without value. Though it would take some years to become clear, there was in fact a place for interferon in the treatment of cancer.

Thanks in part to Zetter's work, angiogenesis was now finally a growing, respectable, even exciting field of study. His success in growing endothelial cells began to attract others who looked at what was going on in the Folkman lab in Boston and decided maybe there was something to this idea after all. By the cusp of the new decade, angiogenesis-related research was getting attention at the National Institutes of Health, the University of Wisconsin, Rockefeller University in New York, and other institutions. It was practically in the mainstream. The results began to look so promising that many former critics were beginning to become competitors, and it was these developments that had finally nudged Folkman to acquiesce to the pressures to step down as surgeon-in-chief and focus on angiogenesis. "You could see that the field was really taking off," Folkman recalls. "I spent a long time deciding whether to continue in the field and also be surgeon-in-chief, which meant you couldn't really devote full time to either one, or just go full time in research, or just stop the research."

But, of course, he had no intention of stopping the research. He needed to continue, now more than ever. Any number of people could be surgeon-in-chief, he believed, but no one else would pursue angiogenesis as avidly as he would. He was heartened that others had finally joined him, but he did not spend much time entertaining the possibility that they could survive without him. "I did not think the field would grow at all unless we were in it," he reflected years later. He knew that any research field needed to reach a critical mass, with enough people working on various parts of the puzzle to keep the enthusiasm level high. If there was no leadership, no one pushing the boundaries, it would become even harder to garner funding, more difficult to get published, and the supply of exciting graduate students and postdoctoral fellows would be even harder to maintain. "If you don't get out and say, 'Here's where it's going, here's where it's going,' all this stuff we could see but couldn't prove—it would just die."

Folkman could not let the field he had nurtured die. One day in 1981, he went into the operating room and hunched over a baby girl whose esophagus had malformed before birth, making it impossible for her to swallow and difficult to breathe. Folkman repaired the damage, reconnecting the esophagus and mending the windpipe, the kind of difficult surgery that had become routine for him during his fourteen years as surgeon-in-chief at Children's Hospital. He sewed her up and sent her on her way. And then he shed his mask and gown, left the operating room, and never performed surgery again.

Chapter Twelve

———

LIKE THE MYTHICAL POT OF GOLD under the rainbow, TAF, the substance that Judah Folkman had been pursuing throughout the 1970s, always beckoned tantalizingly just beyond reach. It did exist; TAF's effects could be seen in various tests Folkman and his corps of researchers conducted both in petri dishes and in animals. But extracting a single, tiny, active protein out of a complex soup of growth promoters, growth inhibitors, enzymes, amino acids, hormones, and other molecules was a goal that for many years even Monsanto's millions and Bert Vallee's expertise couldn't help them reach.

The problem they had confronted from the outset was that the fluid extracted from cultured tumor cells was so chemically complex that TAF—the active agent—could not be isolated. Its effects could be detected in the rabbit eye and chicken egg assays: Fractionated tumor fluid triggered angiogenesis, and other experiments revealed the rough outlines of the molecule being pursued. But none of that was of much use to Vallee's team or to the biochemist then working in Folkman's lab, Michael Klagsbrun.

The problem was that nothing in the fluid could be measured reliably. Dumping tiny amounts of active fluids into rabbit eyes and fertilized chicken eggs would show that the activity existed but offered no precise or reliable way to say how much of the active ingredient there was, nor how long it lasted. Biochemists like Klagsbrun seek precision; they want to know whether they've got exactly 10.4 units of something, or more, or less. Worse, they couldn't tell exactly what was in their fluid along with the growth factor they called TAF. They couldn't purify it far enough—they'd run out of material before isolating TAF. "These assays were, from the point of view of a biochemist, totally impossible," Klagsbrun recalls. "If you put some extract in there you could see something happening. But then you had to worry whether it was real, was inflammation, or something else."

That was the challenge for the biochemists: to try to take the crude fluids from Folkman's labs and separate them into finer and finer fractions to isolate the chemical so it could actually be purified and tested. It was hardly an unfamiliar problem. Doing reliable measurements had always been trouble for biologists and biochemists trying to find and purify the expanding family of growth factors that were being identified in these years. The first of the factors, epidermal growth factor, or EGF, had been discovered years earlier, in 1962; its action was measured in a most imprecise way. Using what its developer, Stanley Cohen at Vanderbilt University, called the "precocious eye-opening test," scientists injected their candidate growth factors into newborn mice. If the tiny, hairless animals opened their eyes a day or two ahead of schedule, it would suggest that the injected substance was active. Although this assay was difficult, often unreliable, and laborious to perform, it was all there was available. And it was good enough to uncover the first tissue-specific growth factor, EGF, the first of a series of discoveries that would earn Cohen a share of a Nobel prize twenty-four years later.

In Folkman's lab, it was Michael Klagsbrun who most directly confronted the challenge of isolating endothelial growth factors, starting with TAF. Klagsbrun had taken his Ph.D. in biochemistry at the University of Wisconsin and had done research at MIT and the National Institutes of Health before joining Folkman as a postdoctoral fellow in 1973. His original research interest had been the tiny viruses that infect bacterial cells, but he eventually changed direction after learning to culture cells from mammals in a summer course at the Cold Spring Harbor Laboratory on Long Island. One of his early experiments involved growing cancer cells and normal cells, and trying to see how they differed. So Klagsbrun was excited when he arrived in Folkman's laboratory at Children's Hospital just as the agreement with Vallee and Monsanto was being negotiated.

Klagsbrun quickly realized that Folkman gave his postdocs remarkable freedom to pursue what interested them. If they found something worthy—and could cobble together enough grant money to support it—Folkman was all for it. By the same token, if a project didn't interest them, they were under no obligation to work on it. Unlike some lab overseers, Folkman did not insist that his postdoctoral fellows work on exactly what he wanted. Of course, he chose them based on their research interests and the overall needs of his lab, and when newcomers arrived he liked to sit down and discuss what they would be doing. But he preferred a soft approach, pointing them in interesting directions, assisting in the pursuit of funds, and offering advice that might keep them from wandering up blind alleys in their research. He also led by example. It was not unusual for the hardest-working postdocs to see Folkman beside them, hunched over a lab bench at two A.M., working with the small petri dishes containing fertilized chicken eggs.

In Klagsbrun's case, although he had hired on ostensibly to help in the search for TAF, his interests changed soon after he arrived and saw that his new boss's efforts to try to isolate the substance were hopelessly ineffective—and that he himself was hard-pressed to come up with a better way.

It was true that by this time biochemical assays were becoming considerably easier and more precise than Cohen's method of watching baby mice open their eyes. But while the new methods were helping researchers uncover numerous growth factors, it seemed to Klagsbrun that TAF would not immediately be one of them. It was just too well hidden, present in too small amounts. So instead of looking for the chemical that tumors put out to stimulate the growth of blood vessels, Klagsbrun decided he would jump ahead and hunt for the opposite: natural substances in the body that *inhibited* blood vessel growth. He looked around the lab and saw the cartilage, tons of it.

Robert Langer was still working on his first project, trying to find ways to apply his training in chemical engineering to the problems of angiogenesis and see what he could discover about cartilage. He chose to look at this plastic-like tissue and see if he could determine what it was that blocked angiogenesis when applied to rabbit eyes. Klagsbrun took on a piece of this work as one of his own projects. Though cancer was relatively rare in cartilage, it was not wholly unknown. There was a variety of tumor called chondrosarcoma that arose in cartilage, and it gave Klagsbrun an idea: Since cartilage is generally the least-vascularized of all the tissues in the body, save the cornea, he wondered whether the complex fluids he could extract from chondrosarcoma cells might contain a substance—an inhibiting molecule—that halted, rather than triggered, the growth of endothelial cells. It might be a long shot, but there was some logic to the idea. After all, it was in the fluids extracted from rat tumors that TAF was detectable, so why not seek a different kind of growth-control agent, an endothelial cell inhibitor, in tissue that was so good at keeping blood vessels out?

To test the idea, Klagsbrun used cultured connective tissue cells from mice, and he employed a relatively new technique to try to detect what was happening inside the cells. This method, which used radioactive tritium (triply heavy hydrogen) to measure the growth of cells, was based on the well-known fact that a cell has to make a complete copy of its genes—new DNA, its chemical blueprint—before it can divide. And to make new DNA, the cell's internal machinery has to pick up hydrogen that is part of the thymidine molecule. In the technique employed by Klagsbrun, tritium, which acts chemically just like hydrogen, is used in the culture medium and, if the cell is beginning to divide, the tritiated thymidine is taken up by the DNA that is being made. So the tritium becomes a built-in, radioactive marker signifying that new DNA is being made and that the cell is setting itself up to divide. If no radioactivity shows up in the cell's nucleus, then the cell must be quiescent. Thus, by watching what happened to the tritium as growth factors were being dumped into the culture dish, Klagsbrun had a precise way to see if the cells were being told to divide, or not divide, while sitting in the petri dish.

Klagsbrun expected the fluid to inhibit growth because it had been derived from cartilage, and all the evidence gathered so far suggested that a substance taken from cartilage should inhibit cellular growth. But instead, he saw a tremendous surge of the tritium signal showing up in the cells' DNA, indicating that they were preparing to divide. That meant that the fluid Klagsbrun was testing actually stimulated growth, rather than inhibited it. Klagsbrun didn't know why he'd get growth when he expected inhibition—"It's hard to understand these things," he reflected later—but it was always great to come upon something unexpected, another clue about cellular growth control. It suggested he might be on to something new—in this case, maybe another of those growth factors that seemed able to spur the expansion of critical tissues. The discovery might put Klagsbrun right into the center of a field that was seething with excitement. Science was showing that it should be possible to begin controlling the production of specific kinds of cells, such as red blood cells, and all across the country, as well as in Europe and Japan, scientists were scrambling to find and identify these new growth factors. Whether Klagsbrun now had his hands on a stimulator or an inhibitor, it could be an important contribution.

Klagsbrun could see the cells in the culture dish begin changing shape, elongating; the dish became more crowded with new cells. Now he had to measure as precisely as possible what he saw. In addition to counting the cells, he also measured the tritium. By calculating how much of the radioactive hydrogen became incorporated into the new DNA, and at what rate, he could determine not only how *much* cell division was occurring but how rapidly.

That single experiment turned Klagsbrun's research back into the search for stimulators. "The inhibitor field was just too complex," he recalls. It was too full of unanswered—and maybe unanswerable—questions that might take forever to work out. His new find, meanwhile, suggested there was not only logic but also a factual basis to support Folkman's long-held strategy of going first for agents that stimulated blood vessel growth, and *then* pursuing those that blocked it.

Klagsbrun's switch paid off in a big way. In the short term, it occurred to him that milk—a food that leads to growth—ought to be a good source of active growth factors. He was right, and in 1978 Klagsbrun won international recognition for finding and purifying special growth-promoting agents found in both cow's milk and human milk. He found that growth factor activity in cows was particularly strong in the first few hours after a calf was born. Soon after he published his work, Klagsbrun was contacted by a team of anthropologists from the World Health Organization, who thought it was an exciting finding for their field, and by people who were trying to promote breast-feeding by new mothers. "I would always be getting these letters from La Leche League," he recalls. The work earned Klagsbrun a strong reputation as a growth factor expert—a standing that put him in position to tackle the single most avidly sought goal in the Folkman laboratory: purifying the first factor known to kick-start the growth of blood vessels.

When he had first joined Folkman's lab, Klagsbrun had taken part in the work to find growth-altering factors in cancer cells and in cartilage tissue using conventional fractionating techniques. But when the research had gone as far as these methods could take it, Klagsbrun moved on to other work. The problem with pursuing growth-altering molecules had always been that measurements were always very imprecise, because finding colorless agents within clear fluids was difficult, demanding, and often unsuccessful. The active agent had to be separated out on the basis of its chemical and physical properties: its molecular size and weight, whether or not it had an affinity for water, its pH, and its electric charge. For a frustrating eight years, from 1975 to 1983, Klagsbrun spent a lot of time trying to purify molecules without really knowing if what he was measuring was a fully purified agent or still a mixture of molecules that would have to be separated and tested further. But now, using new methods such as high-performance liquid chromatography, laboratories around the country were reporting a cascade of discoveries about growth factors. Klagsbrun decided the time was right to get back into the hunt, and to help him, he recruited Yuen Shing, a talented biochemist from Southeast Massachusetts University (now UMass Dartmouth), to work with him part-time.

In 1983, Klagsbrun and Shing saw reports in the scientific literature stating that heparin, a natural blood-thinning, anticoagulation agent made in the liver, somehow enhanced the action of growth factors, including the ones Folkman and his team were pursuing. Heparin had been used for decades, after being discovered by a student who was running experiments while waiting to get into the Johns Hopkins Medical School. Heparin, short for heparin sulfate, is one of the first emergency drugs given to heart attack victims because it acts immediately to keep blood flowing through narrowed arteries, reducing blood's tendency to clot. Now there were clues gathered in experiments in various other labs suggesting that heparin interacted physically to stimulate the work of the growth factors the scientists were seeking—this even though the factors themselves hadn't been isolated. Without heparin, the growth factors, whatever they were, seemed to be much less active, less efficient at stimulating blood vessel growth. This was a vital clue. If the unidentified growth stimulators somehow interacted intimately with heparin, perhaps the two molecules actually *bonded* to each other to create a bigger molecule that worked more efficiently to stimulate blood vessel growth. If that was true, then maybe heparin offered a molecular handle, or connector, that could be used to grab and capture the missing growth factors. That was an idea worth exploring in pursuit of TAF.

Shing and Klagsbrun used chemical-linking techniques to bind heparin molecules to tiny beads of starch and packed the beads into cylindrical glass columns. Then they poured fluids containing their growth-stimulating molecules down through the columns. Now, the real test: Would the assays in the rabbit eyes and chicken eggs show that there was an angiogenesis growth factor attached to the heparin molecules? The results—after all these years—were instantaneous. Angiogenesis! It worked! Folkman and his lab colleagues instantly realized that this was the *Eureka!* moment they had been hoping for. What they had done, finally, was come up with a way to select an angiogenesis growth factor from a complex tumor fluid. It was a huge step forward, a celebratory moment.

The next step was to get enough chondrosarcomas, the cartilage tumors. Now that Klagsbrun and his colleagues knew they could pull an active growth stimulator out of the tumor fluids—by pouring the liquids over starch beads coated with heparin molecules that could grab the growth factor—what they needed was a good supply of these special tumors. "We had to grow five hundred tumors in five hundred rats to give us enough for the final purification, enough so we could publish," Folkman recalls. There wasn't enough room in the lab, so he contracted with a company in Cambridge and shipped the rats there.

Once the chondrosarcomas reached ample size, Folkman's team went over and excised all five hundred tumors in one day, packed them in dry ice, brought them back to the Enders Building, and ground them up. And with further separation work over the next two months to eliminate small amounts of contaminants that were still in the growth-stimulating fraction, Klagsbrun and Shing were able to purify their growth factor. "This stuff had seemed impossible to purify, but it turned out if you put it into a heparin column, you got like ninety-five-percent purification in one step," Klagsbrun later said. And tests in the cell culture system, as well as in the chicken and eye assays, showed that their newly isolated factor did stimulate endothelial cell growth. Shing and Klagsbrun had broken through a barrier that stood in Folkman's way for almost two decades. Folkman was almost giddy: It seemed miraculous.

It took another few months to finish the experiments and write up the details, but Shing, Folkman, Klagsbrun, and three coworkers were able to report in *Science* in 1984 that they had finally succeeded in isolating and purifying the first factor that specifically stimulated the growth of blood vessel cells. They called it cartilage-derived growth factor. As it turned out, the molecule they isolated was the very same agent that Denis Gaspodarowicz and his coworkers in San Francisco had noted years earlier (they had named it fibroblast growth factor, or FGF) but hadn't purified. Because the West Coast team was first to propose that FGF existed, Klagsbrun and Folkman decided to keep that name, even though it actually triggered the growth of endothelial cells better than fibroblasts, and even though the Harvard team was actually the first to nail it down, able to give the agent a chemical identity, rather than having to call it a "factor."

Though FGF turned out to have different chemical properties from the agent Folkman had dubbed TAF, the discovery of any substance that triggered the growth of endothelial cells was a major advance, lending credence—solid, reproducible chemical evidence—to support Folkman's original idea that tumors put out chemical signals that induced blood vessels to sprout branches, grow toward them, and bring in new blood.

———

BACK IN BERT VALLEE'S LAB at the nearby Brigham Hospital, growth-factor work was also proceeding under the boss's rigid research plan. Working independently of Folkman's lab, Vallee's team of biochemists continued trying to isolate and identify a blood vessel growth factor. The two labs were ostensibly partners, but at times they seemed more like competitors—never more so than in 1985, when Vallee and his team announced the isolation of its own extremely potent stimulator of endothelial cell growth.

Vallee and his colleagues had isolated their new growth factor, which they named angiogenin, from human tumors called adenocarcinomas, which were the same kind of tumor President Ronald Reagan had had removed surgically the month before. To a great degree, it was a research process called amino acid sequencing that was crucial to their work. This involved determining the identity and the position of each of the amino acids, each of the building blocks, that were strung together to form the angiogenin molecule.

The arrangement of amino acid links is what gives a protein its identity and specifies its activity, whether it's an enzyme that snips other molecules apart or a signaling molecule that tells particular cells what to do. Scientists had long known that the arrangement of amino acids—how they are linked together, like beads on a string, so they fold up correctly to form a specific protein—is dictated by the chemical "spelling" of a gene in the cell's nucleus. It is through this process, with about a hundred thousand different genes telling the cells exactly which proteins to make, that the business of life is conducted. Indeed, illness strikes when this protein-building process breaks down. If amino acids are left out, or the wrong ones are put in place, a protein such as an enzyme or growth factor is made incorrectly, or not at all, and the result can be the disaster of genetic disease, or cancer. The built-in information system that governs life depends on an amazingly small number of chemical signals: four bases—designated A, T, C, and G—that are arranged in three-letter groupings to specify which of the twenty amino acids is to be put in a particular place in a protein. From that small foundation of chemical information, the living cell can create all of the many thousands of proteins that make up the human body. Based on that simple information system, all of the proteins that make up bone, skin, hair, eyes, and connective tissue are constructed with exquisite precision. The marvel is not so much that the system works so well, but that it works at all.

With this method, Vallee's team was able to decipher the exact arrangement of angiogenin's amino acids and purify the growth factor, and the work reported from his lab, in *Biochemistry* (September 24, 1985), was extremely thorough and detailed. Although they had been quiet for years about what they were doing in the laboratory, Vallee and his staff published three papers simultaneously: one reporting the isolation and analysis of angiogenin, the next describing its exact amino acid sequence, and the third reporting that they had found and copied the gene that makes angiogenin and analyzed it in exact, link-by-link detail. It was a research tour de force that had absorbed the efforts of nine scientists, including Vallee, for many years.

During their research, Vallee and his colleagues had developed a system that would allow cells to grow without needing fetal calf serum, a step that eliminated much of the complexity involved in finding small, well-hidden molecules in clear fluids. They had also tested their new human protein, angiogenin, on endothelial cells from various animals, and it worked as well on other species' cells as it did on human cells. Like the FGF that Klagsbrun and Shing had found a year earlier in Folkman's laboratory, angiogenin's physical and chemical properties were clearly not those of TAF. And, again, like the discovery of FGF, Vallee's analysis of angiogenin strongly confirmed Folkman's long-standing proposal that tumors produce growth factors that can draw new blood vessels in. But neither Vallee nor Harvard went out of their way to take note of that fact.

On the date of the publication of Vallee's results, the medical school issued a press release and held a big news conference, TV cameras and all—and neither invited Folkman nor mentioned his name. Vallee announced that he and his team had found *the* angiogenesis stimulator, even though Folkman's team had found a potent stimulator, FGF, the year before. Given Folkman's role in inventing the field, and his widely publicized partnership with Vallee, it was shocking treatment, especially since the news release did acknowledge with pride the involvement of Monsanto, whose support had marked "the first of such scale between a university and private corporation." Veteran reporters—some of whom mentioned Folkman in their stories anyway—could only guess what behind-the-scenes machinations had brought about such a snub. Folkman was privately furious, especially when he saw Vallee on television explaining his discovery and its significance as a breakthrough in cancer. But he didn't want to get into a public feud with Vallee, and, at the suggestion of one of the senior medical school deans, he simply submitted an overview article on angiogenesis to *Science,* just to put Vallee's discovery in perspective. The episode signaled a further cooling of their relationship.

As it turned out, neither Folkman nor Vallee got to announce the discovery of TAF. Both teams had uncovered molecules that actively stimulated endothelial cell growth, but neither had found a substance with exactly the same properties as were evident in tests of tumor fluid containing TAF. Instead, in 1989 two other researchers working on the body's array of growth factors—one working right across the street from Folkman in Boston, the other across the country in San Francisco—identified the molecule without realizing at first what they had. Both had found an agent that showed activity in tissue culture assays, but until their exact chemical structures could be compared, there was no way to identify either of the new agents. So while they weren't calling it TAF, it was in fact the tumor angiogenesis factor whose existence Folkman had first suspected and begun to hunt for in the late 1960s.

In Folkman's lab, interest in finding TAF had waned by this time, first because the discovery of FGF had given them an agent that worked well in the angiogenesis research—they could now stimulate growth when they wanted—and because after one factor had been discovered, Folkman found it hard to find a postdoc eager to take on the task of finding another. In a sense, the race for an endothelial-stimulating factor had already been won, so whoever finally found TAF would assuredly come in second. But even if purifying TAF no longer had the urgency it once did, Folkman retained a sense of pride about conquering the problem. And by this time, it wasn't the technical challenge it had been throughout the 1970s and early 1980s. A major advance was a new invention called an HPLC—for high-performance liquid chromatography—that used high pressure to force liquids through a densely packed column and then ultraviolet light to detect when the properties of substances were altered by chemical processing. The presence of color in the fluid indicated in which fraction the desired substance was hidden, speeding up the process of sorting through the separated fractions. And the research process called amino acid sequencing, the same one Bert Vallee's team had used to identify the growth factor angiogenin in 1985, was also a critical aid.

That the right tools and techniques had now become available for finding TAF made Folkman even more frustrated. "It was just sitting there," he laments, still annoyed years later. "I couldn't get anyone to work on it." He finally hired a postdoc, Rosalind Rosenthal, specifically to work on the problem, but even then the work went more slowly than he thought necessary. Though he didn't make overt demands on people, he was always in the lab at night and on weekends, and he expected the same from his postdocs. As Bruce Zetter once remarked, "If you're interested in things like how the Red Sox are doing, then you're not paying enough attention to the lab work." That was the culture of the place, and of many such labs. Rosenthal was an able and serious postdoc, but Folkman felt she could have put in more hours to get the job done quickly. Eventually, Rosenthal was able to decipher the exact arrangement of TAF's amino acids and purify the growth factor, though not quite in time for the lab to be the first to do so.

On Memorial Day weekend in 1989, just as Rosenthal was preparing to write up her findings, Folkman got a call from Dr. Napoleone Ferrara, a growth factor researcher at a biotech company in California. He'd heard at meetings that the Folkman lab was close to purifying a new factor.

Ferrara, who trained as a physician in Italy, had begun his research work in the reproductive physiology laboratory at the University of California, San Francisco, a few years earlier, having decided he preferred working as a research scientist to taking care of patients. In San Francisco he became interested in the burgeoning field of growth factors, eventually transferring to the laboratory run by biochemist Denis Gaspodarowicz, where he began poking through the lab's tissue of choice, cow pituitary glands. In 1988, Ferrara began talking to Genentech, Inc., one of the first biology-based companies formed as the biotechnology revolution got under way in the late 1970s. After an explosive encounter with Gaspodarowicz over his relationship with the company, Ferrara left the university, taking his growth factor research with him to Genentech.

Housed in an ultramodern building sitting atop a grassy hill overlooking San Francisco Bay, the company had since its inception nurtured an intense interest in fundamental biological research. As a result of the rapid pace of new discoveries in genetics—especially the so-called restriction enzymes that allowed genes to be snipped out of one organism and put into another—bioscientists all over the world were swapping the genes from humans in microbes such as bacteria and yeast cells, in hopes of forcing the microbes to make products like human insulin, growth hormones, blood-clotting factors, and other proteins that were hard or even impossible to get by other means. At Genentech, where the search for such products was well under way, Ferrara, using cow pituitary glands, found a factor that strongly and specifically spurred vigorous growth of capillary endothelial cells, and he wondered whether it might resemble what was being seen across the country in Folkman's lab. Ferrara had named his factor VEGF, for vascular endothelial growth factor, and submitted a paper on it to *Biochemical and Biophysical Research Communications*, a weekly journal that published findings quickly, as some preferred to do in a field that was so competitive. But first he called Folkman to see if they were looking at the same molecule. "I said sure," Folkman recalls, when Ferrara asked for some sample material. "I didn't think they would be the same. But it was identical."

Ferrara's paper on VEGF came out the following week, and he announced several months later in *Science* that he had also cloned the gene that makes the protein. By this time, the capturing and cloning of individual genes had gone from being high art to a less demanding craft. Once an interesting protein had been found, its amino acid sequence—its structure—could be "read" in the laboratory, and a short piece of genetic material, known in the trade as an "oligo," could be constructed to match part of the gene. Then the short chunk of material could be used as a sort of fish hook that could be dropped into the pool of DNA that had been extracted from human tissue. Because its coding exactly matched part of the gene being sought, the oligo would wander around among the hundred thousand genes in the nucleus and attach itself only to that particular gene. Once it was marked with the oligo, the entire gene could then be extracted from the soup of DNA, and it could be copied many times over by putting it inside bacteria and making them multiply. The process was tedious and time-consuming, but it worked.

Because they had been a bit slow getting off the mark, Folkman and Rosenthal's report was published two months after Ferrara's, much to their chagrin. Folkman was convinced that his team could have found, purified, and published their discovery of the protein four years ahead of everyone else. But since Ferrara was first, Folkman decided to drop the term "TAF" and use "VEGF." That was the end of TAF.

That the Ferrara and Folkman labs had unknowingly purified the same molecule at about the same time was a strange coincidence, but they both soon learned of an even stranger one. Someone else, too, had isolated the substance that Ferrara called VEGF, and that person was working right across the street from Folkman at Beth Israel Hospital. By 1989, Dr. Harold Dvorak had spent a decade trying to isolate a substance that made tiny blood vessels become leaky. A pathologist-immunologist, Dvorak had focused his work on finding antigens, molecules on the surface of tumor cells that might stimulate immune responses against cancer in the body. Looking through his pathologist's microscope as he studied the properties of tumors, Dvorak saw something intriguing and unexpected. He noticed the presence of fibrin—a material in blood that usually stays in the blood—in the tissues around tumors. Fibrin comes from a plasma protein called fibrinogen, and normally separates from the blood only when it's needed in emergencies. In response to injury—a cut, for instance—a fibrin gel quickly forms to create a plug to stop the bleeding. But seeing fibrin surrounding tumor tissue was a big surprise. It had not been reported before. The sight of fibrin told Dvorak that tumor blood vessels had to be leaky, because plasma proteins normally stayed within blood vessels unless there was an injury, with the veins or arteries broken open. The presence of fibrin in the tumor tissue suggested that some kind of agent, a chemical signal, was coming from the tumor itself. Something was causing the blood vessels around tumors to become permeable and leak substances such as fibrin.

As a first guess, Dvorak and his colleagues had proposed that tumors somehow caused specialized immune system cells, called mast cells, to become permeable, inducing them to release histamines, hormonelike agents that open gaps between the endothelial cells that make up the inner lining of blood vessels. That turned out to be wrong. What the tumor was really doing, they found, was releasing a protein that acted directly on blood vessels, making them leaky and also inducing them to grow. In the grand tradition of tagging something with an acronym ending with "factor" before actually purifying it, Dvorak in 1977 postulated the existence of a substance he began calling VPF, for vascular permeability factor. Unlike Folkman across the street, Dvorak was focusing on permeability, and wasn't really concerned with the question of blood vessel growth. Although no one predicted it, in time it turned out that Dvorak's VPF and Folkman's TAF were exactly the same molecule. And both were the same agent that Ferrara had purified and named VEGF, the name that stuck.

THERE REALLY IS NOT MUCH GLAMOUR in day-to-day research. Standing beside a lab bench all day fiddling with glassware is tedious, time-consuming, and sometimes useless. Worse, as American scientists and postdoctoral fellows know all too well, the most necessary and least appealing part of research is the near-constant groveling for money. If the cash dries up, there's no way to keep a lab open. So more time and energy can go into writing grant proposals than into actual laboratory work, and the success rate is often dismal.

What keeps bright and talented people involved in such drudgery is the firm belief that something fundamentally interesting and important will emerge from an arcane experiment no one else ever thought of doing. It's the search for new knowledge, the urge to expand the intellectual frontier. It's opening the door to the next world, if only by a crack. Maybe, given the right combination of drive, ingenuity, and inspiration, one's name will enter the literature as discoverer of a fine piece of scientific knowledge. To be in that position, though, requires the ability to persuade people who have money, or who are in charge of money, to spend it on things they might not understand. Even if they agree that research is valuable, donors and granting agencies have to sort out which research is best, and then dole out the money in ways that are not foolish.

Throughout most of the second half of the century the funding burden had shifted onto the public sector. Who else but the government could afford to send rockets into space? Who else, if not a nation of taxpayers, could support the costs of cancer research? Hence the cash cow for research support was the U.S. government and its long roster of agencies charged with managing the nation's medical and scientific research—everything from the Defense Department's Advanced Research Projects Agency to the National Heart, Lung, and Blood Institute. Each of these agencies within agencies has its own budget, but, of course, there's never enough money to go around. Toward the end of the century, only about 15 percent of the projects approved by scientific review committees at NIH actually received the money. Most grant proposals, however scientifically worthy or artfully presented, simply were not being funded. And the whims of Congress could turn the budgeting process into a high-stakes crapshoot. There were always losers.

Looking outside the government, researchers could seek funding from foundations such as the ultrarich Howard Hughes Medical Institute, or the Rockefeller and Ford Foundations. Elite scientists might get $500,000 to $2 million a year from those foundations to support major research projects. On a much smaller scale, the American Cancer Society, the American Heart Association, and others dedicated to specific diseases also supported research outside the NIH, though they could never come close to the massive amounts of money that came annually from the federal agencies. Corporations, meanwhile, spend a great deal of money on research, but not much of it gets out of their own laboratories. Products generated by in-house research laboratories have been the lifeblood of companies like DuPont, Monsanto, General Electric, and many others large and small. This in-house philosophy is especially strong in the pharmaceutical industry, where biomedical research is the foundation underlying the entire enterprise. And the industry's allegiance to the bottom line is so strong that research tends to focus on near-term results: What can we put in a bottle tomorrow? It's what made Harvard's 1974 Monsanto grant so unusual. Fundamental research—truly creative thinking—is generally left to the government to sponsor. In medical science, it comes down to a partnership. The federal money is vital at the front end, igniting the flames of discovery. Industry is crucial for making real progress toward the clinic, manufacturing drugs, testing treatments, and paying for clinical trials on patients. But partnerships can resemble marriages, sometimes serene, sometimes shrill, some successful, and some not—especially when the partners grow apart.

By the mid-1980s, Folkman was back to being like everyone else, scratching for support. The twelve-year agreement with Monsanto was running out, and the company had informed Harvard that it was not going to extend its backing. Monsanto had given Harvard more than twenty-three million dollars, ostensibly in exchange for the right to license products for commercial use. Monsanto had the rights to FGF and Vallee's compound, angiogenin, but in the end, the company, with a new president, decided to focus on agriculture rather than on basic biology. The original agreement required Monsanto to return the rights to any patentable products if the company didn't intend to develop them vigorously, so the company simply yielded to Harvard the rights to the two angiogenesis stimulators.

Monsanto didn't get a commercial product that could be sold in a bottle, but it did collect something extremely valuable: enormous expertise in biotechnology that set it on a course to survive and prosper in the coming biological revolution. With its newfound experience in growing and separating huge amounts of biological tissues in culture, Monsanto would blossom into one of the world's major players in the genetic manipulation of important crop plants. Bug-resistant cotton and corn, along with plants that resist weed-killing chemicals, are among the sometimes controversial products that have made Monsanto one of the biggest players in early twenty-first-century agribusiness.

But Judah Folkman was left to search for a new partner. His decision to accept his ouster as chief of surgery in 1981 had been a costly one. It had meant a 50 percent pay cut and forced him to cover his lab and office expenses with whatever grant money he could raise. He still held the Julia Dyckman Andrus professorship, whose endowment yielded interest that paid him a Harvard salary of forty thousand dollars a year. Clearly he needed to become a serious and shrewd fund-raiser to build up the lab. "I had to sustain an effort that would be worth the sacrifice of this big clinical career," he says. He had given up a lot to pursue angiogenesis.

Folkman's lab had kept growing because he was able to gradually expand his research effort, hire a few more technicians, and spend more time with postdoctoral fellows who were pursing endothelial cell growth, vascular biology, and related projects. With that expansion he approached a dozen American companies with proposals for support. Only one seemed even mildly interested. Donald Ingber, a researcher who had recently joined Folkman's lab, remembers being in on a meeting with the company's representative—a businessman, not a scientist—and being utterly deflated by his response. "Some guy with a cigar," Ingber recalls. "He sat around and listened to all of our scientific talks; then he said, 'Well, this is all great. But what have you got that's going to be in the clinic six months from now?' That's all they cared about."

To find an interested company, Folkman finally had to go to distant shores. Early in the 1980s, Yukio Sugino, a lead scientist for the Japanese company Takeda Chemical Industries, had visited Folkman's laboratory and announced, "We want your project." Folkman had smiled and said, "Yes, but I'm married now. I'm married to Monsanto." Sugino asked Folkman to call him if he ever got divorced. So when Monsanto decided to dissolve the marriage a few years later, Takeda was waiting in the wings. The company was still anxious to get into angiogenesis research and soon sent a delegation of scientists—with only a few businessmen—to meet with Folkman and his staff. As excited as the Japanese were, Folkman was worried they wouldn't be willing to give him the kind of money he had grown accustomed to getting from Monsanto. He wasn't the only one worrying. Stephen Atkinson, the Harvard Medical School contracts administrator, feared that during negotiations Folkman was getting himself into trouble with Takeda by aiming too low. "He was letting them talk about a small amount of money," recalls Atkinson, who intervened by writing Takeda a firm letter saying that it wouldn't be worth it for either party if Takeda didn't come up with at least a million dollars a year. That was big money—grants from the NIH were rarely that large—but it didn't seem to scare off Takeda. Within two weeks, the company's representatives were in Boston, saying yes. "It was the most startling thing," Atkinson recalls. "In all of the negotiating I'd ever done, I'd never sat at a table where the chief negotiator from the other side said, 'We have reviewed your budget, and we accept it.' Judah and I were so stunned we started arguing with him about it. And he said, 'But we accept it.' "

TAKEDA'S TIMING WAS PERFECT. By pure serendipity, just as it was replacing Monsanto as Judah Folkman's main industrial benefactor, Donald Ingber found something in a petri dish that would turn into a major discovery for the Folkman lab and its new Japanese partner.

Ingber had earned both an M.D. and a Ph.D. in biology from Yale before joining Folkman in 1984. One Saturday afternoon in November 1985, he noticed a strange fungus growing in a culture dish where endothelial cells were living. Contaminants were usually regarded as a potential for disaster and quickly destroyed, tossed out to keep them from spreading to other cultures in the laboratory. But this time Ingber, curious, decided to look at the cultured cells under a microscope, and he saw something unusual. The fungus seemed to be causing the nearby endothelial cells to round up into tiny balls and pull back. Ingber's research was already focusing on why cells changed shape and what it meant, and this action by individual cells suggested that the fungus was somehow controlling the endothelial cells—making them recoil.

Ingber had come to Boston just a year before but was already feeling stretched too thin, having plunged into a dizzying number of projects. Now it struck him that he had stumbled upon one more potential project—and maybe an important one. He turned to a postdoctoral fellow who was working on her own project that Saturday and showed her the fungus. "I bet this is creating an angiogenesis inhibitor that I could culture out of the medium," he told her. "But do I need another project? Do I *want* another project?" The postdoc thought it was unlikely the fungus could be of any value and advised Ingber just to throw it out. After all, there are thousands of kinds of fungi in the world, and airborne mold spores are everywhere. So if you left a petri dish open for very long, it would almost certainly become contaminated by one thing or another. What were the chances that any one of them would turn into something valuable? But Ingber followed his gut instinct. He cultured the fungus in an agar tube (a long tube of gummy growth medium), then closed it up and left it in the incubator. He didn't tell anyone about it for weeks.

Ingber worked next to Folkman many late nights; finally one evening he told him about his cultured fungus. Folkman immediately got excited. He agreed the action Ingber had observed was significant. Normally the cells grew flat on the petri dish, but in rounding up into little balls, they were changing their basic action, and that might very well mean he had happened onto something important. It occurred to him that Ingber's chance discovery was reminiscent of one of the most important events in medicine—the discovery of penicillin. It was a stray organism floating around in the air, accidentally landing in a culture dish, that in 1928 had led a young Scottish bacteriologist, Alexander Fleming, to the most effective lifesaving drug in the world—penicillin.

After pulling his culture vessel from the incubator, Ingber extracted some of the liquid in which the fungus was growing, then dripped it onto endothelial cells growing in other culture dishes. The cells again began rounding up into little balls, indicating that they had suddenly stopped growing. Next they put the same solution into the CAM assay, the embryonic chicken growing in a petri dish. Here, too, it blocked the growth of tiny blood vessels. Hard as it was to believe, it seemed they had stumbled upon a natural agent, coming from a fungus, that could halt the growth of blood vessels. They had yet to figure out why or how it worked, but it seemed that only a small amount was needed to spur profound change in the growing cells. An inhibiting agent had been found in cartilage earlier, but it was too weak to develop into clinical use. This new one seemed far more potent.

When Folkman told the scientists and executives from Takeda about the discovery, they were ecstatic. With its strong interest in things like soy sauce and sake, Japanese industry had become a world leader in fermentation technology, using yeast, bacteria, and fungi to make all kinds of commercial products: foods, antibiotics, enzymes, flavors, industrial chemicals. So Takeda loved the idea of a fungus possibly being the source of an angiogenesis inhibitor. Soon the company grew a huge vat of the fungus in its plant in Japan, where scientists were able to identify and isolate the active compound in the fungus Ingber had found contaminating his petri dish. They named the compound fumigillin, and it turned out to come from a class of fungi called aspergillis, known for causing sniffles in dogs and found on the shellac of antique furniture and in airplane gasoline.

Once fumigillin had been produced in large enough amounts for experiments, tests showed that it inhibited capillary growth in culture dishes. Then came the big step, the injection of fumigillin into live mice burdened with cancer. It was an important test for the aspiring drug, and for antiangiogenesis itself. Success! The tumors in the mice stopped growing. But it was not quite time to jump for joy. There were side effects, including weight loss, which suggested that the drug might be too toxic to ever try on people.

Takeda's scientists embarked on an aggressive effort to find "analogs"— slightly different versions of the fumigillin molecule—that might be effective without being poisonous. Throughout this time, the mid- to late 1980s, Folkman, Ingber, and other members of the lab, along with the Harvard administrator Stephen Atkinson, traveled to Japan to consult with the Takeda people. Atkinson recalls one meeting when a young Japanese researcher nervously— and very deferentially to Folkman, who was "so godlike to these people," according to Atkinson—presented his work to a room full of Takeda and Harvard scientists. The Japanese scientist spoke self-effacingly, apparently embarrassed that what he was about to show was trivial. He apologized for not having examined more analogs of fumigillin—and then went on to present more than *four hundred* analogs. "They had Rube Goldberged a couple of machines so they were doing these assays twenty-four hours a day," Atkinson recalls. The Americans were flabbergasted by the sheer volume of work the Japanese had put out and the cleverness of it.

After trying hundreds of possible molecules, Takeda's people found that their creative diligence had paid off. They settled on one version that seemed to inhibit tumor growth without being so poisonous. They were able to get enough of the substance to begin tissue culture tests, and then experiments on animals. The drug was named TNP-470, and over the next few years, tests in Japan and Boston would show that it slowed the growth of tumors in mice, rats, dogs, and monkeys. It held out the promise of being the first antiangiogenic agent to become available for testing on humans.

It was a pivotal time in the history of angiogenesis. Knowledge was growing exponentially, more people were joining the field, and the work at Folkman's tenth-floor lab at Children's Hospital in Boston was at the hub of it all. It seemed that the time was approaching when someone, somewhere, might be the first person to receive a drug that would starve his or her tumor to death.

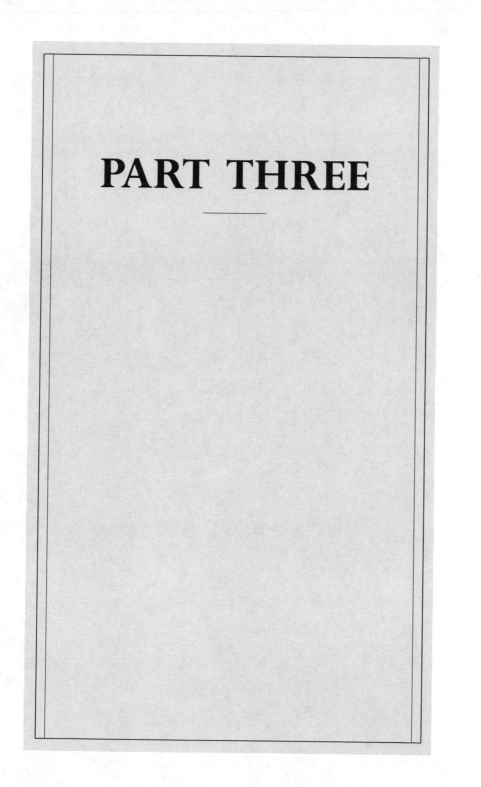

PART THREE

Chapter Thirteen

———

THE FIRST HINT THAT SOMETHING was wrong appeared in Tommy Briggs's fingers. They seemed to have become clubbed, blunt at the tips. It looked a little weird to Tommy, a sandy-haired boy who lived in Aurora, Colorado. It was 1987; Tommy was twelve years old. His parents took him to the pediatrician to have him examined, but the doctor couldn't find any obvious problems. He dismissed the condition as "idiopathic clubbing" and told the Briggses not to worry about it.

But Tom and Judy Briggs couldn't help worrying about their son. Judy was a nurse, and she was aware that clubbing of the fingers could be associated with heart disease or lung ailments. Her concern deepened when Tommy became increasingly short of breath. When he started coughing up bloody sputum, she returned to the pediatrician, who started a series of referrals that eventually brought Tommy to Dr. Carl White, a pediatric pulmonary specialist at the Children's Hospital in Denver. There he underwent a battery of tests. "Treadmill. Tubes. X rays. Skin tests. Catheterization. You name it, I had it," Tommy later recalled. "It was a pretty brutal thing, scary, especially for me at that age."

White and the doctors he worked with agreed that the X rays showed something, but they weren't sure what. Finally, in August 1987, with Tommy coughing up more blood during the night, White decided he'd better take a tissue biopsy from inside Tommy's lungs. He hoped to find something relatively innocent, perhaps a fungus infection. Instead, he found something devastating. Tommy had an extremely uncommon disorder called pulmonary hemangiomatosis, essentially a big, unruly mass of capillaries growing deep inside his lungs. It soon became clear that the options were limited. Tommy had a form of the condition that had been recorded in the medical literature only seven times before—all of them in autopsies.

Hemangiomas themselves are not uncommon, and usually not dangerous. They are ugly, bloodred, uncontrolled clumps of endothelial cells that can show up anyplace, but usually appear on the body rather than inside it. Except in very rare cases, hemangiomas can be ignored; they'll eventually go away on their own. They are fairly common at birth, especially in babies born prematurely, and rarely turn out to be of much consequence. The growths tend to expand rapidly during the first year, then slow down, and begin to regress, finally disappearing by age ten or fifteen. But in about 10 percent of cases, hemangiomas keep growing and cause tissue damage that can be disfiguring. And in about 1 percent of these few cases, hemangiomas arise in a vital organ and become life-threatening. Steroid drugs such as prednisone are effective in approximately a third of these cases, and they help somewhat in another third. But in the remaining third the drugs prove useless, sometimes even making the disorder worse.

Tommy Briggs was one of the unlucky ones. Hemangiomas rarely form in the lungs, and his was especially persistent and dangerous. The bloody mass was disrupting Tommy's airway, and it seemed to be expanding relentlessly. Steroids didn't work. Surgery was impossible. The medical literature offered nothing. Left on its own, the hemangioma would eventually smother Tommy's lungs in overgrown capillaries. By the fall, White had conferred with half a dozen doctors from throughout the country, and all agreed that the tissue extracted from Tommy's lungs confirmed he had a condition that had never before been successfully treated. As time and life seemed to ebb, with Tommy's symptoms steadily growing worse, White had to admit to the Briggs family that Tommy might have only two years to live.

White did not give up, however, and the first whisper of hope came unexpectedly, while he was attending a lecture on pulmonary hypertension at a conference in the Rocky Mountains. Sitting with his fellow physicians, he listened to a specialist giving a talk on the growth-control properties of various biological chemicals. In one of the slides projected onto the screen, White noticed that the new drug called interferon had the ability to stop the movements of blood vessel cells growing in tissue culture. White sat in the darkened room, looking at the diagram, and thought of his desperate patient, Tommy Briggs. Was this significant? Was it a clue? The slide wasn't much to go on, but as soon as he got home White went back into the literature, looking for anything to do with the relatively new, poorly understood drug. What he found excited him: a 1980 report in *Science* by Bruce Zetter, of Children's Hospital in Boston, showing that one version of the drug, interferon alpha, could stop the migration of endothelial cells. Zetter's seven-year-old observation seemed potentially important now, maybe even lifesaving, if White dared allow himself that thought. Hemangiomas are essentially big clumps of endothelial cells expanding inexorably. Could interferon alpha stop the one growing in Tommy Briggs's lung?

Desperate for anything that might help his young, seemingly doomed patient, White dug deeper into the literature on interferon alpha and found another reason for hope. The natural substance had been used to help treat Kaposi's sarcoma, the dark, tumorlike skin blotches that often erupted on the world's growing population of AIDS patients. Kaposi's sarcoma was similar to a hemangioma, except that its tangled mass of capillaries was seen almost solely on the skin. White thought interferon alpha was definitely worth pursuing. For one thing, it was already an approved drug. Discovered in the early 1970s and first tested in humans in 1978, it had shown some effect on a rare malignancy called hairy cell leukemia. But none of the three versions of interferon—alpha, beta, and gamma—had lived up to what had seemed to be their enormous promise as anticancer agents.

White needed to know more, and Judah Folkman was obviously the man to call. No other name was so closely associated with research into the growth of blood vessels. It was in Folkman's laboratory that Zetter, a microbiologist, had spotted interferon's strange ability to stop endothelial cells from migrating in petri dishes. Another scientist who had spent a sabbatical year in Folkman's laboratory, Dr. Robert Auerbach of the University of Wisconsin, had subsequently advanced Zetter's work into living animals, showing that interferon alpha altered the activities of endothelial cells in mice. And then across the street from the Folkman lab, at Beth Israel Hospital, Dr. Harold Dvorak was adding clues about the physiology of blood vessels, such as how those that were associated with tumors appeared to be especially fragile, leaking blood. These were crucial steps. Still, interferon seemed years away, at a minimum, from much use in the clinic.

Tommy Briggs didn't have years. White called Folkman, described his patient, and asked if he thought interferon alpha might, even theoretically, offer some benefit in a case like Tommy's. Folkman wanted to think it might, though he knew that hemangiomas in the lung had always been fatal and it was a long leap from the lab bench to Tommy's bedside. He gave White a short course in his thinking about angiogenesis, then got off the phone and wrote out several pages outlining the issues he thought White needed to explore: Keep the doses low but give them every day. Keep close tabs on Tommy's white blood count and liver function. Make sure to get the proper approvals.

For Folkman, a major moment had arrived. After he had developed his theory in the lab and in his mind for the better part of twenty years, antiangiogenesis was about to be tried in a patient. It wasn't the way Folkman had ever imagined it would happen, but Carl White's alertness, determination, and unwillingness to give up on a patient with no other hope forced the issue.

In Denver, White explained the few options to Tom and Judy Briggs. They could try radiation or chemotherapy, neither of which offered much hope. Or they could experiment with a new, untested treatment, an approach, called antiangiogenesis, based on the ideas of Dr. Judah Folkman. There was only skimpy supporting data—very little work in animals, and less in humans, but Tommy probably had no other hope. The idea was a large and potentially dangerous leap, but Tommy's parents had reached the point of desperation; they were willing to try anything. They gave permission to go ahead.

First, though, White had to work through several layers of bureaucracy. Though interferon alpha was approved by the Food and Drug Administration, he would need permission to try it for an "off-label" use. He had to start by getting the approval of his own hospital's institutional review board, then the drug manufacturer's, Hoffman-LaRoche, and finally the FDA's. There was also an insurance problem: the Briggses' coverage wasn't flexible enough to cover experimental use of interferon. In the end, Hoffman-LaRoche provided the drug for free, and the others also gave the green light. It took half a year, from summer through winter, until finally, early in 1988, White was ready to begin giving Tommy Briggs his first small doses of interferon alpha.

White had to decide how big a dose to use on Tommy. He knew from the medical literature that some leukemia patients saw remissions, at least temporarily, when given ten million international units of the drug per square meter of body area. But they also suffered serious side effects from such large doses. So White decided Tommy should get smaller amounts, starting with one million units for a few days, then two million, and finally settling on three million units daily. And giving the drug more often—small doses daily rather than massive doses once or twice a week—contrasted sharply with the way the drug had been used against cancer and Kaposi's sarcoma.

Immediately after the daily interferon injections began there was trouble. Tommy had an episode of coughing up blood a few days after starting the drug—a few tablespoons' worth, in his mother's estimation—which scared White. Hemangiomas are fragile and tend to bleed very easily, and any bleeding where the lungs are involved is a danger signal. White was also concerned about Tommy's low white blood cell count. On the other hand, it was possible the blood meant that the hemangioma was responding and its blood vessels were being weakened by the treatment. He continued the injections and Tommy stopped coughing up blood. Then White finally began to sense that something was happening in his patient. Tommy's lung function began to improve, along with his tolerance for exercise. He performed better in stress tests, and his white blood cell count was going back up.

Tommy learned to give himself the daily injections of interferon, using a device that shot it in quickly and painlessly. The therapy continued for fourteen months, at which point the daily amounts were cut in half. By then, Tommy had begun to gradually regain normal tolerance for physical exercise, and he felt much better.

By the time he was sixteen, Tommy's life was back on track. He did so well, in fact, that he became a vigorous young athlete, a pitcher for the Stony Hill High School baseball team. The solid thud of a baseball landing in the pocket of a catcher's mitt was the sound of his success. He was perfectly healthy, and his regular doses of interferon had been cut in half. They were finally stopped during his freshman year at the University of Colorado. The hemangioma was gone. He was cured.

Tommy Briggs was lucky at every step. Had interferon been a completely new drug, its toxicities unknown, his doctors would have been subject to standard rules for clinical trials—meaning that he would probably have had to halt the injections before it had a chance to work. With no clear signs of progress seen after a few months, he likely would have been pressured by the drug's maker and his hospital to stop far short of the nine months it took for his health to begin improving, indicating that the hemangioma had begun to shrink. But because interferon was already an approved drug, whose toxicities were known, White and his colleagues could continue giving it even when they couldn't report immediate signs of efficacy.

Folkman's advice about dosage was also vital. Giving relatively small amounts every day, rather than large jolts spaced out over long periods, ensured that the interferon level in Tommy's blood would remain high, somehow and for reasons not yet known constantly telling the blood vessels in his hemangioma to shut down, shut down, stop growing. So it took patience and perseverance on the doctor's part, and courage from Tommy and his family.

Tommy ultimately owed his life to a piece of serendipity and to his doctor's attentiveness. Had White not attended the conference on pulmonary hypertension, and noticed the role of interferon in stopping the movement of blood vessel cells, Tommy Briggs would in all likelihood have died.

TOMMY'S SURVIVAL DID NOT GO unnoticed in Boston. White's report appeared in *The New England Journal of Medicine,* accompanied by an editorial letter written by Folkman. Then Folkman quickly teamed up with two colleagues at Children's Hospital—Alan Ezekowitz, a pediatric hematologist, and John Mulliken, a plastic surgeon—who were determined to try interferon alpha on the severely sick hemangioma patients being sent in from other hospitals around Boston. They hoped to match, and thus confirm, what had happened with Tommy in Denver. They also wanted to start a larger study. But to begin that, Folkman, Ezekowitz, and Mulliken had to spend a year trying to win permission from their own hospital's review board and approval from the Food and Drug Administration and Hoffman-LaRoche, the drug's maker. The problem they faced was that they could not say in their applications exactly *how* interferon alpha worked on hemangiomas. They really didn't know. But they could point to Tommy Briggs as a good result justifying further clinical study, and finally, in 1991, they got the go-ahead to treat their first hemangioma case.

It was a small child with problems somewhat similar to Tommy Briggs's, a two-year-old girl burdened with a massive hemangioma growing on the back side of her liver. All attempts at treatment had failed, and she was bleeding to death by the time Folkman and his team were called in. The doctors immediately got going with interferon alpha, but they were too late: The child died. Their next desperate patient arrived in late spring, a terribly sick baby girl just a year old. She had been rushed to the hospital with a hemangioma growing inside her heart. It was obvious she was slipping into heart failure; a cardiac surgeon assigned to the case announced that it was absolutely hopeless. Still, Folkman, Mulliken, and Ezekowitz began regular, frequent infusions of interferon alpha, hoping they could somehow beat the odds. Not much had changed by September, but they considered that good news: She still clung tenaciously to life. Then, in October, the little girl's hemangioma began to shrink. And within weeks it had actually disappeared. She went home healthy.

The third emergency case was an external hemangioma, a huge red blob growing like a camel's hump on a year-old infant boy's back. It had grown so large it was about half the size of the baby himself. The poor child was bleeding severely, and heart failure seemed imminent. When Folkman and his colleagues got to the emergency room, the doctors on duty were standing glumly around the dying child; there seemed to be nothing they could do. Folkman ordered immediate infusions of interferon, and they continued for several weeks before the huge hemangioma finally began to blanch, lose its deep red color, and stop growing. Gradually it withered and disappeared. This child, too, went home well.

With these almost miraculous successes, the Children's Hospital team found more and more dying children being sent their way from outlying hospitals. But as they tried to expand the use of interferon to treat these stricken children, they encountered a serious supply problem. There wasn't a big market for the drug yet, so production hadn't been scaled up. Moveover, Hoffman-LaRoche, concerned about liability, was being very careful about how much interferon it supplied, and to whom. At Harvard, it was the job of Stephen Atkinson to work out the complicated agreements with the drug company to get the supplies the Children's team needed. But as the delays continued, Folkman became increasingly frustrated. Children's lives were at stake.

Atkinson had worked with Folkman ever since the Monsanto agreement many years before and had seen him face obstacles of every sort. But he had never seen him as emotional as he was the day he showed up in Atkinson's office wanting to know what the problem was. "I said, well, you know . . . and I started talking the way people in my field talk, about problems with the terms in paragraph 6a," Atkinson recalls.

Folkman looked at Atkinson hard. "We've known each other a long time, right? Do you have a minute?"

"For you, Judah, I always have time," Atkinson said.

"Well, come with me."

Folkman took Atkinson across the street to Children's Hospital, up an elevator, and through a maze of corridors and doorways, all the while hammering away at how important it was to get these agreements worked out. They arrived at the door of a hospital room. There was a baby in a crib, and the baby's mother sitting in a chair next to him. "You're probably wondering why I want this so much," Folkman told Atkinson. "So I want you to see this baby."

From the angle Atkinson first saw the baby, he couldn't see the hemangioma; he saw a beautiful baby in a crib. "I remember the lighting in the room;

it was not typical of a hospital room, more like being in a home. I took a look at the mother and she was one worried individual. She'd been there for several days. Then Judah picked up this baby, and showed me a huge red growth on the side of its face. It had closed the ear, and the eye." Atkinson and his wife had a baby less than a year old at the time, and he was speechless. "I can shrink this down to nothing—if I can get this interferon alpha," Folkman told him.

"You will have your agreements," Atkinson promised. And he got them. "Judah is not given to dramatic acts," Atkinson later reflected. "That's the only time I've seen him do something like that. But, boy, it got my attention."

Folkman, Mulliken, and Ezekowitz had originally expected to publish results based on just the first four children treated, but within two years, they had more than twenty cases to describe, almost all of them successful and some positively astounding. The doctors published their results as a series of case reports in *The New England Journal of Medicine* (May 28, 1992), and that opened the floodgates still further. Within six months Boston's Children's Hospital was inundated with dire hemangioma cases. Envelopes with X rays and Polaroid photos of stricken children poured in from just about everywhere, along with urgent requests for consultation. They came from all over the world, even from such prestigious pediatric hospitals as the Hospital for Sick Children in Toronto and Children's Hospital of Philadelphia, where Folkman had trained under C. Everett Koop (by now a former surgeon general) twenty-five years before. Many of the doctors asked if they could send their patients to Boston—far more than the hospital could handle.

Instead of bringing all the children to Boston, Folkman and his colleagues decided to export the treatment, sending the protocols out so doctors elsewhere could begin using interferon alpha in their own hospitals. A special committee—the Vascular Anomalies Program (VAP)—was set up to handle pleas from doctors and hospitals all around the world and to give quick and accurate advice. Each Wednesday at five-thirty in the afternoon, the seventeen members of the committee met in a conference room to discuss the cases that came in from Europe, Africa, Asia, and all across North and South America.

The meetings would begin with one of the doctors, such as radiologist Patricia Burrows, handing out a description of each case and then using an overhead projector to display the patient's X rays on a screen. Each case spoke of untold suffering, enormous disability, and often the dark prospect of death: a four-year-old burdened with a massive growth in her stomach, chronically losing blood through gastrointestinal bleeding; a teenage girl suffering with blue rubber bleb nevus syndrome, which included lifelong eruptions of hemangioma-like growths on her skin, neck, lungs, liver, spleen, and gastrointestinal tract. As each patient's condition was discussed, the doctors—Folkman, Mulliken, Burrows, and others—examined the X rays in detail and sometimes asked for more data: Do we need an MRI scan? What about a gastrointestinal workup? What advice can we offer? Should the referring physician watch the patient a while longer to see what develops? Is there danger in that?

Each case got careful scrutiny and assessment, some of it disappointing: "He's going to have a miserable time; we have nothing to offer. " The atmosphere was intense and highly focused as the complex images of body parts were projected onto a screen across the darkened room. The sessions continued for hours, and Folkman, always on the lookout for new knowledge about blood vessel growth, would sometimes spot something. "We've got something sitting here looking at us," he might say. "Wow, this could be hot." His idea would become another piece of the picture, perhaps be posted on the board in Folkman's conference room, listed along with other "burning questions" he hoped to see answered—maybe even becoming a research subject around which a graduate student or postdoctoral fellow would build a career.

TOMMY BRIGGS and the children who followed him were the first patients whose survival demonstrated that Folkman's long-held ideas about angiogenesis were on target. Even if it wasn't cancer they were treating, the successes offered evidence at last that drugs could be used to block abnormal blood vessel growth—the first destination on the long and tortuous route from the laboratory bench to the clinic. But it wasn't a clean victory for Folkman.

About six months after the Children's Hospital report on hemangioma treatments appeared in *The New England Journal of Medicine,* two members of the hospital's medical staff complained to Dr. David Nathan, the chief of medicine, that some of the numbers in the research paper published by Folkman and his colleagues didn't quite add up. There was no question about the overall results—most of the patients had indeed survived and recovered—but there were problems with the accuracy of the report. The complaining doctors, who had been involved in the care of some of the patients, told Nathan they were bothered by some of the data used to demonstrate the effects of interferon alpha. In one case, for instance, a hemangioma that Folkman's team said had regressed 100 percent had actually gone down 95 percent—a small but potentially significant error. In another case, they had failed to report a patient's side effects: The interferon had made her irritable. And an examination of the treatment records raised still other worrisome questions. One baby was said to have been given a dose of interferon on a date that preceded her birth. Did the problems result from sloppiness—or something worse?

The allegations were serious, especially because they surfaced at a time when suspicions about fudged data were running deep throughout the world of science and medicine. Even hints of error or miscalculation—to say nothing of suggestions of fraud—could instantly ruin careers. Nathan had to decide what to do about it. He could call the researchers in and ask them to address the criticisms, then determine whether errors had been made, and if so how, why, and in what manner they should be corrected. But Nathan was uncomfortable handling it on his own. He felt he had no choice but to bounce it up to the hospital administration, which—because federal money was involved—then had to report it as possible misconduct to the National Institutes of Health. A special hospital committee was appointed to investigate the episode.

But even before the committee began its work, Folkman and his team undertook their own review. They spent four or five months, every night, going through the charts, and they found even *more* errors. The result was a long correction that *The New England Journal of Medicine* published in 1994. But it, too, turned out to be less than perfect: The data contained some mathematical errors in the percentages of hemangioma regression and some problems in the toxicity data. "I begged them to do nothing until the committee met and told them what to do," Nathan recalls. "But Judah said, 'Oh, no, we're going to correct it ourselves, and do it right away.' Goddamn him, you couldn't talk him out of it! He just went ahead and did that, and of course he did it wrong too. And that just created hell." It also created the need for an embarrassing second correction that ran in the *Journal* (August 31, 1995)— three years after the original paper had been published. The second correction included a statement that a final review by the Harvard faculty committee had "concluded that ambiguities in method, presentation and conclusions should be clarified, and that errors remained that should be corrected." Their correction ended with the statement: "We are embarrassed by our errors and regret them. We apologize to the readers for any misunderstanding, and thank our colleagues for their assistance in correcting our report."

The problem, in the end, was the kind of carelessness that Folkman's critics had long felt was his weakness. There was no doubt that the interferon treatments had been followed by the shrinking or disappearance of hemangiomas. But the details of the treatment were fuzzy: Folkman and his colleagues had been scrambling to save children and didn't tend to their data nearly as well as they did their patients. They relied on hospital charts for the numbers they reported in their paper. And the hospital charts, it turned out, were riddled with errors. They also had no data manager, no funding, and had not originally planned to do a clinical trial.

As Folkman explained it, with young lives hanging in the balance, harried nurses often didn't have time to fill in each patient's chart moment by moment. Later, when the nurses finally did get a chance to come back and record what happened, they were sometimes less than accurate about when a dose of the drug was given. Maybe a treatment was ordered at one time—as shown on the chart—but the patient wanted to go home, and the doctors agreed it would be all right to give the treatment two days later. The change might have been noted by a nurse but was overlooked as the research paper was being prepared. "So we had, my gosh, these errors of two days," Folkman recalls. "And when we started to look at them, adding them up, there were a lot of these little errors. And the dates of birth, they would be a day off, so we had patients being given the drug before they were even born."

David Nathan says, "The word 'fraud' was all over the place. But this was not fraud; it was carelessness, which is a big difference." The problem, Nathan concluded, was partly the fault of the medical school and hospital. It might have been avoided had the hospital had a system like the one across the street at Dana-Farber. There, a squad of data managers supervised the preparation of all clinical studies. That suggestion, though, raised another criticism of the research. Unlike clinical researchers conducting a formal, double-blind study, the doctors at Children's had no randomly selected patient population, with half being treated with the drug and a control group getting placebos. "We were doing these as cases, not as a clinical trial," Folkman says. But Nathan argued that Folkman and his colleagues could have—should have— conducted a rigorous clinical trial, setting up a separate control population for comparison with a treatment population, to make absolutely sure the interferon was responsible for the successes, rather than natural regression of the hemangiomas. Folkman and his colleagues could have treated the life-threatening cases as emergencies, excluded them from the study, and then used the remaining patients who were in less serious trouble in a clinical trial.

Though the hospital's investigating committee found that Folkman,

Ezekowitz, and Mulliken were guilty only of sloppiness, there was more trouble when the scientific journal *Nature* heard about the episode and published an article in which Nathan was quoted as saying there had been numerous allegations of fraud against Folkman and his colleagues. Folkman, who was still upset with Nathan for his decision to pass the complaints up to the hospital administration and then the NIH, was stung by these remarks. That would make the relationship between the two doctors difficult from that point forward.

Academic squabbles notwithstanding, there was little arguing about the benefit for patients. Before the treatments with interferon alpha started, 60 percent of the half-dozen or more very severe hemangioma patients who arrived each year at Children's Hospital didn't survive. In 1992, the year of the *NEJM* paper, the mortality rate was down to about 40 percent. By 1993 it would drop to just 9 percent, staying at that level until 1997, when only one child—who had a liver hemangioma and came in very late—died. And by 1998, there would be no hemangioma deaths at all. Similarly dramatic improvements, based on antiangiogenesis treatments using interferon, would be reported at major medical centers in Milwaukee, Montreal, Rome, and other cities.

EVEN AS ANTIANGIOGENESIS was finally being brought from the lab into the clinic, research continued apace. There was much more to be learned about why interferon alpha worked—and this new knowledge would help pave the way toward figuring out the mechanisms of tumor angiogenesis.

It was soon discovered, for example, that many hemangiomas seemed to be dependent on fibroblast growth factor, or FGF, the natural and potent growth-stimulating agent that had been identified and isolated by Michael Klagsbrun and Yuen Shing in 1984. Now, several years later, FGF offered a valuable yardstick in treating hemangiomas. By measuring how much FGF was present in a patient's urine, the Folkman lab could gauge how aggressively the hemangioma was expanding. In patients whose hemangiomas were starting to shrink, the level of FGF dropped as the clump of tissue got smaller. Thus, when big hemangiomas were treated with interferon alpha and started to regress, the amount of FGF they produced showed a similar decline. So it seemed likely that a cause-and-effect relationship existed, and that interferon alpha stopped hemangioma growth by somehow blocking or shutting down production of FGF, the growth factor. That didn't explain *how* it worked, but the discovery of the relationship was so important it was published in 1994 as a cover article in *The Journal of Clinical Investigation.*

The scientific spin-off from the hemangioma work, and the use of FGF as a marker for aggressive blood vessel growth, began to generate a lot of new excitement among research physicians. As usual, Folkman was on the road, giving talks in the United States, Canada, Europe, Japan, and elsewhere, sharing his work and gathering more ideas about angiogenesis from fellow researchers he was meeting. At a technical meeting in San Francisco, Folkman was to be followed on stage by Isaiah Fidler, a respected cancer researcher from the M. D. Anderson Cancer Center in Houston. As Folkman was finishing his talk, he remarked that despite the exciting results with interferon alpha against life-threatening hemangiomas, he and his colleagues were still puzzled, having no idea how it actually worked. Fidler sat in the audience, chuckling to himself. After Folkman finished speaking, Fidler stepped to the podium and announced: "Judah, if you will have patience to sit through my presentation, I'll show you the mechanism."

Fidler and his colleagues had discovered, through their own research into the intricacies of tumor growth and the problems and causes of drug resistance, that interferon actually shuts off the production of the growth factor b-FGF (the *b* stands for basic, as opposed to acidic). Fidler discovered that interferon alpha is made in huge quantities by normal skin cells, so it is always present in the skin, ready to go into action. It was still not known exactly what role interferon alpha played in normal metabolism, but a strong suspicion among researchers was that it is a natural antiviral agent that stands by, ready for battle in case of a viral infection.

Fidler subsequently showed that in the bloody growths called hemangiomas, interferon was actually the missing ingredient; the serious trouble arose because, for some reason, too little interferon was present. His discovery meshed nicely with the notion that hemangiomas, like tumors, resulted from a loss of control, like a truck storming downhill after its brakes have failed. Thus hemangiomas, without enough interferon present, reacted as if there were some kind of damage, say wounding or an infection, and increased production of their own growth stimulator, FGF, to cope with the emergency. The excess FGF, in turn, stimulated further abnormal growth of capillaries, and this was what kept the hemangioma growing. As Fidler explained it, "A hemangioma is the most angiogenic tumor you can think of. It's a tumor of the blood vessels." It turned out that injecting interferon—restoring its natural presence—caused the growing hemangioma to stop making FGF. And once that happened, the tumorlike mass couldn't call in new blood vessels, and cells in its interior began to die for lack of oxygen. As the cells died off, the mass gradually shrank. And Tommy Briggs had survived.

Because of all that followed Dr. Carl White's fortuitous decision to take a desperate gamble on a dying child, Folkman had gained proof that the body produces substances capable of slowing down or stopping the growth of blood vessels, and that those substances could be introduced to attack abnormal cell growth. Now, trying to exploit the discovery that interferon was one such agent, he and several colleagues would make the leap into cancer research. They initiated a major new study at Children's Hospital, measuring the levels of FGF and a similar growth stimulator, VEGF, in the urine of more than two thousand young cancer patients. They hoped to see some correlation between growth factor levels and patients' tumors.

The results were startling. So much so that soon the study was expanded to include adult cancer patients at two neighboring Harvard-affiliated medical centers, the Dana-Farber Cancer Institute and the Brigham and Women's Hospital. Patients with all kinds of cancers participated, and by 1993 the study began to yield exciting data. In patients with bladder cancer, for instance, the amount of FGF found in the urine turned out to be an eerily accurate predictor of cancer recurrence. The doctors discovered that a patient's FGF level in urine begins going up about a month before other signs indicate that the tumor is growing again. In childhood tumors, the FGF level, very high with the tumor in the body, drops precipitously as soon as the tumor is removed. For Folkman, these links between growth factor levels and tumor activity offered the most important concept to come out of the hemangioma work. And it eventually led to an exciting and wholly unexpected discovery.

The idea that leukemia needed angiogenesis seemed on its face counterintuitive. After all, leukemia is a disease of the bloodstream. The aberrant cancer cells are awash in blood all the time, so it wouldn't seem likely that they'd need more. But in the study of growth stimulator levels among cancer patients, it turned out that at least half of all leukemia patients had abnormally high levels of the angiogenic proteins in both their blood and urine. In fact, the leukemia patients seemed to have the highest levels of growth factors of all the cancer patients, often ten times higher than the others. A detailed, two-year survey of bone marrow samples taken from young leukemia patients at Children's Hospital produced a second surprise: Tests showed that the marrow of many of these patients had been infiltrated by tiny capillaries, suggesting that leukemia was also dependent on angiogenesis, the growth of new blood vessels. Perhaps the new capillaries were needed to support the rapid, abnormal production of white blood cells so characteristic of leukemia.

In contrast, there were few or no blood vessels detectable in the bone marrow of a control group—children with other kinds of cancer and other diseases. It was also noted that after the leukemia patients were given thirty days of therapy with five or six combined drugs, the tiny capillaries in their bone marrow began to disintegrate, and then recede back to normal. So it began to seem likely that leukemia, like other forms of cancer, was in fact angiogenic, though not necessarily dependent on new blood vessels.

Hoping for some clarification, Folkman and his colleagues began running leukemia experiments on mice. First they injected the animals with aggressive leukemia cells and left them untreated. The mice died in about three weeks. Then they tried treating their poisoned animals with agents known to be antiangiogenic. To begin, they chose TNP-470, the drug that had been derived from the fungus that Donald Ingber had found sitting in his petri dish that day back in 1985 and had later been developed by Folkman's Japanese partner, Takeda Chemical Industries. TNP-470 was slowly emerging as potentially the first major antiangiogenic drug. The drug had been shown to block the growth of dozens of kinds of tumors in mice, rats, dogs, and monkeys. But would it work in humans? The answer was a long time coming.

TNP-470 seemed ripe for clinical trials within a couple of years of its early development by Ingber and Takeda. But then it hit a web of delays. Takeda and the NIH became bogged down in the question of who to test the drug on and how to use it. Worse, Takeda found itself in a cumbersome business entanglement. Takeda had a standing agreement with a large Chicago pharmaceutical firm, Abbott Laboratories, requiring that any product Takeda wanted to bring into the United States be developed and marketed by a subsidiary, TAP Partners, formed by the two companies. With a lot invested in TNP-470, Takeda was excited about its potential, but the Abbott people seemed to give the drug a low priority. Ingber believed that corporate indifference delayed the drug's development, which frustrated him a great deal. He felt that Takeda had essentially ceded control of the drug to Abbott. Ingber, meanwhile, was kept out of the information loop, so he could keep track of his drug's progress only through the research grapevine. It took until 1992, seven years after it was discovered, to get TNP-470 into clinical trials.

That October, the tests began at the M. D. Anderson Cancer Center in Houston. But even then, the design of the trial seemed wrong to Ingber, who opposed the NIH's requirement that the drug be given daily for four weeks straight, followed by four weeks off. "The whole concept was to give it con-tinuously, long term," Ingber later said. "What we knew from the heman-giomas was that you can go for six months and have no effect. Zero. But by nine months it's shrinking, and by a year it's gone. So that was kind of crazy." Because of the dosage protocols, Ingber wasn't surprised when the early re-sults were not promising; the drug didn't seem to prolong the lives of the first patients to take it. But by the mid-1990s, when TNP-470 began to be used in combination with chemotherapy or with radiation, results began to improve dramatically. For reasons unknown, TNP-470 seemed to sensitize tumors to the cell-killing effects of radiation. It also seemed to improve the effectiveness of chemotherapy agents such as Taxol. One speculation was that the antian-giogenesis agent altered or opened up the blood vessels feeding a tumor, al-lowing a greater flow of the chemotherapy poison to get into the tumor itself.

Folkman, meanwhile, wanted to see what TNP-470 would do in mice with leukemia. He found that it seemed to extend the lives of the sick lab animals by about 40 percent. That was an impressive start, suggesting the drug could become part of the antileukemia armamentarium. If TNP-470 could be com-bined with chemotherapy agents that were known to be effective, at least tem-porarily, they might get closer to cures. Could it do the same for humans? The Food and Drug Administration granted permission to begin a drug safety trial at Children's Hospital, using TNP-470 on patients who had failed all other treatments. But the doctors were unable to recruit enough patients for a solid trial. The good news was that it was because so few children were failing all other treatments; the five-year survival rate had passed 80 percent. Ulti-mately, though, the discovery at Children's Hospital that capillaries invaded the bone marrow in many leukemia patients and in animals made the idea of antiangiogenesis far more visible among blood disease specialists, triggering a significant increase in angiogenesis research in more laboratories. Indeed, by decade's end, a large number of the papers published in the journal *Blood* would be angiogenesis papers, a remarkable turnaround for a subject that had been almost taboo years earlier.

Virtually all these developments, all these ideas and advances and hopes, could be traced in some way to the day Tommy Briggs arrived at Children's Hospital in Denver in 1987. The use of interferon to save the life of this one child was the spark of a small medical revolution. Over the next ten years, the use of interferon alpha against hemangiomas would spread worldwide, saving the lives of hundreds of children every year and leading to many new avenues of research. By 1998, Folkman's home institution, Children's Hospital in

Boston, one of the world's centers for treatment of hemangiomas, would reach a landmark: It would get through an entire year without a single hemangioma death. By then, Tommy Briggs was a healthy young man of twenty-three, a recent graduate of the University of Colorado working for an investment company, a victor. "I was the first person to survive this horrible disease," he wrote in his college application letter. "I was overcome with a feeling of absolute joy and personal pride. I had defeated something that had almost taken my life."

And he had provided a vital catalyst for the drive to make antiangiogenesis a major weapon in the cancer wars. With reports of the success of interferon in the early 1990s, Judah Folkman and his wild ideas were scorned no more, and his lab was no longer a place for bright young biomedical researchers to avoid. Now, in fact, the competition was fierce for a slot on Folkman's team. Brilliant young researchers with blue-chip credentials were routinely turned away. Like many great team builders, Folkman has a gift for looking beyond the résumé to the intangibles that produce groundbreaking work. Happily, his antennae were working the day he fielded a less-than-stellar initial application—and letters of support—from a young doctor who would produce some of the field's most momentous achievements.

Chapter Fourteen

———

ONE OF THE FUNDAMENTAL LESSONS Judah Folkman passed on to young people joining his laboratory was that success can often arrive dressed as failure. Success is great—satisfying, good for the ego, capable of bringing reward and prosperity—but doing experiments that invariably bring the expected results may mean the questions aren't tough enough. To fail, then struggle to understand why, may offer more insight and greater learning. Asking "Why not?" is often an important and productive stop on the way to learning "why."

Generations of surgeons had been frustrated by occasional cases—about 4 percent of patients—in which surgery to remove a tumor was successful but the patient still died. Extra care would be taken to cut nice, wide margins around the tumor tissue to get it all. No signs might indicate that the tumor had spread to distant organs. The patient would go home, scarred but optimistic about recuperating and getting life back on track. But disaster followed, in the form of tiny, hidden tumors that seemed to erupt like black magic in the bones, the brain, lungs, or liver and grew with unrestrained vigor, finally killing the patient.

How did this happen? Why did patients perish despite what seemed to be successful surgery? If all those tiny metastases had already scattered throughout the body before surgery, why had they remained so small that they were invisible? Why did they wait to grow until after the operation? Several generations of doctors had been unable to answer these questions.

The problem of postsurgical eruption of metastases was well documented in the medical literature. Pictures of satellite tumors growing after the removal of a primary tumor could be found as far back as 1900, and scientists had varying interpretations of what might be going on. Maybe a primary tumor caused some sort of immune reaction, generating antibodies that prevented the secondary tumors from growing. Maybe a tumor caused growth resistance, or some unknown form of tumor suppression, in its cousins. What was especially baffling was that of the more than one hundred kinds of cancer, only a few seemed to have an ability to keep their own metastases under control. One commonly held view was that metastasis was, in effect, the surgeon's fault. By trying to remove the tumor, the surgeon allowed a few cancer cells to escape and begin their lethal growth in distant tissues.

By the time Folkman began considering the question, there was no evidence to support the idea that bad surgery was to blame. It was fairly clear that in some cases, as long as the big primary tumor kept growing, the tiny metastasizing "seeds" that had migrated through the bloodstream to other organs were somehow kept from growing beyond microscopic size. So why did these dangerous metastases wait to grow until after surgery? Within that disarmingly simple question—why *then*?—was hidden the answer that Folkman had begun pursuing as a navy draftee three decades earlier. Within that question lay the riddle of tumor dormancy—and perhaps the future of cancer treatment.

As early as 1985 Folkman began assigning some of his surgery trainees to explore the question of why removing primary tumors seemed to leave distant metastases free to grow. His students found no plausible answers. Their best guess was that the conventional wisdom—that metastatic cancer cells were released as a surgeon was cutting away a primary tumor—was right. But Folkman wouldn't buy the idea that metastases were a by-product of surgery. He was convinced they were actually present elsewhere in the body at the time the primary tumor was removed.

The first real insight had come one night in 1987 when Folkman and Harold Brem, one of his postdoctoral fellows, were staying late in the Enders Building to study the activity of the new drug, the fungus-derived TNP-470, that Donald Ingber had discovered. In animal experiments, TNP-470 was showing exciting promise as the first antiangiogenesis agent potent enough to slow or even stop the growth of large tumors. These signs of success were encouraging, but incomplete. Although regular doses of TNP-470 could inhibit the growth of an animal's tumor by 70 percent or more, the experiments were running into strange complications. In their tests in mice, the researchers could see that as repeated doses of the drug gradually slowed a tumor's growth, in some cases even shrinking its size, the invisible metastases lurking in distant organs suddenly erupted, growing aggressively. And just as was seen for so many years in cancer patients, this release from dormancy came only if the big, primary tumor was receding. Folkman and Brem talked about what might be going on. Were they overlooking some innate mechanism?

One possibility was that the drug itself was somehow driving the action of metastasis, maybe even causing it. But to Folkman and Brem that seemed unlikely, because there were no signs that TNP-470—an angiogenesis inhibitor—could stimulate tumor growth. So it was an enigma, but one pregnant with possibility. One of those "Aha!" moments came that night in the lab, when Brem was grumbling to Folkman that his newest experiment with TNP-470 wasn't going very well. The drug was working on the primary tumor, but that strange, vexing pattern—the sudden eruption of metastases—was being seen again. Brem didn't like it; he hoped to show that TNP-470 was a pure cancer fighter.

Folkman thought about it for a moment. Could it be that the vigorous primary tumor was producing some unknown inhibiting agent that kept the metastases from growing? And could it be that as the big tumor was being defeated by TNP-470, its shrinkage reduced the output of that inhibiting agent? Such a scenario might explain why TNP-470 was strong enough to drive the big primary tumor down but couldn't seem to finish the job. Maybe TNP-470 didn't have quite enough power to kill off both the primary tumor and its metastases. Perhaps before treatment with TNP-470 began, the big tumor had been leaking some substance of its own into the bloodstream, an unknown angiogenesis-inhibiting agent that was keeping the small, distant tumors from growing. And as the big tumor was killed off, maybe the loss of the mysterious inhibitor released the brakes on the metastases.

This notion, though sketchy and speculative, seemed to fit with one of Folkman's favorite ideas. He had thought since the early 1960s that no tumor could grow beyond a tiny size until it sent out a chemical message to recruit an ample blood supply. For that chemical signal to be sent out, Folkman believed, an angiogenic switch had to be flipped—a switch that turned on the tumor's production of a growth-promoting agent such as b-FGF (basic fibroblast growth factor), or VEGF (vascular endothelial growth factor), which Folkman had long referred to as TAF. It was this angiogenic switch that made nearby blood vessels sprout and grow new branches and kick-started the rapid growth of tumors.

The problem, of course, was that no such angiogenic switch had been identified. Several growth factors, including FGF and VEGF, had been discovered, and their involvement was clearly crucial. But exactly how they worked—when and why a tumor began to produce a growth factor—was anything but clear. Even more opaque was this fresh, new idea that tumors themselves sometimes made yet another agent, a substance that turned *off* the angiogenic switch.

The picture was either complicated further, or clarified somewhat, by research done jointly by Folkman and a colleague, biologist Douglas Hanahan of the University of California, San Francisco. While working earlier at the Cold Spring Harbor Laboratory on Long Island, Hanahan, a lanky, silver-haired scientist with an easy grin, had created his own special breed of "transgenic" lab mice. He had used gene-splicing technology to endow the animals with a special gene that ensured they got cancer. The tumors caused by the inserted gene almost invariably arose about six weeks after birth, in the insulin-producing beta cells, the islet cells of the pancreas. Even at that young age, the animals' tumors were well vascularized (well fed by blood vessels), indicating that the angiogenic switch had been tripped quite early.

Hanahan's engineered mice were especially valuable for cancer studies because experimenters could accurately predict exactly when and where their tumors would arise. The predictability made it easy to monitor step-by-step what was happening to the animals as they approached their date with cancer. Blood tests and biopsies could be taken to follow what was happening in the pancreas, in the blood, or in the rest of the animal's body, as the time for tumors to erupt drew near. But the results revealed something baffling: Repeated tests on the mice showed that their incipient tumors typically turned on production of the growth factor VEGF, as expected—but fully two weeks before there was any sign of excess blood vessel growth near the small tumors. Similar tests showed that production of the other potent growth stimulator, b-FGF, also started weeks before angiogenesis began. Hanahan and Folkman couldn't understand why there was this two-week delay between the upsurge in growth factors and the onset of tumor angiogenesis. Why didn't new blood vessel growth begin immediately, once the growth factors were present in measurable amounts?

The phenomenon offered an important clue. It suggested that something else, maybe some other factor that played an inhibiting role, was temporarily holding back the growth of blood vessels. But where might it come from? And how did it work, if it existed at all? No good evidence existed to support such a scenario, but it was an intriguing avenue of inquiry.

The solution finally came into focus almost by accident, through the brilliant work of cancer researcher Noel Bouck, a molecular biologist at the

Northwestern University School of Medicine in Chicago. Attending the annual meeting of the American Association for Cancer Research in 1987, Bouck was meandering through the big hall where hundreds of scientists were standing by elaborate posters, some earnestly explaining their results. By then, Bouck was tired, most interested in finding a quiet place to sit down to rest her aching feet. She managed to slip into a darkened, vacant meeting room at one side of the hall, where she kicked off her blue high-heeled shoes. But just as she was beginning to relax and feel comfortable, the lights flashed on, and the room suddenly filled with eager people heading for vacant seats. It was too late for her to collect herself and scramble out. "I was trapped in the middle of the row, and I couldn't get out without making a commotion," Bouck recalls. "And then I overheard that the speaker was a surgeon. Oh, that would be so dull."

The surgeon was Judah Folkman, who gave one of his enthusiastic talks about the phenomenon called angiogenesis, exploring his ideas about the growth of tumors, discussing the latest evidence, and suggesting that tumors might be controlled if blood vessel growth could be stopped. Bouck had never heard of Folkman—as a surgeon, he was not well known among people doing fundamental genetic and biological science—but she found his message and his enthusiasm about angiogenesis almost overwhelming. By the time he was winding up his talk, Bouck remembers, "I was ready to jump up, wave my arms, and yell, 'I believe! I believe!' "

So strongly did she believe that the experience turned her cancer research in a new direction, toward angiogenesis. And within two years she and her colleagues at Northwestern would make an invaluable contribution, discovering the first natural angiogenesis-inhibiting substance created by a growing tumor. Working with animal tumors in a tissue-culture system, she devised a way to engineer a gene so it would work only at a certain temperature; to switch it on or off, all she had to do was change the temperature. The cells growing in culture were constantly releasing factors that stimulated endothelial cell growth. But when the gene was turned off, the cells began pouring out a compound that seemed capable of keeping distant tumors from growing. Bouck found through biochemical tests that the compound was thrombospondin, a known chemical, and that it was being released from the tumor itself in very small amounts—barely enough to be detectable in the bloodstream, but maybe just enough to keep any metastases from growing.

For Folkman, Bouck's discovery was a *Eureka!* moment. He thought about Bouck's work every day for months, pondering what it meant that tumors put out both angiogenesis stimulators and inhibitors. One day that September, sitting in a back row of Temple Israel in Boston during Rosh Hashanah services, it finally hit him: It was a balancing act! Blood vessels grew toward tumors when stimulating molecules began to overpower inhibiting molecules. A teeter-totter—maybe that was the answer to the riddle of the angiogenic switch. The Hebrew prayers for the Jewish New Year filled the sanctuary, and Folkman was playing out a refined theory of angiogenesis in his mind: *Blood vessel growth is controlled by a balancing of opposing factors. A tilt in favor of stimulators over inhibitors might be what trips the lever and begins the process of tumor angiogenesis.* "I remember exactly the seat, the row, everything," Folkman later recalled. "It was ten-thirty in the morning. And the whole idea came that this was the way. Then I understood what her paper meant. She said there was a net balance between stimulators and inhibitors, and that's the first time people had said that." Folkman made Bouck's 1989 paper in *Cell* required reading in his lab.

As it happened, that very idea was also in the air in Bouck's lab. A graduate student, Sara Tolsma, illustrated it with a diagram resembling a seesaw. Blood vessels tended to grow toward tumors when stimulating molecules began to overpower inhibiting molecules. Tip the balance one way, and the tumor grows. Tip it the other way, and growth stops, or even regresses. The discovery and the thinking that flowed from it laid the foundation for an elegant new notion of human biology: that even under normal circumstances in a healthy body, angiogenesis promoters and inhibitors coexist as part of the body's natural emergency defense system. Both are made in advance, kept in storage, ready for action in case of trouble. In response to a wound, for example, the growth-promoting factors immediately begin calling in new blood vessels to help repair the damage. Then, as the wound-healing process continues, the inhibitors are released to keep blood vessel growth from going too far. And, more to the point, it seemed logical to Folkman that a disruption of this fine balance was one of the abnormal conditions of cancer. The tipping of the balance in favor of blood vessel growth could, in fact, be the fundamental event triggering the wildfire progression of a tumor.

A number of studies now offered evidence in favor of a scenario involving a seesaw of growth factors. It was known, for instance, that the inhibitor TNP-470 could shrink a tumor in size, driving it toward dormancy, presumably because it was causing the tumor's access to blood to be restricted. But once the primary tumor got small enough, the distant metastasized tumors would then begin to grow. It was also clear from Douglas Hanahan's specially

engineered mice, which were programmed to come down with pancreatic tumors, that production of the stimulating agents alone was not enough to get
cancer going strongly. And then Noel Bouck's work suggested that the stimulating molecules were ineffective until production of another agent, the inhibitor thrombospondin, declined enough to let tumor growth begin. This
growth-control scenario suggested a natural system that was carefully bal-
anced, poised for action, but kept in check. The stimulating molecules could
be present, urging blood vessel growth to go. But blood vessels ignored it until
the balance was tipped by the slowed production of the inhibitor. Bouck
showed that tumor growth began when the amount of thrombospondin was
reduced to only 4 or 6 percent of normal.

As the evidence for this scenario accumulated, Folkman and his staff came
to the working hypothesis that even a very small percentage of inhibitor was
enough to keep distant tumors, metastases, from growing. A key ingredient of
this theory was that the stimulators, VEGF and FGF, lasted in the bloodstream only briefly, about three and a half minutes, while inhibitors lasted for
hours. The stimulators didn't survive long enough to reach the metastases, so
they lost their growth-stimulating power almost immediately. In contrast, the
far more durable inhibiting molecules kept their potency while coursing
through the bloodstream, easily reaching the distant metastases. This difference in molecular survival time seemed critical. So with the primary tumor
growing in the body, the balance was tipped in favor of the inhibitors, preventing new blood vessels from forming, keeping the mestastases dormant.
But in the big primary tumor's immediate neighborhood, Folkman hypothe-
sized, it was a very different story. The short-lived growth-stimulating factors
coming from the tumor lasted just long enough to stimulate vigorous blood
vessel growth nearby. At that close distance, the plentiful stimulators easily
overpowered the flow of inhibitors, tripping the angiogenic switch, calling in
new blood vessels and allowing the tumor to grow.

So why, in that small number of cases, did metastases grow after the primary tumor was surgically removed? After all, without that primary tumor,
production of both inhibitors and stimulators ceased. Folkman suggested that
those metastases, having taken root elsewhere in the body, began developing
their own ability to make stimulators, such as VEGF and FGF. Then they
drew in their own new blood supply, enough to take on independent growth.
In fact, Folkman suspected, if a metastasis got enough of a head start and produced enough inhibitor, it could keep its neighbors from growing. It was a

phenomenon that Folkman and Michael O'Reilly, a postdoctoral fellow, would later harness to find new inhibitors.

It was a grand idea. And, like most grand ideas, it was going to require grand proof. As he did with other big ideas or tough problems, Folkman scribbled the big, overarching question—How does a primary tumor keep its metastases at bay?—at the top of the "burning questions" list that covered the big message board in the conference room. He hoped one of his more ambitious postdoctoral fellows might take on the challenge and devise experiments to find out whether and how primary tumors used inhibiting agents to control the angiogenic process, keeping metastasized tumors from luring in an ample blood supply of their own.

Intriguing as it was, nobody in Folkman's lab wanted to work on it, much to the disappointment of the boss. The proposition that natural angiogenesis inhibitors might be found inside the body was still new and not well tested, despite increasing successes of interferon alpha against hemangiomas. The notion that really potent, cancer-blocking antiangiogenesis agents might actually be hidden within the body marked a major change even in the Folkman lab's thinking; it was a hard sell even at home. Some in the lab were clearly uncomfortable with that, particularly since the proposal was essentially devoid of any firm evidence. The hypothesis struck many as too broad, too poorly defined. Among the new postdocs who joined the lab each July, trying to track down such putative inhibiting agents was seen as a complex, high-risk project, a gamble that was likely to consume a lot of time, perhaps yield nothing, and even harm a young scientist's career. Though there had been a quantum leap in the development of analytical tools and separation techniques, looking for these molecules in tumor tissue, blood, or other bodily fluids was a challenge reminiscent of the long, frustrating search for TAF—not very appealing to someone who hoped to spend a couple of years working on something publishable before moving on to a career in medicine or science.

So for two years the denizens of the Folkman lab left the looming question untouched, ignoring the silent challenge they walked by every day. "I thought, 'God, I'll have to do this myself,'" Folkman recalls. "But that meant I would have to stop writing grants. And I can't keep the lab open and also do these kinds of experiments, which take eight to ten hours a day." And then, finally, someone took the bait.

It wasn't someone Folkman was originally very optimistic about. When Michael O'Reilly arrived in July 1991, he had so little research experience that he'd just barely managed to win a spot in the lab. He wasn't an obvious candidate to take on one of the biggest challenges facing Folkman's team.

By this point, the competition for the half-dozen postdoctoral fellowships chosen annually in Folkman's lab had become downright fierce. Folkman had finally reached the point where extraordinarily well qualified young people from all around the world were vying to work with him. Hundreds of applications came in every year, so many that Folkman couldn't even answer them all. Only the people who tried over and over again even got replies. In making his selections, Folkman tried to identify young people who not only had solid research experience, but who had already done something extraordinary—young M.D.'s or biomedical scholars who had gone beyond superior academic work. "Good grades are important, but they don't show you somebody who will move out and away from the ordinary," Folkman says.

At first glance, O'Reilly seemed to be a fine young physician but not a strong contender for one of the coveted research fellowships. O'Reilly's father, a financial consultant with the accounting firm Coopers & Lybrand, had served as chairman of the board of trustees at the Dana-Farber Cancer Institute. The younger O'Reilly, a Tufts medical school graduate, had done well in a surgical training program at the University of Massachusetts Medical Center. He hoped to go into pediatric surgery, but his mentors at UMass advised him to get some research experience first. Folkman's lab at Children's Hospital seemed ideal—if he could win a spot. But his application for a fellowship didn't impress Folkman. "I had him way down on the list," Folkman recalls. "He had terrific letters, but he had no research experience, and we rarely take anyone with no research experience." But it was one of those letters—actually two sentences in the letter—that saved O'Reilly from the reject pile, giving him a fighting chance.

The letter was from Dr. Al Wheeler, chief of surgery at the UMass Medical Center, promising that O'Reilly was someone special. "If there's something no one else can figure out, he figures it out," Wheeler wrote. O'Reilly had figured out, for instance, that a mixture of saline solution and dextrose kept intravenous tubes open when blood cells tended to clump together and clog them up. Wheeler also advised Folkman that O'Reilly "is a guy who cannot be outworked." That, too, caught the attention of Folkman the workaholic. It was reminiscent of his own inclinations when he was a fledgling physician working in the surgical laboratory with Robert Gross. So Folkman gave O'Reilly an interview, and he liked what he heard. He decided to give O'Reilly a shot.

Joining the incoming class of postdocs in summer 1991, O'Reilly met with Folkman his first day in the lab to discuss what he would be doing. Folkman had a number of possible projects laid out, but O'Reilly had his eye on something else: the top of the "burning questions" list, the enticing problem of how tumors suppressed their metastases. Well, said Folkman, that one's no sure bet, but it's definitely the most interesting. If you're up to the challenge, sure, give it a go.

O'Reilly started by going back to the fundamentals, diving first into the medical literature, which showed that doctors had first recorded this enigmatic relationship between primary and secondary tumors as far back as 1895. By now, a century later, the effect was well known, almost taken for granted as a problem that probably couldn't be solved. O'Reilly had seen the phenomenon himself during medical school; he even remembered the cases. Now he found himself considering all the speculations he found in the literature: the idea that cutting the primary tumor out allowed some cancer cells to escape to distant parts of the body; the possibility that an immune reaction was at play; and the notion that the tumor was releasing a substance that inhibited growth of the metastases, somehow keeping cancer cells from dividing and forcing them to remain quiescent within the small tumors that had settled in distant organs. This was close to Folkman's theory, except that Folkman wasn't talking about the primary tumor's ability to stop the growth of cancer cells; he was talking about its ability to stop the growth of blood vessels—of angiogenesis.

O'Reilly read Noel Bouck's *Cell* paper and saw, as Folkman did, how beautifully it demonstrated that a small residue of thrombospondin leaked out of mutant tumor cells even after they had turned down production of the supposed growth-inhibiting molecule. That small amount of inhibitor was enough to keep the metastases from growing. To Folkman, it meant that in some cases when surgeons excised a big, primary tumor they were actually removing the only source of inhibiting molecules that were keeping metastases under control. That realization became a vital piece of the puzzle. Angiogenesis researchers were seeing the outline of a whole new physiological phenomenon. The obvious task for anyone who wanted to conquer that entry at the top of the "burning questions" list was to track down and identify those inhibitors. Surely there were others, maybe more potent than Bouck's thrombospondin. What were they? *Where* were they? And, for that matter, what was thrombospondin?

O'Reilly realized quickly that the literature offered him very little to go on, and that he would have to break new ground and devise experiments that would help point him in a direction that would uncover one of these purported growth-inhibiting factors. It was a tall order indeed for someone so inexperienced in the lab—especially after the National Cancer Institute summarily rejected a grant proposal Folkman had written to support O'Reilly's work. Folkman was convinced the idea was right, and he saw that O'Reilly understood the concept and was as hard a worker as he'd seen. O'Reilly was already deep into mouse tumor fluid, using separation columns to try to find an inhibitor. Though he couldn't isolate the factor from the special tumors that seemed to inhibit their metastases, he did demonstrate in the special assays—the rabbit eyes and the chicken embryos—that the inhibitor was present: It blocked the growth of blood vessels. Now he had to find it.

Few researchers outside Folkman's laboratory had even heard of the new thesis that there was a balance between growth-stimulating and -inhibiting factors, so it failed to resonate strongly with review committees at granting agencies. "We wrote a beautiful grant," Folkman says. "We said we had an inhibitor, and we described how it worked. But they turned it down completely, saying it was impossible." The reviewers at the NCI had a logical argument: They contended that if there was a protein circulating in the body that could inhibit tumors, then there shouldn't be *any* tumors. They didn't buy the teeter-totter idea.

Being turned down by the NCI was something of a disaster, because O'Reilly's research had proceeded while the grant request was under consideration. In fact, Folkman and O'Reilly were burning money on the project, trying to purify the unknown inhibiting molecule without actually having the money to do it. The work was expensive—hundreds of mice were needed, and it cost three thousand dollars a month just to keep them alive and healthy, while the separation columns could cost as much as four thousand dollars each—and Folkman was using funds from his other grants to support O'Reilly's research. This tactic worked only until the hospital administration got wind of it. Having already spent two hundred thousand dollars from other accounts, Folkman realized that O'Reilly's work would soon grind to a halt.

Desperate to keep it going, Folkman contacted everyone he knew at the top of the major pharmaceutical companies. He went to Merck. No. He went to Upjohn. No. Hoffman-LaRoche. No. Everyone. They all knew him, and they gave him appointments, but they simply weren't interested in angiogenesis. It was more of the same what-have-you-got-that-we-can-put-in-a-bottle-in-six-months? syndrome. The landmarks of the previous decade—the discovery of the growth factors FGF and VEGF and the inhibitors TNP-470 and thrombospondin—had gotten serious attention for angiogenesis from research scientists but little interest from anyone who had anything to do with patients. The notion that this field might have any immediate practical use was simply not on the radar screen in mainline cancer research. Almost all the effort and money were still being poured into finding better chemotherapy approaches, improved delivery of radiation, and new diagnostic means to find tumors earlier. Companies and clinicians were still viewing angiogenesis—and antiangiogenesis—as another laboratory curiosity: interesting, but not ready for prime time. "The pharmaceutical companies had not accepted it, and no oncologist had accepted it," Folkman later said.

Folkman next decided to try the flock of small new biotechnology companies headquartered around Kendall Square in Cambridge. Several of them understood exactly what Folkman was trying to do and said they loved it. What they didn't do was write a check. They had limited amounts of venture capital, and were already spending what they had on their own high-risk projects. They couldn't afford another. But Folkman found it refreshing at least to be rejected for practical reasons, not because of doubts about the merits of the research. He decided to widen the search to other companies that might have a few dollars to spare. He and O'Reilly wrote to just about every major biotechnology company in America—nearly one hundred letters in all. The response was lukewarm, at best. Ultimately, in fact, the only company that had any real interest at all came in through the back door, with neither a great deal of money nor a whole lot of experience.

The connection came through Robert D'Amato, a young research ophthalmologist in Folkman's lab who was working on ways to use antiangiogenesis to prevent blindness. A decade earlier, after winning a high school science contest, D'Amato had worked for a neurophysiologist, Dr. John Holaday, at the Walter Reed Army Medical Center in Washington. They had become friends, and years later Holaday started a biotech company in Rockville, Maryland. Its first project was aimed at developing a vaccine against high cholesterol.

Catching up on the phone one day a few months after Holaday started the company in 1991, D'Amato offhandedly mentioned that Folkman was having trouble getting financial support for his latest project, the pursuit of angiogenesis inhibitors. The work so far was promising, but neither the government nor any of the large pharmaceutical companies—Merck, Upjohn, and the rest—was interested in supporting it. "I can't believe these big companies aren't showing any interest," Holaday told D'Amato. Then Holaday asked, somewhat sheepishly, "Do you think Judah might be willing to talk to us, even though we're small?" D'Amato said he wasn't sure; he knew Folkman was looking for "big-time support"—he was used to dealing only with companies like Monsanto and Takeda—and that negotiations, though tenuous, were still semiactive with several companies. Holaday's company, EntreMed, meanwhile, was less than a year old and had limited venture capital to support its own work in vaccines, as well as anything else it wanted to do. Still, D'Amato thought, you never know. He agreed to arrange a meeting between Holaday and Folkman.

Holaday and a few of his executives flew up to Boston in April 1992, but they realized quickly that Folkman was not thinking seriously about hooking up with EntreMed for the major work of the lab. "Judah's attitude was that maybe they could do some work with him on a small project, and we started thinking about them giving us a grant to work on that," D'Amato recalls. But over the next few months, it became clear that Folkman couldn't afford to be too choosy. "The negotiations with the big companies just got even more sour," D'Amato says. "They were all starting to leave the table." And as everyone else's interest waned, Holaday's rose. Over the summer, he and Folkman exchanged letters that made it clear that Holaday was moving toward an offer Folkman might find hard to resist. "We talked about a million and a half dollars annually, when we only had between three and five million for the company," Holaday says. "So we were betting the store on this. We realized that it was a real opportunity."

Still, Folkman was skeptical that EntreMed had the wherewithal to support O'Reilly's ambitious project. Later that summer, Folkman went to Toronto to give a talk; from there he was going to fly to Europe to visit several large drug companies he hoped might be more interested than their American counterparts. Holaday decided to fly to Toronto, and he met with Folkman in a hotel room. "We went there to convince him we were serious, to convince him we had the moxie to get into this," Holaday said. He believed so strongly in the search for antiangiogenesis agents that he would raise additional capital to fund much of the laboratory.

Ultimately, Folkman agreed: EntreMed would supply Folkman's lab with two million dollars a year for three years. Holaday and EntreMed were in fact betting the store. But they would own the rights to develop and market any antiangiogenesis agents that emerged.

O'REILLY DUG INTO THE PROJECT with all his energy. He first set out to develop a reliable living system in which the proposed tumor-inhibition phenomenon could be clearly observed. The way to start, he decided, was to develop a mouse in which a primary tumor was especially good at blocking the growth of its own metastases. To find that mouse and that tumor, O'Reilly began what was to become a year of screening different kinds of tumors to find just the right one. It was a rather informal search: He nosed around Folkman's big research department and other laboratories, asking everyone about the tumors they were working with, collecting samples of tumor tissue for his own studies. His quest was to find especially aggressive primary tumors that would not only grow well when implanted into mice, but—more important—had the ability to keep their tiny metastasized seeds from sprouting. Using various staining techniques, he could spot the dormant metastases, as well as the blood vessels that sat nearby but didn't sprout branches toward the tumors.

Most of O'Reilly's initial experiments were flops. Standing at a high laboratory bench, he would implant aggressive tumors in the animals. The tumors grew, but they failed to inhibit their metastases. The work was repetitive and time-consuming—and the mice bit. Finally, after many months of searching, O'Reilly tried a variety of lung cancer called Lewis lung carcinoma and hit upon a way of measuring its activity on metastases. He implanted the tumors onto the mice's backs and waited for the cancer to metastasize to the lungs and begin growing. Then he'd euthanize the mice and weigh their lungs to see which tumors had been most effective at inhibiting the growth of their metastases. Eventually, he found a Lewis lung carcinoma that blocked its metastases by about 70 percent. But it wasn't enough. He wanted a tumor that kept its metastases completely dormant—pouring out enough of the mysterious substance to inhibit them not by 70 percent, but by 100 percent.

O'Reilly had an idea. He implanted ten mice with the Lewis lung carcinomas and identified which one best kept its metastases under control. Then he removed that tumor and implanted pieces of it in ten more mice. Each of those tiny slices became a new, individual tumor—with its own, individual properties, with genes constantly mutating—so that O'Reilly again could identify the one among ten that was best at inhibiting its metastases. By going

from generation to generation—like trying to improve corn by always re-
planting only seeds from the previous year's tallest plants—O'Reilly was able
to identify a promising tumor after a couple of months. (He also did the opposite, selecting some tumors that were less and less able to block their own
metastases, using them as a kind of negative control.)

The Lewis lung carcinoma that best controlled its metastases behaved exactly the way O'Reilly wanted. Every time one of these tumors was implanted
in a mouse, it grew aggressively—while the flood of metastatic cells it released
into the bloodstream remained dormant. The tiny satellite tumors settled in
the lungs and remained, doing nothing, as the big primary tumor grew dramatically on the animal's back until it overpowered it. The carcinoma was so
lethal that it killed a mouse within twenty-one days of implantation. Meanwhile, the metastases were so small that they remained almost microscopic,
even up to the moment of death. So now the question was what would happen
if the mouse was saved by surgery. If the primary tumor was removed, would
the metastases remain dormant as before, or would they be unleashed?
O'Reilly cut the big, implanted tumor off the first mouse's back, and the news
was big: The dormant metastases suddenly blossomed, overwhelming the
mouse's lungs within two weeks! So O'Reilly had found his first mouse
model. Now he could begin exploring the inhibition phenomenon. He could
start the search for the inhibiting factor that seemed to block blood vessel
growth.

To begin the hunt, O'Reilly put these aggressive metastatic tumor cells
into tissue culture and searched through the liquid growth medium, the fluid
in which the cancer cells were multiplying, hoping to find the mystery factor.
No luck. O'Reilly couldn't detect any inhibitor molecules present when he
tested the growth medium in the lab's angiogenesis assay systems. Only later
would O'Reilly realize why simply studying cells growing in culture dishes
wouldn't be the answer: Their action too closely resembled what happened in
the mice with primary tumors. In culture, as in a mouse, the big primary
tumor made a vast excess of stimulator, overpowering the inhibiting effect. So
O'Reilly wasn't able to find any signs of the inhibitor molecules.

Stumped, O'Reilly decided to take advantage of his surroundings. He solicited the help and advice of the many researchers who worked throughout
the lab. Postdoctoral fellow Rosalind Rosenthal, biochemist Yuen Shing, and
biochemist Helene Sage were particularly helpful, and eventually O'Reilly
decided to give up on tissue culture and scour the mice's blood. Maybe the
elusive inhibiting factors could be found there. He began drawing blood both

from mice burdened with huge tumors and those that were tumor-free. He soon found that there was a difference—not only between the healthy and sick mice, but among the mice with tumors. If he took blood circulating far from the tumor, say in the tail, and then tested the serum with bovine endothelial cells growing in a culture dish, he found that a factor in the blood inhibited the growth of the cells. Conversely, blood from near the tumor seemed to contain stimulating agents. The tests indicated, as Folkman had suspected, that short-lived stimulating agents were effective close to the tumor, but not far away.

There had to be something in the blood coming from the tumor that could block the formation of new blood vessels, something potent. It not only inhibited new blood vessel growth, it stopped it cold. What was it?

O'Reilly put the serum through several purification steps and began testing the fractions on endothelial cells. He did this week after week, month after month, hoping—as Folkman had hoped years earlier when he was searching for the angiogenesis-stimulating factor TAF—that he could isolate the inhibiting factor. Eventually O'Reilly concluded that he was headed down a blind alley. After about a year and a half of collecting serum and trying to purify it, he had to concede that the serum had too many proteins in it. He sent off a sample for an analysis of the proteins, in the hope of deciphering the arrangement of amino acids and perhaps getting enough information to identify the protein molecule and its function. But if too many proteins are present in a sample, such a protein sequence analysis gets terribly messy. Sure enough, the information was essentially useless. As O'Reilly recalls, "You go from having an overwhelmingly large number of proteins to a bit less overwhelmingly large. We were able to get down to not-quite-clean-enough; we couldn't get it to a hundred percent pure."

The messy sequencing results were a blow, but O'Reilly found a new possibility one day when he attended one of the regular grand rounds lectures, a periodic seminar on a given topic presented at Children's Hospital. The speaker's topic was cellular growth factors, and he touched on techniques that could be used in searching for growth factors in live animals. At one point, he began talking about purification methods and brought up urine as one place to start. O'Reilly sat up. Could the inhibitor he had been searching for in the mice's blood serum also be found in their urine? He loved the notion. In his words, "You would get the mouse's kidney to do the work for you." It would be a kind of natural, built-in filtration system helping him extract the mystery fluid from the blood. O'Reilly headed immediately for the library to do more learning—this time about all the techniques and pitfalls of isolating specific proteins from urine. What he read convinced him that it could be done. Molecules of the mystery inhibitor might well be ending up on the bottom of all those mouse cages.

As it turned out, collecting a little mouse urine was not hard at all. But collecting *a lot* of it was a real problem. O'Reilly was able to devise special cages with mesh bottoms and funnels to collect extremely clean mouse urine. Trouble was, mice are small, and don't pee a lot. The little urine that did trickle down through the funnels tended to evaporate too quickly; the samples often dried up before they could be used. To solve that problem, O'Reilly began feeding the animals large amounts of sugar water. The mice began urinating prodigiously, enough so that the fluid could finally be collected and O'Reilly could begin his experiments.

There had to be two collection systems, one for the mice dying of cancer, one for those spared. Testing in the cell culture assay revealed that, yes, the urine of mice that were growing tumors contained an inhibitor of endothelial cell growth. And no sign of an inhibitor was found in urine from mice that were not burdened with tumors. O'Reilly thus had his biggest triumph since joining Folkman's lab. The work was obviously worth pursuing further, even though the costs were high. The next step was to begin scaling up his urine collection system, stacking cages together and running collection tubes down to a big container. O'Reilly got the idea for his drainage apparatus from a maple syrup farm he remembered visiting in Vermont. Instead of using buckets, the farmer put tubing on the spigots and ran the tubing all the way downhill into the sugar shack. O'Reilly jury-rigged a similar system. He ran plastic tubing down into a Styrofoam box chilled with ice, because warm urine can serve as a growth medium for bacteria.

Once the system was up and running with forty mice, O'Reilly collected urine three or four times a day, sterilized it, and stored it in plastic bags for the separation process. Collecting all of this urine did not make O'Reilly especially popular among the three dozen researchers in Folkman's increasingly crowded tenth-floor lab; fresh mouse urine exudes a most unpleasant odor. O'Reilly found that after a while he got used to the stench, and it was not without its upside. "I found it was a great way to get space," he recalls. "Dr. Folkman attracts so many people that his laboratory is always crowded, and for the first couple of years—before I was ever working with mouse urine—I had a box I would carry around, and I would just find a space and start working. But then I found if you come in with a big vat full of mouse urine and plop it down, people tend to move out of the way—and they don't come back for a while."

Trying to extract a very tiny amount of inhibitor from a vast amount of mouse urine was an extraordinarily time-consuming task; it was a harsh introduction to day-to-day research for O'Reilly. Using separation columns and other methods, doing the work step-by-step and over and over, each stage taking hours and each mistake setting the process back, O'Reilly took a full year to collect the first ten liters of mouse urine and process it to extract the unidentified inhibiting factor. The work finally yielded about two hundred nanograms—two hundred billionths of a gram—of the inhibiting protein, enough to send out to a specialized laboratory for analysis of its amino acid sequence, and perhaps identification. Such labs existed because of the burgeoning revolution in molecular biology, which was making it possible to read the molecular structure of a protein, such as a growth factor, and determine the exact arrangement of the amino acids, its fundamental building blocks.

When the data came back, O'Reilly was surprised to learn that his mystery substance was not unfamiliar: It was plasmin, a fragment of a larger, relatively well known protein molecule called plasminogen, a product of the liver. This was good news: Plasminogen had already been carefully studied, so the information available in the literature gave O'Reilly a head start in understanding the role it might have in angiogenesis. Plasminogen is normally found in the blood, where it is an "inactive precursor" for plasmin—essentially a form in which a necessary molecule can be stored dormantly as part of a bigger molecule. When needed, as in response to injury, special enzymes snip the precursor molecule into fragments, which are ready to go to work immediately to help repair the damage. It offers the body a quick way to respond when it would take too long to turn on a set of genes to make a necessary molecule—like having an ambulance warmed up and ready to go, rather than taking the time to build an ambulance while a person is bleeding. For plasmin to be activated, it must first be snipped out of the larger plasminogen molecule. Once it is free, plasmin's role in the bloodstream is to break up the gluelike structure of blood clots, a mechanism that is vital to ensure that blood always keeps flowing throughout the body, especially to vital organs such as the brain.

Although the new sequencing data and the research that produced it seemed clean, O'Reilly had some qualms about its accuracy. It was not impossible that what he and his colleagues had isolated might just be a stray contaminant that had inadvertently slipped into their protein sample. Even some people in the laboratory that did the sequencing advised O'Reilly against assuming any conclusions about plasmin and plasminogen based on a single test. Uncomfortable with such doubts, and hoping to avoid the quibbling that so often accompanied the novel reports from Folkman's laboratory, O'Reilly scaled up his mouse urine factory, processed another forty liters, and sent a larger batch of the protein—a few micrograms—out for reanalysis. The new data was the same as the first: The protein's biochemical structure was unmistakable. It consisted of "kringle loops," each resembling a pretzel-shaped European cookie of the same name. It was the structure of plasmin.

The discovery that the angiogenesis inhibitor is chopped out of plasmin offered the first insight into a new, unifying concept: that the human body gets much more bang from its bucks by using a large molecule for one function, then—like using the change from a dollar bill—breaking the molecule down into fragments that perform other functions. "It showed us that the body is storing two functions in one protein," O'Reilly says. It was too soon to say that the molecule they were chasing would be a potent anticancer weapon, but the discovery did suggest that there were more places to look for angiogenesis inhibitors than they thought. It suggested that even fragments of proteins ought to be studied.

The identification of the inhibiting factor as a part of plasmin was also very good news from a practical standpoint. Now that they were satisfied that the protein isolated from the mouse urine was a fragment of plasminogen, O'Reilly and Folkman realized they didn't have to go through all the time and effort to collect, purify, and analyze the growth-inhibiting protein. It would be much simpler just to go out and buy human plasminogen from a commercial lab and use chemical processing—mixing in enzymes that acted like chemical scissors—to produce the plasmin.

After running numerous experiments to prove that the protein isolated from mouse urine and the protein produced from commercial plasminogen were essentially the same, O'Reilly and Folkman set out to squeeze enough of the molecule from plasminogen to plan the most important experiments yet. They wanted to see whether their new purified substance would actually do anything in cancer-bearing animals. But first they had to decide what to call the agent they had separated out of the plasminogen. At one of the regular Friday lab meetings in 1994, two dozen names were debated for an hour— "That sounds like a shaving cream," someone said of one of the contenders— before one of Folkman's suggestions was adopted. The molecule would be called angiostatin, a combination of word fragments meaning "to stop blood vessels." Now they were ready to see if it was worth anything—to see whether it would block angiogenesis, and cancer.

THROUGHOUT MICHAEL O'REILLY'S FIRST three years in Folkman's almost frantically busy laboratory, where experiments were under way on bench tops, in incubators, and lab dishes all around him—and with Judah Folkman looking in occasionally to see how he was progressing—O'Reilly had encountered persistent doubts and even disparaging remarks about the idea he was pursuing. At the lab bench, he would occasionally be advised by a neighbor that it was useless, he was wasting his time, he should get on with something that might actually be productive. Outside the laboratory, too, there were abundant doubts about the wisdom of his quest. Some of his fellow postdocs considered his research a doomed venture. The problem was that few thought that inhibitors would be produced by tumors. If they were, wouldn't tumors inhibit themselves? Folkman was impressed that O'Reilly carried on despite such a discouraging atmosphere. "Anybody else would have given up," he later reflected.

So now it was time to see if the doubters were right—time to test angiostatin on animals. It had to be done with extraordinary care, not only because O'Reilly needed thoroughly documented and repeatable results, but also because he had only a tiny amount of the drug and couldn't afford to waste a drop. If he ran out of material in mid-experiment, it could set his work back by months, maybe longer. Of course, there was no way to predict if the experiments would work at all, and there was always the risk that his animals would die. Then O'Reilly would have to try to figure out why.

To get started, O'Reilly implanted large, metastasizing Lewis lung tumors on the backs of fifteen mice and watched the cancers grow. Then, after a little more than two weeks, he removed the massive tumors surgically and divided the mice into three groups of five. The first group would get small daily injections of angiostatin. The second group would get shots of the bigger molecule, plasminogen. The third group would get no treatment at all, only injections of saline solution. And then the hard part began: the waiting. Everyone in the lab was aware of O'Reilly's apprehension. They saw him make trip after trip into the mouse rooms to check out his animals, make sure the injections were being given, and watch, and watch, and watch. The plan was to wait until the untreated mice began to die, and then to euthanize and cut open all fifteen subjects to compare what happened to their lungs. O'Reilly couldn't predict how long the experiments would take, but he hoped to avoid setbacks that might push them past 120 days. That's about how long the supply of angiostatin would hold out.

O'Reilly knew from previous experiments that the Lewis lung tumors' metastases were surely growing wildly in the lungs of the untreated mice. But what was happening inside the bodies of mice that were being given angiostatin? Were their lungs filling with metastasized tumors, or was the angiostatin inhibiting new blood vessel growth and keeping the metastases dormant? O'Reilly and Folkman got their first clue about ten days in. The untreated mice were slowing down. They were less active than normal, short of breath. The mice in the angiostatin group looked normal. Folkman had worked with mice for so many years that he he could almost sense what was going on in the animals. He taught O'Reilly all the signs of a healthy mouse: nice pink ears, a coat with a glossy sheen, vigorously active inside the cage, a hearty appetite. Folkman picked up a mouse by its tail, and it urinated down his sleeve. Folkman smiled. "Yeah, if they do that you know they're healthy," he told O'Reilly with a laugh.

The other ten mice, meanwhile, were getting sicker and sicker. O'Reilly suspected they would begin to die in a few days, so he started visiting them every few hours, and came in to check on them several times at night. The worst thing would be to arrive in the morning and find the mice dead, before the research team had a chance to look for differences between the control animals and those getting regular doses of angiostatin. O'Reilly and Folkman wanted a clean experiment, and that meant dissecting all fifteen mice at the same time to minimize the variables.

One Thursday afternoon, O'Reilly looked in on the mice and saw that one of the untreated ones was about to die. He ran into Folkman's office and told him the time had come. "Oh, everyone's going to want to see this!" Folkman said excitedly. He went around the lab announcing, "If you want to see how well angiostatin works, come on down." After three years of struggle, of pouring urine day after day, of caging mice and implanting tumors, and now of two weeks of angiostatin injections, O'Reilly's work was reaching its climax. With a horde of excited researchers jam-packed into a small laboratory room, Folkman euthanized all fifteen mice, then began handing them one by one to O'Reilly to dissect. O'Reilly took the first mouse, made an incision in its chest, and removed the lung. The organ was overwhelmed by cancer. Folkman checked a notebook to see which group the mouse had been in. It was one of those that had gotten only saline. O'Reilly cut into the next mouse and removed its lung. It was perfect. What treatment had it gotten? The notebook revealed it was angiostatin.

The excitement was building. The murmuring hubbub in the little room got louder as Folkman picked up the mice and handed them off to O'Reilly, who would open their tiny chests and pass them back for others to see. Mouse by mouse, minute by minute, the results were stunning, far outrunning even Folkman's eager optimism. He and O'Reilly had been expecting there would be some differences between the treated mice and the control mice, but the results then passing through their hands were almost overwhelming. The lungs from the mice given angiostatin were pristine. Just as clear was that the angiogenesis-inhibiting drug worked—it blocked metastasis, at least in mice. Here, for the first time, was the solid, convincing evidence that he had sought for almost half a lifetime. It was a strange and wonderful thing to be nose-to-nose with reality, not speculation, and to see that he had been right all along.

As the lab members talked excitedly, speculating over the amazing results, O'Reilly kept going through the mice one by one, weighing their lungs, counting the metastases to provide good, firm data to report in research papers. He was trying to concentrate on what he was seeing, no easy thing while everyone else was buzzing in celebration, spouting ideas and theories about what had occurred, offering suggestions for what to do next. The gleeful scientists knew the results meant antiangiogenesis worked. By struggling together and never giving up, Folkman and the people who worked with him had kicked open the door to a new world of biomedicine. When O'Reilly came to the Friday lab meeting the next morning, Folkman smiled, told him, "Good job," and patted him on the back. Later, he handed O'Reilly a big bottle of champagne and told him to go celebrate with his wife, and to tell her all that work with smelly mouse pee was worth it.

And when he was sure of what he had, Folkman called John Holaday at EntreMed and told him his investment was beginning to pay off.

FOR THE FOLKMAN TEAM, and especially for O'Reilly, the real payoff—the kind that puts academic careers into overdrive—came in fall 1994, when a major peer-reviewed report detailing O'Reilly's experiments was published as the cover article in *Cell,* one of biology's most prestigious journals. O'Reilly, of course, was listed as first author, followed by seven colleagues and, last, by Folkman as the laboratory's chief. "It was the equivalent of seven papers in one," Folkman said, and indeed, there was enough work in it to sustain several reports.

The paper was big news in the science world—a wake-up call for the cancer establishment. It contained clear evidence that Folkman and his colleagues were on to something big that had to be taken seriously. Theories that had been dismissed over and over again as mere laboratory curiosities were beginning to take on real shape and substance. And even though O'Reilly's paper got very little public notice—the news media mostly ignored it—workers in other laboratories began taking angiogenesis seriously. The number of research papers on the topic would jump from a handful to hundreds within the next few years, and requests came in to Folkman's laboratory daily asking him to share research materials. For Folkman, the sudden popularity of angiogenesis as a research topic was in itself a major milestone.

O'Reilly, meanwhile, was enjoying the benefits of getting the cover of *Cell* his first time out. It meant instant credibility for a young doctor who was an unknown in the world of scientific research. It was to be the first in a series of high-profile publications for O'Reilly, whose achievements would attract many job offers from other medical centers over the next few years—offers of tenure-track positions, along with huge, well-funded laboratory facilities. But O'Reilly hoped to remain at Harvard and stay with the man who gave him his chance. Soon Folkman would begin including in his presentations a slide of O'Reilly, accompanied by a wry tribute. "When people first come to the laboratory in July," he would say, "I sit down with everybody and say that our goal for you, for your career in this lab, is to increase your scientific self-confidence as soon as possible. That's our overriding goal, no matter what it requires. How to pose a testable question. How to give a talk. What to do when the slides fall out, all of that. O'Reilly's first paper in his life got the cover of *Cell*. His second paper was in *Nature Medicine*. His third paper in *Cell*. His fourth in *Science*. So his self-confidence has reached unmanageable levels."

Despite the excitement of the success with angiostatin, however, Folkman knew well that when it came to angiogenesis, even the most solid results would face doubts. Critics would argue that finding this particular agent was a fluke, that it was "a special case" that could not be repeated in other animals, in other laboratories, by other researchers. And indeed, reports began to surface that other labs were having trouble making angiostatin. It turned out to be a fragile molecule that had to be handled properly. Folkman blanched at this convention of science that held that if someone couldn't immediately duplicate a piece of work, it meant the work was wrong or even dishonest. He called this the Stradivarius Syndrome. Stradivarius made magnificent violins; that others couldn't make equally magnificent violins didn't mean Stradivarius was a fraud.

But it also meant that Folkman's lab would have to refine or standardize the experimental system so everyone could use it and no one could doubt it. Because critics were also likely to argue that the new results were limited to mice and should not be extrapolated to humans, Folkman suggested that O'Reilly develop another system using tumors taken from humans. It would at least answer half the question: He would be working with human tumors, even if they were still extracting the angiostatin from mice. The goal, of course, was to make angiostatin in its human form, and then try it as an anti-cancer drug. But first, they needed to learn how to make more angiostatin. A lot more.

Several months before, after he had first purified angiostatin from those vats full of mouse urine and discovered it was a normal fragment of plasminogen, O'Reilly had taken another look into the literature and found that angiostatin, which he was cleaving out of plasminogen, had actually been described back in the 1970s. At the time, of course, no one knew what the nameless molecule was or what it did. He also found several reports in the literature about how to make the molecule the Folkman team was now calling angiostatin. The reports were written mostly by Lars Sottrup-Jensen, a Danish biochemist at the University of Aarhus who was working on the subject of plasminogen because of increasing interest in the blood clotting system as it related to heart attacks and circulatory problems.

In those early papers exploring the properties of plasminogen, Sottrup-Jensen had suggested that the plasminogen molecule could be cleaved by enzymes into smaller pieces, and he had advised researchers to look at each resulting fragment and study what its activity might be. It seemed possible that a chunk of protein liberated from a larger molecule might be active, either performing some function or doing harm. O'Reilly had pursued Sottrup-Jenson's suggestion and referenced the Danish work in his *Cell* paper. Seeing that, Sottrup-Jensen sent him a copy of an older paper on the subject, and a congratulatory note saying he was pleased that the protein fragment now named angiostatin had such potent activity against tumors.

Now that O'Reilly had done just what Sottrup-Jensen had advised—had identified angiostatin and sorted out what it was—the next step, a crucial one, was to locate and copy the genes that make angiostatin so that the drug could be naturally manufactured in large enough amounts to run major experiments. Biotechnology had reached the point where the easiest, cheapest, and most reliable way to obtain proteins such as angiostatin was to engineer living microbes to make it, rather than trying to isolate it from complex fluids such as blood or urine. By using gene-splicing technology to engineer the angiostatin-making genes into bacteria, yeast, or cells from insects or mammals, they could be coaxed into producing an endless supply of the drug, far more than could be extracted from even the largest vat of mouse urine.

The process was relatively quick. The genes involved in making the parent molecule, plasminogen, had already been found, so it was easy for one of Folkman's postdocs, Li Jin, to scan through the chemical coding of the large gene that makes plasminogen and identify the specific portion that makes the smaller fragment, angiostatin. With a gene-cloning technique called the polymerase chain reaction, which can be used to easily copy a gene in unlimited numbers, the team could get enough copies of the gene to use in their cell-based production system and accelerate the testing of angiostatin. Then, once they had the mouse version of the gene, the researchers could go after the human and dog versions to expand the research.

At EntreMed, the discovery of angiostatin was the biggest moment in the company's brief history. But as EntreMed's technicians began trying to scale up production of the drug by putting the gene into *Pichia pastoris* yeast cells, John Holaday had some serious thinking to do. He was, needless to say, feeling very good that EntreMed had been the one company among hundreds to take a chance and support Folkman's laboratory. But now he and his colleagues realized their small company might need some help moving the research along, and he began to pursue partnerships with major pharmaceutical firms. One that was interested was the big German firm Boehringer Ingleheim, which was strong in the production of protein products such as antibiotics and other medicines but had little experience with cancer drugs. Another was Bristol-Myers Squibb, the world's leading manufacturer of cancer drugs. But after some talks, Bristol-Myers decided against teaming up with EntreMed, apparently because its top executives, like those at many other pharmaceutical giants, weren't convinced, even by the results with the mice, that antiangiogenesis had much future.

At least they weren't convinced by EntreMed. As it happened, Judah Folkman was a member of the Bristol-Myers scientific advisory board, and the company's new president for research, Leon Rosenberg, had nominated him for the prestigious General Motors Prize for cancer research. Soon after

Bristol-Myers decided against a partnership with EntreMed, Folkman won the 1997 award and went to Rockefeller University in New York to accept, bringing with him a talk explaining his research. Folkman gave one of his trademark lectures, a fascinating and optimistic presentation of the work that was under way, its scientific background, his thinking about cancer, and a few glimpses of the latest encouraging results from his laboratory, especially the successes of angiostatin. The talk was a revelation, even to Leon Rosenberg.

Soon thereafter, John Holaday found a helicopter descending on EntreMed in Maryland, and Rosenberg and a squad of executives piled out. Over dinner in Holaday's small executive dining room, the Bristol-Myers people made it clear they were interested in EntreMed, Judah Folkman, and angiogenesis. The deal that was eventually worked out called for Bristol-Myers to buy an equity stake in the young company in order to gain access to some of the rights to angiostatin. The five-year deal called for Bristol-Myers to make standard annual payments to support research and development, plus pay so-called milestone fees when EntreMed achieved certain goals. Bristol-Myers also won the right to license other molecules of interest that might emerge in such research. Because the research was so new, EntreMed was sublicensing discovery not of an actual drug that might soon be given to patients, but of a biological molecule that was not yet well defined or close to being understood. So the discovery of angiostatin was akin to finding a new insulin, or a new growth hormone, without knowing how it might work. In fact, it was similar to the deal Harvard and Monsanto had made two decades earlier, when Folkman and Bert Vallee were chasing a molecule that was still mostly an idea, the long-elusive angiogenesis stimulator, TAF. But this was much less risky for Bristol-Myers: Angiostatin was more than an idea. The big task was to find an efficient and economical way to produce large enough amounts of the drug to make it clinically—and commercially—viable.

EntreMed and Bristol-Myers weren't the only ones pouring money into angiogenesis inhibitors however. Now they were joined anew by an institution that had been a key supporter of angiogenesis research over the years for Folkman: the federal government. His lab's original request for support of O'Reilly's work had been turned down cold, but now things were suddenly different. After that glorious day when they'd found that angiostatin blocked lung cancer in mice, and after O'Reilly wrote up the results and had them accepted by *Cell,* the National Cancer Institute took a different view. Folkman submitted an updated grant proposal and included a prepublication printout of O'Reilly's paper. This time the grant committee decided that maybe it was worth funding the work after all. "Of course when it's in *Cell*, they'll accept it," Folkman later said derisively. "That shows the great wisdom of the review committee, how much vision they have. They have zero vision. They have trouble dealing with new ideas."

Folkman wanted to keep the momentum going. Specifically, he wanted to find another similar factor, and maybe more. He was already hearing, as he knew he would, that the success of angiostatin was a special case, peculiar to only one kind of tumor, Lewis lung carcinoma. The obvious thing to do was find at least one other factor from another kind of tumor and show that it, too, blocked angiogenesis. Maybe angiostatin was just one member of a whole family of inhibiting molecules. O'Reilly had a big head start in trying to find them. After several years of collecting mouse urine, he knew how to avoid most of the pitfalls and dead ends he'd experienced in the search that led to angiostatin.

Folkman suggested O'Reilly try a special hemangioma he had in his storehouse of tumor samples. This one grew as a big blob of tissue surrounded by "sentinel" tumors that were all the same small size. "Why aren't there two or three big ones?" Folkman asked, the kind of question he'd been posing for decades. "Why is there one big one and ten little ones? And why all the same size? They shouldn't be." Because of the work of Folkman's lab, it was now fair to assume that the central tumor was releasing an inhibitor that blocked angiogenesis and kept the small tumors dormant. It was a matter of finding it.

O'Reilly began building another mouse system. In less than a year, as opposed to the three years it took to find angiostatin, he was able to isolate a second inhibiting molecule. Soon he demonstrated that the drug had the same inhibiting effect on metastases as angiostatin. At another Friday lab meeting, the new molecule was christened endostatin.

Not even Folkman and O'Reilly had grasped the power of the agents they now had in hand however. At first, they were ecstatic that angiostatin, and then endostatin, could keep small metastatic tumors from erupting and growing in the far reaches of the body. Understanding and controlling metastases, after all, was what O'Reilly was trying to do when he attacked the top of Folkman's "burning questions" list. And the results so far indicated that lives might be saved by beating back metastasis, the phenomenon that kills about 90 percent of cancer patients. But no one, not even Folkman, was thinking that angiostatin or endostatin might also be effective against *primary* tumors. The most they could hope for, Folkman was convinced, was to find agents that could be used as adjuvant treatments, drugs that would hold cancer back after primary treatments with more established therapies such as surgery, chemotherapy, and radiation. That was a big enough goal. But once O'Reilly discovered endostatin, people both inside and outside the laboratory began to ask, What about the primary tumor?

To see what might happen, Folkman and O'Reilly decided to give small daily doses of endostatin to four mice *before* rather than after the big tumors growing on their backs were surgically removed. The results were cause for jubilation: The massive tumors implanted onto the mice suddenly stopped growing, began drying up, shriveled down, and ultimately disappeared. The response went far beyond what anyone expected, showing vividly that the two anticancer agents had unprecedented power to attack and conquer even the most aggressive tumors. Folkman had only wanted to show that the agents could keep metastases from growing. Nothing in his and O'Reilly's previous experiments indicated that they could actually make primary tumors regress. Had he even raised that possibility, he surely would have heard the old mantra: Your conclusions go beyond your data.

The Folkman lab was definitely on a roll, but there was still a nagging worry that the tumors that were falling to angiostatin and endostatin might, like tumors treated with chemotherapy, develop resistance and no longer respond to the drugs. Folkman wanted to explore that possibility, and at the same time see what might happen to the mice if their tumors were driven into dormancy and then the doses of endostatin were stopped. So the researchers gave daily doses to a handful of mice, stopping once the tumors had regressed. Without treatment, the shrunken tumors began to regrow rapidly and within days had ballooned to their original size. Additional doses of endostatin were given, continuing long enough to drive the tumors down again. Then the treatments were stopped again. The tumors grew back once more. "We took it up and down, and after the fourth time everyone was saying, 'Why aren't you publishing this?' " O'Reilly recalls. "But I had noticed that on the fourth cycle not only were we not seeing any [drug] resistance, but the tumors seemed to be slowing down on the way up. I remember at lab meetings everyone saying, 'Oh, you're crazy! Just publish!' Except for Dr. Folkman, who said, 'No. No. Let's go on with this,' and he gave one of his motivational speeches about discoveries being missed because of what you've assumed. That quieted people down, except for Thomas Boehm, who was making all of the endostatin at that point. So we kept going, and sure enough after the fifth cycle it was even more dramatic in slowing down. And after six cycles, not only did it slow down, it didn't come back. We were getting self-sustained dormancy." In other words, it looked like a cure.

O'Reilly's presentation of his latest results at a lab meeting was a defining moment. He began showing his slides, mostly graphs and figures, punching through the images one by one and explaining the details. Then he put up one he quietly described as "an interesting graph." Its import didn't sink in immediately. People were chatting about previous meetings where O'Reilly had shown the tumors shrinking, then growing back again as angiostatin was stopped. They were well aware that the tumors could be shrunk, would grow again, and then be shrunk again. But the new graph went beyond just another up-and-down. Now the tumors went down—and stayed down. But such dramatic results could be a hard sell to researchers more used to incremental advances. These seemed almost too clear. Maybe it's an artifact, someone said—say the mice are starving. Or maybe the tumors are just coming back slowly. Folkman liked his postdocs to take their best shots at these meetings— "If you can defend your work at our fighting lab meetings, you'll do much better outside," he liked to say.

O'Reilly survived the in-house onslaught, but he wasn't through yet. He and Folkman wondered what would happen if they treated a cancerous mouse with both angiostatin *and* endostatin. Again, it took about two weeks for the tumor to regress and disappear. But instead of suspending the treatment to see if the tumor reappeared, Folkman wanted to keep going as long as possible—to the consternation of some staff members who pointed out how hard it was to make angiostatin. He urged them to keep giving the new agents for two more days, two more days, jesting at one point that if they wanted their salaries that week, they'd better keep the experiment going. Finally, after twenty-five days, they stopped. "We all bet twenty-five cents on when we thought [the tumor] would come back," Folkman said. "Everybody thought it would be one week, or ten days. I bet it would never come back." And it didn't. "The lesson here," Folkman told his colleagues as they paid their quarters, "is don't bet against the house."

The executives at EntreMed, of course, were thrilled with their gamble. The small start-up company had invested six million dollars in O'Reilly's work, and now they were anxious for the payoff. They wanted the work applied in the clinic. In mice, angiostatin and endostatin seemed to be 100 percent effective, vanquishing tumors with ease, and without the side effects that might have been expected of such potent drugs—not even inflammation at the injection sites. Nothing like this had ever been seen before, even in mice that had been cured with chemotherapy in other research laboratories in the past. The tumors on O'Reilly's mice were massive, making up 2 or 3 percent of the animals' body weight, and even with the most effective conventional treatments, they would not survive such a cancer load.

Remarkably, O'Reilly's experiments also showed that it didn't even matter what kinds of tumors were involved. The new antiangiogenesis treatments drove them all into dormancy and kept them there. Cancer of the breast, the colon, prostate, bladder, the brain—the results were always the same. "We don't even ask what kind of tumor it is anymore before we go down to give the treatments," Folkman said. It made sense to him because these antiangiogenic drugs were aimed not at the tumors themselves but at their life support systems, blood vessels. And all these blood vessels were the same. "We haven't lost a mouse yet," Folkman liked to say.

Then again, it is a long leap from mice to men. As one leading brain cancer specialist at the Dana–Farber Cancer Institute, Dr. Howard Fine, put it, "We've been curing *mice* of cancer for fifty years."

Chapter Fifteen

———

LATE ONE JUNE NIGHT IN 1994, five-year-old Jennifer LaChance appeared at the foot of the stairs in her home in Rhode Island and told her parents that her ear hurt. Her mother, Lillian LaChance, called her daughter's pediatrician, who prescribed antibiotic ear drops over the phone and instructed her to bring Jennifer in a week later. A week passed, and Jennifer hadn't improved. The pain persisted, and a little lump appeared on the left side of her lower jaw. Her doctor thought Jennifer, who had been in a pool, might have a case of swimmer's ear. The dose of antibiotics was doubled.

A week later, Michael and Lillian LaChance returned with their daughter. The lump had started getting bigger. Now the pediatrician was concerned and referred them to Hasbro Children's Hospital in Providence. There, X rays were taken, but they were inconclusive. Jennifer was next referred to an oral surgeon, Dr. Al Carlotti, who said he could probably remove the growth but wanted her to see Dr. Leonard Kaban instead. Kaban, at Massachusetts General Hospital, specialized in pediatric oral surgery and had recently moved from the University of California Medical School in San Francisco to become chief of maxillofacial surgery at Mass General, where he had earlier trained. The LaChances were told that Kaban ranked among the best oral surgeons anywhere, and his new corner office on the twelfth floor of the hospital's Warren Building, with a sweeping view of the Charles River and Cambridge to the north, suggested as much. When the LaChances went to see him, they noticed awards and mementos from his distinguished career in maxillofacial surgery lining the shelves near his Harvard Dental School diploma. Among them was the program from an Eagle Scout award ceremony Kaban had attended for a young boy whom he had treated successfully a dozen years earlier.

The LaChances found Kaban friendly and sympathetic but not as definitive as they hoped. He thought Jennifer's problem was a relatively common swelling that might regress on its own, and he told them he wanted to wait and see. "Come back in a week," he said, "and we'll devise a plan of action." But Jennifer's parents were beginning to fear they were being shuffled among doctors who seemed unsure what was wrong with their daughter. Their concern heightened when, a few days later, Jennifer was running a fever, losing weight, and having trouble sleeping. The swelling was now the size of a large orange, disfiguring the left side of her face, and though there was little pain, she could feel the sensation of pressure.

Back at the hospital, Kaban examined Jennifer and decided to operate. He saw how scared Jennifer's parents were, but he wasn't particularly worried. He had seen a fair number of children with a rapidly progressive swelling of the jaw, and he judged this one to be an aneurysmal bone cyst, a swelling that was vascular in nature. Such cysts are commonly treated successfully with surgery. The growths are removed, and 90 percent of them don't come back.

Kaban removed the growth from Jennifer's jaw, and the pathologist who examined the tissue supported his diagnosis of an aneurysmal bone cyst. The surgical procedure was called an enucleation, which basically meant that Kaban opened up the tissue, stripped out the lining around the growth, and washed it clean. He expected that with the pressure reduced, the tumor site would collapse and fill in, beginning to heal. And that's what happened: Jennifer responded as everyone hoped. "A month later, she looked pretty much okay," Kaban recalled.

But Jennifer was not really okay. A few months later, her face began swelling again—she was apparently among the unlucky 10 percent. Kaban judged that the bone was the problem, and that it should be removed. This second, more aggressive round of surgery required removal of about half of Jennifer's lower jaw and replacing the missing bone with a titanium plate. By then the growth was so large—almost the size of her father's fist, Michael LaChance remembers thinking—and had caused so much deterioration of bone that Kaban thought it was amazing Jennifer's jaw hadn't broken. But he was still confident it was just an aneurysmal bone cyst, if one with some so-called giant cells—oversized cells with more than one nucleus, but not malignant—mixed in. "I told them again it's not a problem," Kaban recalls. "We do see these occasionally, and we were actually writing a paper on the subject. So not to worry." But Kaban could see Jennifer's parents were still very worried, her father particularly. "We'll stick with it," Kaban told him assuringly. "We will get it taken care of." There was even a small chance the bone would grow back. That happened on occasion, though it was more likely that they would eventually want to replace Jennifer's missing lower left jawbone by taking one of her ribs and implanting that bone as a substitute. But don't worry about that for another year, Kaban told Jennifer's anxious parents.

Kaban's advice proved impossible to follow: Three months later, the tumor came back. Once more, Kaban operated to remove the tissue mass. But now, for the first time, he was worried about his diagnosis. Was it a solid tumor—a common form of cancer called a sarcoma—that was behaving more like a local hemangioma than a truly malignant tumor? Was it something else he wasn't picking up? Puzzled, Kaban went back to all the slide-mounted tissue samples and made sure all the pathologists studied them in detail to see if something had been missed. But everyone said the same thing: This was a giant-cell lesion that was benign, not malignant. But Kaban wasn't satisfied, and he decided to take Jennifer's case to the hospital's weekly pediatric sarcoma conference. There to share their expertise were top specialists in radiation therapy, pediatric hematology, oncology, pediatric orthopedics, and radiation oncology. Kaban waded through all his materials—the X rays, the pathology reports, the previous consultations. The consensus: Jennifer's tumor, whatever it was, seemed to be behaving like a sarcoma, even though the pathology studies didn't show it. So the answer if the growth came back a third time was to hit it with radiation, chemotherapy, or both. In other words, attack it as if it *were* a sarcoma, a true malignancy.

Almost as if on schedule, the tumor again ballooned up to about the size of an orange, distending the left side of Jennifer's face. It was distressingly clear that she was in deep trouble. Kaban tried a drug called calcitonin for a few months but without success. The only known option left, then, was to use a massive dose of radiation to the left side of Jennifer's face, which might finally eradicate the tumor. But there would be dreadful side effects. The radiation would stop the left side of the little girl's face from growing, but not the right side, resulting in a grotesque distortion. But Kaban felt there was no choice. Without treatment, the tumor's growth would probably be unstoppable. Kaban had seen it happen. "Rapidly progressive giant-cell lesions grow locally and usually invade up toward the skull base, and eventually the children die," he would say later. "So the thing had to be treated. The choices were radiation and/or chemotherapy. Neither of these was very attractive."

With these grim choices facing the LaChance family, Kaban thought of one more possibility. Jennifer's tumor had come on suddenly and proliferated rapidly, and it was loaded with blood vessels. In essence, it occured to Kaban, it was behaving like an expanding hemangioma. He decided to take the case over to Children's Hospital to discuss the details with the country's top hemangioma experts, John Mulliken and Judah Folkman.

Mulliken was not optimistic when Kaban presented his case. He wasn't convinced that bone growths like Jennifer's were the same as hemangiomas, though they could be related. Folkman, however, was eager to explore that option. His two very potent inhibitors, angiostatin and endostatin, were still confined to the lab bench, and the prospects for TNP-470 were uncertain. But the rousing success with Tommy Briggs and the other hemangioma patients who followed had led him to wonder whether interferon would be as powerful against some solid tumors. Now he would have a chance to see. Folkman had seen cases in which children's faces had been left terribly disfigured by antitumor treatments, and it seemed their lives had been simultaneously saved and destroyed. These disfigured children lived in isolation. Some even tried to commit suicide. He would do everything possible to help Jennifer LaChance avoid such a terrible prospect. Take a urine sample from Jennifer, Folkman urged. See if the tumor's putting out an excess amount of a growth factor. If her FGF level is elevated, treat her with interferon alpha.

Kaban thought it was definitely worth a try, and Mulliken finally agreed. There really was nothing to lose. Interferon alpha was already an approved drug; it had been established as safe. And if it didn't work, they could still try the other treatments. The only question was whether Jennifer's parents would agree to let their daughter become the first patient with such a tumor to get the experimental antiangiogenesis treatment.

Kaban told the LaChances about Folkman and his work. This was no ordinary doctor, he assured them. Someday, people would speak of him as they speak of Jonas Salk. But Kaban also warned the LaChances that the proposed interferon treatment was brand-new and might not work. But at the very least it was worth exploring. Sure enough, the urine test revealed that Jennifer's level of fibroblast growth factor was extraordinarily high—twenty-eight times above normal. The LaChances didn't need to be convinced. Though Kaban had failed to cure Jennifer with surgery, they had never stopped regarding him as the best in the business, a doctor whose word was gospel. So when radiation seemed the only other option and Kaban said, "You know, you really don't want to do that," the LaChances unhesitatingly agreed to allow their daughter to be given the experimental treatment.

Michael LaChance, a tool-and-die-maker, prepared himself to give his daughter the daily shots at home. He first did a little practicing on a ripe orange to get used to the feeling of breaking the skin with a needle and delivering the injection. Then he began giving Jennifer the low-dose shots. She didn't like it much, and would squirm and become cranky when she saw the shot coming. Lillian LaChance, who worked as a meat wrapper in a Providence supermarket, used an ice cube to cool the injection site and let Jennifer lie on top of her for comfort. "I would do the loving. Mike would give the shot," she said. Their oldest child, eight-year-old Christine, would be there for moral support.

As expected, the drug gave Jennifer high fevers—"She started seeing Gummi Bears running around in the house," her father recalls—but her body soon adapted to it and the fevers went down. And that wasn't the only thing that went down. Within about three weeks, it seemed that the tumor had stopped growing. And then, soon after, it started shrinking. That was great news, but it was short-lived. After a few months, Lillian called Kaban and said the tumor seemed to be growing again, and that Jennifer wasn't feeling well. To see what was going on, Folkman suggested that Jennifer's urine be tested again for FGF. It showed that her levels of the growth factor were going back up. Folkman thought the problem might be with the dosage. Jennifer was growing—and outgrowing the low dose of interferon alpha. So her doses were increased, and it worked: Her FGF level came down, and the tumor began to shrink again. A few months later the same thing happened again. Lillian reported that Jennifer was doing okay, but that the tumor had stopped shrinking. So the dose of interferon alpha was increased once more. The tumor began to shrink again. This time, it kept shrinking. And then, after nearly a year of daily shots, the tumor was gone.

Kaban and Folkman kept Jennifer on shots; they thought she should get them for a full year to make sure the tumor didn't come back. For Jennifer, it wasn't easy. She was wiggling more each time her father prepared the shot, and sometimes she tried to hide. Then, one day during their regular appointment at the hospital in Boston, Kaban told Jennifer he'd stop the shots if she'd give him a hug. He got his hug—a huge one.

The year was up, a cause for celebration in the LaChance home in Rhode Island. "You took the shots," Lillian said to her daughter, "and we made the year." They put her to bed that night and prayed the tumor wouldn't come back.

The three doctors didn't announce the success immediately because they wanted to make sure Jennifer was really cured. Kaban knew that giant-cell tumors like Jennifer's had occasionally been seen to recur within two years of surgical removal. So he watched her for another two years. The tumor never reappeared. In April 1998, nearly four years after the tumor was first noticed, Jennifer, at nine, was pronounced cured. She still had to face some serious dental work to replace all of the lower teeth on the left side of her jaw. But her jawbone had grown back, and Kaban expected that tooth implants, which would be screwed into the bone, would work just fine. Otherwise, she looked terrific—full of energy, giggly with a mischievous grin, thrilled to have overcome the ordeal that had dominated her childhood. She told her parents, "If I helped another kid not have to go through what I went through, then it's worth it."

Kaban knew the experience with Jennifer was a major advance for his field. He believed that a number of vascular tumors could be treated with interferon or with some other angiogenesis inhibitor. And he expected that in the future doctors who saw children with rapidly growing jaw growths would immediately test their urine and then treat them with interferon if the FGF marker was elevated. He and Folkman were also surprised and delighted that the bone that Kaban had taken out before interferon was tried had replaced itself. That eliminated the need to take one of Jennifer's ribs to replace her jaw structure—a great relief, of course, to Jennifer and her parents.

For Folkman, it was a major triumph—the first solid tumor eradicated by antiangiogenesis treatment. Later, he would make Jennifer's case a routine part of his lectures, a human success story he could talk about while explaining the even more promising research that had not yet made it into the clinic. He would flash slides of Jennifer's face showing her tumor gradually shrinking— "This is after one year on interferon, and it's still coming down. This is four months off therapy, and her face now has normal symmetry."

The LaChances' only disappointment was that they never got to meet Folkman face-to-face. During her course of interferon treatments, they made several trips to Boston to drop off Jennifer's urine samples at Children's Hospital, and they had hoped to be able to thank him in person. But each time he was out. "But he did call me one day," Lillian LaChance says. "And he told me, 'Mrs. LaChance, I'm calling to say thank you for letting Jennifer try this drug.' "

"SHE WAS THE FIRST CASE," Folkman says of Jennifer LaChance, and he was determined that she would be the first of many patients whose growing tumors might be erased by antiangiogenesis treatment. It would take time—major trials involving thousands of people would still be needed before angiogenesis-based treatments would ever become routine—but this was a promising start. For now, though, he hoped interferon alpha could be used in other desperate pediatric cases, children whose tumors had become totally resistant to chemotherapy and radiation and couldn't be helped by surgery.

The year 1997 brought another patient, a two-month-old boy whose hand was being destroyed by an aggressive tumor called an angioblastoma, a horrible growth that looked like a big red baseball expanding at the end of his arm. His condition had progressed so far that the tumor had already eaten through half his hand, completely dissolving two bones, the fifth and fourth metacarpals. Until now the only way to save the baby's life would have been to amputate his hand. But even then, the long-term prognosis would not be encouraging. Experience had shown that the surgeon's cut might release cells from the tumor, cells that could migrate through the body and eventually lodge in the lungs, where chemotherapy would be unable to stop them.

As in Jennifer's case, Folkman suggested testing the baby's urine to see if the expanding tumor was making one of the angiogenesis-stimulating agents, either FGF or VEGF. It turned out that the tumor's output of FGF was huge, about fifty times higher than normal. So at age four months the little boy began getting regular low-dose infusions of interferon alpha. Once again, the results were stunning. By the time the little boy was eleven months old, the angioblastoma was completely gone. More amazing, the bones that had been eaten away by the tumor were being replaced, having regenerated while his hand was returning to normal. Folkman felt the baby's hand. Almost normal, he thought, except that the boy's little finger had been amputated because it had been shoved aside by the tumor.

With this and similar cases, Folkman found that he and his colleagues were expanding the possibilities for antiangiogenic treatments. The challenge was on: How many different kinds of abnormal growths could successfully be attacked? How effective would the treatments be, and how far could they safely press the boundaries?

Bianca Denis was born with a strange, dark marking on her right arm, a condition her doctors originally called a "port-wine stain" birthmark. But her condition was far worse than that. When she was a few months old, Bianca's father, Taso Denis, felt her wrists and noticed that the right was thicker than the left. "I mean, I'm not crazy; there was something not normal there," he would recall thinking. The Long Island family was sent to a specialist at New

York University Medical Center, who announced it was not a birthmark. It was a hemangioma, and Bianca was in need of serious help.

Taso, a CPA, did some quick research on the Internet and concluded that the place to go was Boston's Children's Hospital. Before Taso took Bianca north, however, Dr. Alexander Bernstein and his colleagues at NYU did numerous tests, and raised the possibility that Bianca might have something even more serious than a hemangioma: a dreadful bone-destroying disorder called an arteriovenous malformation, or AVM. All the textbooks on the subject had been written by Dr. John Mulliken at Boston Children's. "I'm going to Boston to see Dr. Mulliken," Taso Denis told the NYU doctors, and they agreed it was the right thing to do.

In Boston, Mulliken called in several colleagues to look at Bianca's arm. As the diagnosis was firmed up, Bianca's situation seemed increasingly grim. One very abrupt physician told the Denises there was no hope for Bianca's arm, and they should think about having it amputated right away. But then Mulliken introduced them to a radiologist, Dr. Patricia Burrows, a physician whom Folkman liked to call "the Michelangelo of interventional radiology." Unlike many of their other appointments with a range of doctors, both in New York and Boston, the Denises first session with Burrows left them cautiously optimistic. She thought she could save Bianca's arm, perhaps by getting very detailed images of the existing blood vessels and doing delicate surgery to improve blood flow. "We left with hope," Elena Denis, Bianca's mother, recalls. But not much more than hope.

Bianca was admitted to the hospital, and her parents spent the first night with her in a small, dark room. With Elena trying to doze nearby, Taso reclined as best he could while cradling baby Bianca against his broad chest, with her IV tubes dangling and stretching away into the dark. In the middle of the night, Taso saw a weak beam of light approaching slowly through the darkness. As it got closer, he realized it came from a small penlight carried by a nurse, a young man who tiptoed in to see how they were doing. "Mr. Denis, let your wife hold Bianca for a while now," he whispered. "I've set up a cot for you in the next room, and I'll come get you if anything happens. You get some rest."

In the days that followed, the New York doctors' suspicions were confirmed: Bianca's condition was worse than a hemangioma. Her arm was actually being destroyed by an arteriovenous malformation, a condition in which the arteries and veins fail to make the proper connections and everything in the surrounding tissue goes haywire. Blood doesn't flow properly, tissues are starved for oxygen, and waste products can't get out quickly enough. Enzymes begin to dissolve bone—Bianca suffered a broken arm three times—and no form of surgery offers much relief. Although her arm looked as though it was being damaged by a hemangioma, the effects were more like that of the bone-eating tumor, the angioblastoma, that had been consuming the hand of the baby boy who had been treated earlier. In fact, Bianca's condition is known among doctors as disappearing bone disease. The damage was clearly visible in X rays. Bianca's doctors could see that her arm bones were simply disappearing, apparently being dissolved. But, fundamentally, it was abnormal blood vessel structure and growth that were doing so much harm. So Patricia Burrows called Judah Folkman in to consult.

As several doctors had advised, Folkman knew that the only known treatment would be to amputate the arm. But even if Bianca's arm were to be amputated, there was still the chance that surgery might stimulate regrowth of the malformation in the remaining stump, then in her chest and lungs, and grow to become life-threatening. Standard chemotherapy, such as steroids, might control inflammation. Delicate operations to improve blood flow in her arm, and to strengthen her thinning bones, had already helped. Neither could solve the underlying problem, though, and meanwhile, Bianca was in terrible pain. Folkman thought first about interferon, but tests showed that Bianca's tumorlike tissue wasn't putting out either FGF or VEGF. That seemed to rule out interferon.

Despite Burrows's initial confidence, Bianca's prospects were looking grimmer and grimmer. One day, while discussing the case, Burrows, Mulliken, and Folkman grasped at a new idea. What if Bianca's bone was being eaten by the enzyme collagenase? Collagenase had recently become a hot topic in angiogenesis research. Blood vessel cells secrete it as a tool to chew their way through tissues, providing a way to get the new blood vessels they're making into new areas where oxygen is needed. The medical team in Boston was aware that a small firm in the United Kingdom—British Biotech, Ltd.—was experimenting with a drug called marimastat, a compound that seemed to block blood vessel growth by interfering with the activity of collagenase. British Biotech was among the handful of research companies that were now beginning to seriously explore both angiogenesis and antiangiogenesis research. At this point, there were several smaller companies in the game as well: Sugen, Inc., Collateral Therapeutics, and Ixsys, Inc., plus the much larger Genentech. And, of course, still hoping for success with TNP-470, the first antiangiogenic drug, was the Takeda–Abbott Laboratories partnership.

Folkman called British Biotech in Oxford and asked if he could get the drug for Bianca. On what basis? the company asked. The Boston doctors had to admit they had very little data to even suggest it might work; they hadn't even done animal experiments. Their strongest argument was simply Bianca, a toddler in deep trouble. What they were seeking was "compassionate approval" to try the drug on an emergency basis. British Biotech's executives were not thrilled. The company hadn't planned to treat any children, at least not so early in the research process. The last thing they wanted was a bad result that might derail approval of the drug. The odds were certainly strong that something might go wrong, and everyone involved would get burned. So the word came back across the Atlantic: It was too big a risk for the fledgling company. The answer was no.

But Bianca's team of doctors wouldn't take no for an answer. Folkman, Burrows, and their colleagues embarked on a six-month campaign to change British Biotech's decision. They became nuisances, bombarding the company, the FDA, and anyone else they could think of with pleading letters, phone calls, and e-mails. Finally the relentless pressure paid off. The FDA ruled in favor of the trial, and British Biotech yielded. The little yellow marimastat pills were sent from Oxford to Boston, a label on each plastic bottle warning bluntly: CAUTION. NEW DRUG. LIMITED BY FEDERAL LAW TO INVESTIGATIONAL USE ONLY. BRITISH BIOTECH, OXFORD, U.K. TO BE USED BY DR. FOLKMAN ONLY. There was also a serial number, and a warning that the pills could be taken by only one patient: Bianca Denis.

Bianca's treatments began almost as soon as the pills arrived, even before her doctors had sorted out what the best dose might be. Starting cautiously, they gave her a single two-milligram pill in the morning and another each evening. They stuck with that regimen for a month but saw that nothing was happening. Bianca's parents were getting more and more distressed as they saw that even doubling the dosage to four pills a day did nothing. But then the doses were pushed higher, to six pills per day, and Bianca finally began to respond. The first sign was that her pain stopped. Overjoyed, the Denis family called Boston to say their little girl had slept clear through the night, without morphine. And, they noticed, she began to use her damaged arm, even picking things up with her right hand, something she had never been able to do. The arm itself was beginning to look normal: The swelling was coming down, and its ruddy color was fading. For Bianca and her family, and for Burrows, Folkman, and the other doctors, it was a wonderful moment. Skeptics might have argued that it was a spontaneous regression, a waning wrought by natural changes in Bianca's body, but X rays soon showed that something bigger was happening. After Bianca had been on marimastat for four or five months, Burrows showed Folkman the latest X-ray images. They could see that new bone was gradually growing in, rebuilding itself in Bianca's fragile arm. As treatment continued, her bone growth kept improving, and then the tumor-like tissue itself began to self-destruct, growing softer and shrinking.

After two and a half years on the drug, what was left of the bloated-looking tissue was detectable only in Bianca's right hand. By that time, she was in school, enjoying a relatively normal, pain-free childhood. But she was not free of problems. One night, Bianca tripped and fell onto an overturned chair and broke her arm exactly at the point where the old abnormal-tissue growth had been. It was late on a Sunday night, and Bianca's parents rushed her to Long Island Jewish Hospital, where the emergency room residents were faced with a patient with a large, red, swollen hand at the end of her broken arm, who was taking a drug they'd never heard of.

Taso insisted they call Folkman, who explained that Bianca's arteriovenous malformation made her arm especially fragile. Then he called the chief of pediatric surgery, Dr. Alberto Peña, at home. Peña summoned a member of his staff to immediately come over to set Bianca's arm. The next morning, the Denises went to Peña's office and saw a photo of him with Judah Folkman on the wall. Peña had been trained by Folkman at Harvard Medical School. "Let me know if there's anything I can do," Peña told the Denises. "If there's a door not opening for you, you come and see me. I'll get you to the right person."

Bianca's broken arm marked a turning point in her treatment. Because marimastat was meant to block blood vessel growth, the drug's maker, British Biotech, worried that it might also keep Bianca's arm from healing. The company informed Folkman that it would immediately stop supplying the pills, and the FDA agreed with the decision. But Folkman and the Boston team vehemently disagreed. Their progress would be reversed, they argued, if they stopped the drug that seemed to be making her better. Their deepest fear was that without regular doses of marimastat, the activity of the collagenase would resume and the disappearing bone disease that was destroying Bianca's arm would begin to get worse, rather than better, and her arm bones might be weakened further. They were not convinced the drug would block the blood vessel growth needed for healing.

As before, though, their position was very weak, and they knew it. Folkman and his colleagues had only one similar case they could point to—the little boy with the bone-eating angioblastoma in his hand. He had been treated with interferon alpha, which shut down production of the blood vessel stimulator FGF, not marimastat, which shut down the action of an entirely different agent, the enzyme collagenase. Once again, Bianca's doctors lobbied hard with the FDA, and the agency and the company finally agreed to allow Bianca to keep getting the drug.

It was the right decision: Bianca's broken arm healed beautifully. British Biotech now seemed to have a winner in marimastat. It became the first drug ever available for the treatment of arteriovenous malformations. Bianca's arm was still somewhat swollen, but she hadn't lost the limb, and she was living a normal life. Her doctors kept her on the drug; they were afraid to take her off.

Folkman was delighted to add Bianca to the list of successes, but he was thinking beyond her. Interferon alpha and marimastat, though fine first steps, were relatively weak inhibitors of angiogenesis. Other drugs, more potent ones, were on the way. One of these was TNP-470, developed by the Folkman lab's Japanese partners. It had finally made its way to clinical trials in 1992. One of the first patients to receive the drug was a forty-nine-year-old Houston woman with cervical cancer. Her cancer had initially gone into remission after radiation treatments, but after three years, X rays showed that the cancer was back and had metastasized to her lungs. With no other treatment options, she agreed to join the TNP-470 trial. Beginning in 1995 she was given intravenous doses every other day for four weeks, followed by two weeks of nontreatment. She then went through a second course, and at that point the tumors in her lungs showed signs of shrinking. After a third round of TNP-470—twenty-two months after the beginning of the first one—the tumors were no longer detectable. "That woman was on the drug for a year and a half, had no side effects, and there was complete regression," Donald Ingber, the doctor whose serendipitous discovery of a fungus in a petri dish had ultimately led to TNP-470, said in 1999. By this time Ingber was running a large laboratory of his own in Folkman's department. "Now she's been off the drug for two years. She's cured."

That success, published in *The New England Journal of Medicine* in 1998, wasn't the only one. Three other patients responded well—"all end-stage people," said Ingber. But fourteen others could not be saved. Their cancers progressed, unchecked despite the treatments. These results led Ingber to take exception to the protocols calling for the drug to be given in large jolts, with relatively long delays between treatments. But the mixed results also raised the possibility that the type or number of angiogenesis-stimulating factors a given tumor was making could make a critical difference. It also seemed from the outset that TNP-470 could inhibit substantially but not totally, which could explain why it looked so much more promising when combined with traditional chemotherapy agents or radiation. Unlike angiostatin and endostatin, which seemed potent enough to erase tumors by themselves, TNP-470 seemed to need a little help. And with the results of trials being conducted in Houston, Washington, Los Angeles, and Boston still to be reported, the jury was out on TNP-470.

TOMMY BRIGGS IN DENVER, Jennifer LaChance in Rhode Island, Bianca Denis in New York, and the few successful TNP-470 patients all heralded the arrival of the era of antiangiogenesis. It was no longer just theory. It worked. How *well* it worked—that was the real question now. Folkman and his colleagues were eager to find out. That meant getting their most potent antiangiogenesis drugs, angiostatin and endostatin, out of mouse cages and into hospital rooms.

It was true, as Dana-Farber's Howard Fine had said, that researchers had been curing mice of cancer for fifty years. What few people outside Folkman's laboratory could yet see, however, was that curing mice using antiangiogenesis therapy was fundamentally different from any previous treatments that had worked in mice but not in people. Never before had anyone been able to cure mice whose tumors were so far advanced, or so massive that their relative weight was equal to a two-pound tumor in an average person. It had never before been possible to cure the animals without causing deleterious side effects. And it had never been possible to cure mice by treating their blood vessels instead of their tumors. This was different—a new world.

Word of the difference was getting around. O'Reilly's 1994 paper on angiostatin had won wide notice among cancer biologists. Folkman was talking about it regularly and showing slides of the afflicted and cured mice at major conferences. The excitement in the laboratory had doubled after O'Reilly found endostatin, which gave Folkman even more to talk about on the lecture circuit once it turned out to be as effective as angiostatin.

One of his best opportunities came on May 20, 1996, when he gave the prestigious Karnovsky Lecture at the annual meeting of the American Association for Cancer Research, in Philadelphia. Before a huge audience that included many leading cancer doctors and cancer biologists from around the world, Folkman painstakingly and clearly outlined his three decades of thinking and experimentation, and illustrated the latest achievements with the stunning pictures of mouse tumors shrinking and then disappearing. The room was electrified, and as Folkman finished his last slides by showing photos of O'Reilly, Thomas Boehm, and other laboratory members, the applause rose like thunder. Whereas in the past researchers wandered out of the room when Folkman got up to discuss angiogenesis, now most remained glued to their seats through the question-and-answer session. When Folkman left the podium he was surrounded by researchers eager to ask questions and learn more. What had once been an obscure subject was finally coming into its own, blossoming into a field requiring major conferences. Within a couple of years, the American Association for Cancer Research would draw five hundred scientists, doctors, biotechnology executives, and government research administrators to a special meeting devoted to angiogenesis.

Nonetheless, despite excitement among cell biologists and the attention of a few science reporters, most major news organizations were still concentrating on the hot news in molecular biology, on cancer genes, including the accumulating evidence that cancer is caused by a loss of genetic stability. There was news about telomeres—the small chunks of DNA that keep chromosomes from unraveling—and how they're related to cancer and aging. Angiogenesis, and Folkman, remained largely overlooked by the mainstream media.

That began to change in fall 1997, when Folkman was invited to give the Director's Lecture at the National Institutes of Health. There, in addition to the spectacular pictures of mice and their disappearing tumors, Folkman showed photos of Jennifer LaChance. He told her story: how, as a last resort before radiation, he and her doctor had used antiangiogenic interferon to try to eradicate a large growth on her jaw that kept growing back, and how it had worked. Folkman was able to show the huge audience of doctors in Bethesda pictures of the tumor getting smaller and smaller. Folkman closed his talk with some thoughts about where the work seemed to be going. Angiostatin and endostatin had done the job in mice. Now, he said, he hoped to try them in dogs—and not just laboratory dogs. Folkman's mice all had borne implanted tumors. Now he wanted to see whether the drugs were as potent against a natural tumor. The answer would bring him a step closer to human trials.

Folkman finished, and the audience remained still for a moment. Then a roar of applause erupted from the hundreds of doctors and researchers in the room. It was clear, then and there, that angiogenesis research was on the front burner and that Judah Folkman's long-pursued idea was ready for prime time.

A few months later, Gina Kolata, a noted science reporter for *The New York Times*, was in Los Angeles for a banquet, and got a seat next to James D. Watson, the Nobel laureate who with Francis Crick had found the structure for DNA. So what's new? Kolata asked at the dinner table. Watson was then the president of the Cold Spring Harbor Laboratory on Long Island, and the lab had recently put on a small symposium on angiogenesis. Folkman had spoken, and afterward he and Watson had gone off and talked into the night.

What's new? Judah Folkman and angiogenesis, that's what's new, Watson told Kolata. "Judah is going to cure cancer in two years," he said offhandedly.

Chapter Sixteen

———

THE NEW YORK TIMES dropped with its usual heavy thud in front of Judah and Paula Folkman's home in Brookline on Sunday morning, May 3, 1998. Paula freed the paper from its blue plastic wrapper, then glanced at the top of the front page. She was floored and quickly called her husband. There, in big, bold type, Folkman saw the headline: A CAUTIOUS AWE GREETS DRUGS THAT ERADICATE TUMORS IN MICE.

The story itself seemed to display more awe than caution. It reported—not for the first time—the discovery of angiostatin and endostatin, and their almost miraculous success in blocking angiogenesis in tumor-ridden mice. But that wasn't what gave Folkman a queasy feeling. What did was a quote near the top of the story. "Judah," said James D. Watson, "is going to cure cancer in two years."

Flabbergasted, Folkman read on. Watson's quote was the most stunning, but only the first in a series of laudatory comments from Folkman's fellow scientists—remarks so energized with admiration and excitement that he was sure to be pilloried by his colleagues at Children's Hospital and Harvard. The antiangiogenesis results coming out of Folkman's lab, said Dr. Richard Klausner, director of the National Cancer Institute, were "remarkable and wonderful . . . the single most exciting thing on the horizon." He added, "I am putting nothing on higher priority than getting this into clinical trials." Dr. James Pluda, who was in charge of the NCI's drug tests, told Kolata that researchers at the institute were "electrified" when they heard Folkman deliver a lecture on his lab's latest results: "People were almost overwhelmed. The data were remarkable." And, Pluda said, there was much more in Folkman's research that hadn't yet been published. He was talking about the triumph of

Jennifer LaChance, and the recent discovery of additional antiangiogenesis factors.

Folkman knew instantly that the expectant tone of this story, and its placement at the top of the front page of the Sunday *New York Times*—equivalent to shouting from the rooftops—was likely to bring far more aggravation than gratification. But even Folkman couldn't have predicted the frenzy that would immediately engulf him, Children's Hospital, the Harvard Medical School, the National Cancer Institute, and doctors and patients throughout the world.

Gina Kolata's story was accurate and contained all the right caveats. She had carefully repeated *mouse, mouse, mouse* throughout, and pointed out high in the story that many promising cancer treatments had produced remarkable results in animals but failed in humans. But she also reported, "Some cancer researchers say the drugs are the most exciting treatment that they have ever seen." And so even as Folkman himself was reading the article, thousands and thousands of people were leaping past the literal news about cures in mice and assuming that the end of cancer was now at hand. Or at least hoping. At the New York *Daily News*, columnist Mike McAlary sat down at his computer and wrote: "On Sunday we opened the paper and there was hope on the front page. Maybe we don't have to die." McAlary, age forty, had colon cancer.

McAlary's interest was painfully personal. But all across the media world that Sunday, editors seized on a big story on a quiet Sunday in spring. Bess Andrews, the director of public affairs at Children's Hospital, was still in her bathrobe when the first call came. It was nine in the morning, and a woman in the CBS planning unit in New York was on the phone asking Andrews about the story in *The New York Times*. Andrews hadn't seen it; she had to go out and buy the paper. Meanwhile, the calls kept coming. She tried to get Folkman through his beeper but couldn't. She was perplexed that the story was getting so much attention. After all, it was not really new. *Newsday* had reported on angiostatin, endostatin, and the mice fully two years earlier. *Business Week* had recently reported on it, and the *Times* itself had run an article on the same lab work the preceding November. But that story appeared inside the paper and was decidedly more muted than Kolata's. Quotes like Watson's put the story in a whole other category of news—news that took on a life of its own, spreading like a virus onto the news budgets of virtually every major media operation in America, as well as many outlets abroad. But that was just the beginning.

When Folkman arrived at his office on Monday morning, he found the tape on his answering machine completely full with messages from frantic patients, their families, and members of the media, all wanting to talk to him personally, now. All night long the tape had been taking messages from everywhere, in every language. The story was especially big in Italy, it seemed. Some of the callers—pleading, crying—said they were flying to Boston right away. Could they get into the hospital? How soon would treatments start? What would it cost? Did it hurt? Were there side effects? Meanwhile, outside the hospital on Longwood Avenue, local and network television crews were staking out Children's Hospital. Folkman was declining all requests for interviews, so he was ambushed by reporters and cameramen each time he left the building. As the week wore on, so many crews staked out the hospital that it was sometimes hard to get in or out.

Folkman was astounded by the coverage: "Peter Jennings talking about a cure in Boston! Jim Watson saying it's like Einstein!"—Darwin, actually—"so by the second day there's anger from Dan Rather, anger from Ted Koppel, calling me, asking why I won't go on camera. They were calling me at home, everywhere. I had to go to the NIH, and when I came out there were cameras. I had to go testify about NIH funding before Senator Kennedy and they picked that up; there were hundreds of cameras." Folkman decided to back out of giving the keynote address at a prostate cancer conference that week at a Boston hotel. He didn't want to feed the fires or look like he was seeking or even enjoying the attention. The fact was he had mixed feelings. He was thrilled to have arrived at this point but extremely uncomfortable with the public notice, wishing it would go away until there was something real to celebrate—a headline, for instance, that said, DRUGS ERADICATE TUMORS IN HUMANS. He also fretted that all the publicity suggested that angiogenesis was his work alone, especially after Andy Rooney, on *60 Minutes,* proposed a Judah Folkman Day should the new drugs work on people.

Folkman had always been reluctant to have his picture in the papers, and now his unwillingness stiffened. He refused to be photographed by either print or broadcast media, which only intensified the demand. Some photo agencies tried to make money selling the few pictures available. Meanwhile, the hospital gave a photo of Michael O'Reilly to the Associated Press, hoping that would ease the pressure. And still the demand for news, information, and photos kept coming in, from Chile, Brazil, Greece, and even the Vatican. Bess Andrews saved a newspaper from Rome in which the story of Folkman's work shared front billing with the first murder in the Vatican.

At Andrews's urging, Folkman agreed to do "background" interviews—

no direct quoting allowed, and definitely no pictures—with the major networks and three major newsmagazines, *Time, Newsweek,* and *U.S. News & World Report.* He hoped it would help keep the news in perspective and dampen the rampant optimism. But the strategy didn't work. All three newsweeklies ran cover stories that touched off another round of calls from desperate patients. As promised, some would-be patients really did arrive at Boston's Logan Airport and find their way to Children's Hospital. Some tried to get beds next door at Dana-Farber. The hospital had the difficult job of turning them away, and the doctors—especially the oncologists—were extremely upset.

And still the pleas continued to come. These were dying patients, people who needed the drugs immediately. Some had only weeks to live. They didn't care that the drug had been used only in mice; they wanted it. Dana-Farber was also swamped with calls; and in Bethesda, so was the National Cancer Institute. Children's Hospital had to assign someone to spend eight hours a day just fielding phone calls. The calls didn't abate and the lab found itself with a new permanent position. Meanwhile, Folkman decided to recruit a corps of surrogates to give interviews to explain about cancer and the reality of antiangiogenesis research. These weren't professional spokesmen—flaks, as they are sometimes known in the news trade—but rather people like the president of the American Cancer Society, David Rosenthal. For the high-profile network anchors, top officials of the National Cancer Institute subbed for the man of the hour. For Ted Koppel's *Nightline,* it was the institute's director, Richard Klausner. For Dan Rather, it was James Pluda, the chief of the drug-trials unit. "So all of these people are suddenly drafted into it, and they've become the experts," Folkman said. "Pluda's giving the best talks on angiogenesis he's ever done."

The story of angiogenesis was also big news on the stock market. The Friday before the *Times* story, stock in EntreMed, the small biotechnology company that had supported Folkman's work and held the licenses for both angiostatin and endostatin, closed at twelve dollars on the NASDAQ list. On Monday morning, EntreMed's shares leaped immediately to eighty-three dollars. Two days later it was down to forty-three dollars a share (which was still more than three times its value before the publicity). It was only the beginning of what would be a long roller-coaster ride for the company's stock. It would remain highly volatile for two years, jumping up and down with each tidbit of information announced or leaked from EntreMed and its partners, from Folkman's laboratory, or from other sources.

Inevitably, the scent of money raised suspicions among some of the reporters whose requests for interviews were being rejected. "When you've turned them down, they come back with pejorative questions," Folkman recalls. " 'Isn't it working? Why can't I get anybody to talk about this? What are you hiding?' " Some assumed that Folkman was making money on the upsurge in EntreMed's share price. But Folkman had always made sure to avoid all perceptions of conflict of interest, and he held no stock in companies that were supporting his work.

If the furor was awkward for Folkman, it was embarrassing for James Watson, the man whose dramatic—and incautious—prediction was as responsible as anything for getting the story so much attention, first from Kolata, then from her editors, and then from the rest of the world. A few days after the story was published, Watson wrote a letter to the *Times* claiming he'd been misquoted, though the letter itself was anything but restrained in its enthusiasm for antiangiogenesis. Not many people believed Watson's claim that he'd never made the "two years" comment; though it started out as an offhanded remark over dinner, a few scientists who had visited at Cold Spring Harbor in preceding weeks remembered him repeating it several times.

The thrust and impact of the story came as a shock to Folkman because he had assumed it would run in the *Times*'s Tuesday science section and would draw about as much reaction as the other stories that had been written in recent years—which is to say, not a lot. After all, the discoveries of angiostatin and endostatin had been published in major journals, and stories about the mouse tests had appeared in the mainstream press. So when Kolata had phoned Folkman for an interview soon after her encounter with Watson in Los Angeles, he reminded her that the *Times* had run essentially the same story the previous November, after his Director's Lecture at the NIH. Kolata had been undeterred—she had the Watson quote, and that in itself was news—but she had said nothing to Folkman indicating the story would get such major play. She herself didn't know it at that point. In any event, Folkman, sensing Kolata's excitement, had urged her to make sure the story—especially the headline—made clear that the results had been seen in mice, not people. Kolata had pointed out that reporters generally have no control over headlines on news stories. "You're a famous science writer," Folkman had replied. "You've got to get mice into the title. And you've got to get this quote in: 'If you have cancer and you're a mouse, we can take care of you.' " Kolata used that quote, and the headline was indeed about mice. But it hardly mattered.

Over the next weeks and months, oncologists across the country continued getting calls from patients wanting this magical drug. Most of the physicians hadn't a clue, having seen little on it in the clinical literature. Feeling ignorant, unable to give their patients any useful information, they looked to the National Cancer Institute. But the NCI was also unprepared for the onslaught and it could offer little help because treatment with angiostatin and endostatin still seemed far from the clinic. "Klausner kept saying they couldn't understand this massive number of calls," Folkman says. "I said, 'What do you think? It's because our existing treatments are so bad. It's because we have great science and no real applications. These calls represent our ignorance.' "

Overcoming that ignorance was fast becoming a hot priority. One of the things that did happen, with little notice and no ballyhoo, was a complete turnaround by the National Institutes of Health on the question of angiogenesis. On July 30, 1998, just three months after Kolata's explosive story, three branches of the National Institutes of Health released a program announcement calling for research proposals for studies in blood vessel biology. The National Heart, Lung, and Blood Institute, the National Eye Institute, and the National Cancer Institute had decided "to encourage the translation of basic knowledge of the angiogenic process into therapeutic applications." In other words, these three leading federal research agencies were announcing it was time to take Folkman's work seriously—very seriously. All researchers—public, private, foreign, domestic—were invited to submit research proposals. The agencies made big money available to support research in colleges, universities, hospitals, state agencies, and federal research centers. One paragraph in the seven-page document said it all:

Cancer and cardiovascular disease, two entirely different diseases, account for nearly three quarters of all deaths in the U.S. New strategies for treating these diseases are beginning to emerge that are surprisingly similar, and involve regulating angiogenesis, the process by which new blood vessels arise as outgrowths of existing vessels. In addition to these potentially fatal diseases, other less life-threatening diseases involving uncontrolled angiogenesis, for example neovascular eye diseases causing blindness, may also be amenable to this type of treatment. Therefore, controlling the angiogenic process may prove effective as a treatment paradigm for a wide range of cardiovascular and pulmonary diseases, for inhibiting tumor growth and metastasis, and for preventing and treating certain eye diseases.

That statement could have flowed directly from Judah Folkman's pen a decade earlier. It was vindication, published and backed by money. Angiogenesis and antiangiogenesis could no longer be denied, even though skeptics were still complaining about too much optimism and too much publicity for treatments that, after all, had only been tried in mice. The NIH program announcement was so important, such a big moment, that Folkman promised to frame it and hang it up right next to his first grant rejection notice, from the National Cancer Institute in the early 1970s. He would have to find a place to hang them among the dozens of major awards he was now receiving.

What Folkman found particularly gratifying was a paragraph in the announcement that took note of how quickly angiogenesis had risen to prominence in recent years: "The NCI has not previously targeted angiogenesis research as a special priority. However, it has become a field of immense opportunity because of the acceleration of developments that demonstrate the profound dependence of tumor growth and metastasis on the generation of new blood vessels. The results of this research have gone beyond the initial promise of understanding the regulation of vascular growth to the creation of a new era of cancer therapy."

Indeed, even before the NIH program announcement, the spread of Folkman's ideas was becoming a phenomenon, with a number of companies preparing to begin clinical trials of antiangiogenesis agents that had been developed in labs other than Folkman's. California's Genentech, for example, had begun exploring the potential of antiangiogenesis almost as soon as Napoleone Ferrara discovered the endothelial cell stimulator VEGF in the late 1980s. Over the next few years, Genentech and other companies began developing prospective drugs that took a different tack than the Folkman lab's angiogenesis inhibitors, angiostatin and endostatin. They focused on antibodies, the body's main defense against infection, a line of research that could be traced back more than two decades. In 1975, César Milstein and Georges J. F. Köhler, in Cambridge, England, had learned how to make specific antibodies in unlimited amounts. Researchers soon devised ways to make large doses of highly specific antibodies that would attack any particular protein they chose and began to use these "monoclonals" to attack the action of growth factors and, thus, tumors.

This approach took advantage of the fact that all animals have an immune system that regards the arrival of any protein it doesn't already know as "self" to be an enemy that must be eliminated. Whatever comes along and looks threatening—a virus, bacterium, fungus, or even a protein from another animal—triggers an immune reaction. As an enormously powerful defensive system, immunity is constantly on a hair-trigger setting, always making thousands of different kinds of antibodies that wander around in the body, alert for foreign invaders, ready to raise the alarm. What Milstein and Köhler did was to find a way to exploit this alarm system. They created odd cell cultures called hybridomas—fusions of cancer cells with an antibody-making B cell. Because it can grow forever, the cancer cell brings immortality to the mixture. Thus by choosing which B cell to force into the hybridoma, scientists could choose which antibody the hybridoma would make in unlimited amounts. And because the immune system has a built-in gene-shuffling mechanism that allows it to make millions of different antibody molecules, each tailored to recognize and grab on to a specific protein, they could be designed to inhibit factors that trigger blood vessel growth to tumors.

By the late 1990s, several companies had drugs developed under this line of research in the works. Genentech had a trial under way testing its own agent—a monoclonal antibody meant to grab on to molecules of the growth factor VEGF to keep it from stimulating blood vessel growth. Two more California companies were also becoming players in antiangiogenesis drugs: Ixsys, Inc., was testing another monoclonal antibody meant to keep endothelial cells from getting a "grow" signal by blocking a molecule called Alpha-v, Beta-3. Sugen, Inc., meanwhile, was already into clinical trials and hinting about success with its own version of a monoclonal antibody, which it called SU6668. So Judah Folkman might not quite cure cancer in two years, but enough people were working on antiangiogenesis to perhaps even beat him to the punch.

IN LATE JUNE 1998, only weeks after *The New York Times* turned Folkman's life upside down, he traveled to Burlington, Vermont, to deliver a lecture on interferon and its power against some giant-cell tumors. He showed the slides of Jennifer LaChance's gradually improving face and talked hopefully about a future in which interferon would be just one drug among many that might cause tumors to starve to death. In the audience, Dr. Alan Homans listened with more than casual interest. When Folkman finished his lecture, Homans approached and asked for some advice. He had a patient with an incurable giant-cell tumor in her abdomen. Did Folkman think interferon could help? Folkman told him to send a urine sample.

Homans's desperately ill patient, Tonya Kalesnik, had actually been a patient at Folkman's home base, Children's Hospital, and on this day was in Boston, getting bad news at Dana-Farber. But when she returned home to Vermont, Homas called and told her, "We're going to try something."

Tonya was just about at the end of her rope. Her doctors at the university's medical center in Burlington and at Dana-Farber had tried every treatment known to defeat the tumor that was growing in her lower abdomen, and they doubted she would survive more than a few more months. She had a rare tumorlike growth called a giant-cell sarcoma that had expanded almost to the size of a basketball and defied treatment. Surgery, and then a month of daily doses of radiation, had failed. The pain in her lower back was excruciating, almost constant. Her "sweet" sixteenth year of life was spent in agony.

Her ordeal had begun one night in fall 1997. She was helping scare the wits out of children going through a haunted house on Halloween when she felt a sharp pain in her backside, just above the tailbone. Tonya thought she'd hit something in the excitement, but the pain didn't go away. She went to the doctor, who told her she probably had a fractured tailbone that would heal itself. But the pain persisted. "I kept going in about every two weeks, and I'd get the same answer," Tonya says. "The pain was getting worse. Then I had a spell in school, and I couldn't move. No one could touch me. It was pain from the sacrum area [the lowest bone in the spine]. It was excruciating. I went to the doctor again and got an X ray, and all they could see was a hairline fracture that looked really old. I had fractured my tailbone in 1992 when I hit the gym floor. So I thought that was acting up again."

But acting up was not the term for it. By February 1998, Tonya began going numb in the saddle area and in the back of her thighs. Her doctor thought she might have a ruptured disk and ordered a CAT scan, but it showed nothing. "She did it in the middle of my back," Tonya later said. "If she'd gone a little bit lower she probably would have seen something." The physician prescribed a cortisone shot—"Pretty much to shut me up," Tonya decided, after the doctor called her mother and asked if Tonya was just seeking attention and might be faking. The doctor offered Patricia Kalesnik the phone number for a mental health center. "No!" Tonya's mother retorted. "I'm up all night with her since October, screaming. This is not imaginary."

When Tonya got to the New England Spine Institute for her cortisone shot, the doctor there thought the pain she was describing didn't sound like a fractured tailbone, and he ordered additional X rays. The new images finally made clear that Tonya had a huge growth in her abdomen. A week of tests—MRI, CAT scans—revealed the worst. Tonya had cancer. The doctors suspected it was a sarcoma, but they were unsure which of the five known kinds it was. A needle biopsy determined it was a rare and hard-to-treat giant-cell sarcoma. The doctor said he was sending her to Boston's Children's Hospital. "We've never dealt with a giant-cell tumor," he said. "Boston will be able to handle you better."

Tonya and her mother expected to go to Boston just for a consultation, but she wound up being admitted and staying for a month. By then, the tumor was pressing so hard on Tonya's nerves that she had lost some control of her bladder and bowels. The sciatic nerve pain was so severe she couldn't walk to the bathroom. She had a catheter instead. But Tonya had remarkable spirit. When the nurses came in her room, they almost always found her smiling. "My whole outlook on this thing is that you've got to stay happy," Tonya said later. "If you get depressed, it's just going to eat you up; you're pretty much willing yourself to die."

Tonya's good cheer was tested by one ghastly procedure after another. "I had a couple of needle biopsies—they wanted to make sure what they were really dealing with—and I had four surgeries," Tonya recalls. "In the first one they did an embolization, where they tried to cut off as much of the blood supply [to the tumor] as possible. I was in there for six hours because they kept finding more and more blood vessels they wanted to block off. The next day, I had an open biopsy, where they tried to take a little of it out to see how it's doing. Then the next week I had the debulking surgery, where they tried to remove everything. But they couldn't. I started hemorrhaging, and they almost lost me in there."

The last operation only succeeded in removing a small portion of the tumor, but it did seem to help relieve the pressure enough to allow her to start walking again. Tonya went home, but just for a few days. She had to come back so surgeons could reposition one of her ovaries so it would be out of the way of the radiation treatments they were scheduling. They brought it up into her liver and gall bladder area, and they took X rays that showed that the tumor was as big as a soccer ball. "How pregnant did I look?" Tonya asked a doctor later. "About five months," the doctor replied.

Toward the end of April, Tonya finally got to go home again to Vermont, and a month later she began a monthlong series of daily radiation treatments at the Children's Specialty Clinic for Pediatric Oncology in Burlington. About halfway through that grinding ordeal, her doctors took more images and could see that the tumor wasn't responding anymore. It was still growing. The decision was to double the radiation dose, giving the blasts of energy twice a day instead of once. But more scans showed the tumor was still growing inexorably, though more slowly, squeezing tighter and tighter in her crowded abdomen. "That's when I started really getting scared," she says, "when they told me it didn't look good. When they told me I wasn't going to make it." Tonya's pregnant sister was with her, and when their mother asked if Tonya would live to see the birth of her niece, the doctors were unable to answer.

Tonya and her mother decided to go back to Boston for a second opinion about her prognosis. What they heard from a doctor at Dana-Farber was of little solace. Since there had been a partial response to radiation, they could try that again, at an even higher level. They could explore chemotherapy, though that was unlikely to work. They could do more surgery, but the outlook for that was no better than the last time. There was nothing new.

But fate interceded, just as it had for Tommy Briggs. On the very day that Tonya was in Boston hearing the bad news, her oncologist in Vermont, Alan Homans, was back in Burlington hearing Judah Folkman talk. What he heard came as a complete surprise. When Folkman showed the slides of little Jennifer LaChance and described interferon's power against giant-cell sarcomas—results that were not yet published but which compellingly illustrated the promise of antiangiogenesis therapies—Homans couldn't wait to collar him at the podium.

Tonya left Boston that day trying to cope with the strong probability that she would be dead in a few months. But when she got home, there was the phone call from Homans. "We're going to try something else," he said. "Something experimental. There's a doctor in Boston who's been using a drug that seems to work with certain large-cell tumors. Let's not get our hopes up, but it's worth seeing if it could help."

Tonya came in, and Homans told her all about Folkman and interferon, the lecture he'd attended while she was in Boston, the brief conversation he'd had with Folkman, and Folkman's request for a urine sample to see if she had high levels of something called fibroblast growth factor. What a coincidence of timing, Tonya thought. Maybe there was a reason for it. She gave Homans a urine sample and prayed it would show elevated levels of FGF. It did: Tonya's tumor was making twenty times more of the growth factor than normal. Folkman told Homans that experience recommended daily doses of interferon alpha.

Tonya's mother began giving her the injections right before the Fourth of July. As with Jennifer LaChance, the side effects—nausea and high fever—were immediate, but the intended effects were not. But after two months of anxious waiting, an X ray finally showed that Tonya's tumor had begun to shrink. The interferon was working.

Through these months, Tonya and her family were anxious to meet the man whose lab had pioneered the treatment that seemed to be saving her life. They were unaware how famous he was—they had somehow failed to notice the media eruption that spring, and so were not among those who called Boston, trying to get on a list that didn't exist. Now, months later, Tonya picked up a tattered magazine in a doctor's office. "It was an article in *Newsweek* about this angiogenesis thing," she recalls. "And I said, 'This is the guy!' It said all of the broadcasters wanted to get interviews with him, and he declined. I said, 'We're meeting him. Forget Tom Brokaw. I'm meeting him!' "

Tonya's mother called Folkman's office, and Susan Connors, his patient-liaison specialist, arranged for them to come in and meet him. On the appointed day, they drove down to Boston and met Folkman in an oak-filled conference room across a hall from his office, in the old part of Children's Hospital. Tonya expected Folkman would be dignified and businesslike—a big doctor. But he was the opposite, friendly and warm, totally without airs. And Folkman found Tonya spunky and determined, remarkably brave. He felt good to have met her. Tonya's mother took a picture of Tonya with Folkman and Dennis Hughes, the oncology resident in Vermont who worked under Homans. ("Take me with you," Hughes had said to Tonya when she told him she was going up to Boston to meet Folkman.) As he does with other patients, Folkman gave Tonya his home phone and beeper numbers, and urged her to call any time, anywhere, if she had any problems. "We can get him anywhere in the world," Tonya's mother said.

Tonya's tumor continued to shrink, and by the end of 1999, eighteen months after daily interferon treatments began, X rays showed it was 90 percent gone. Her urine samples, meanwhile, showed that her FGF levels were down to normal, indicating that the interferon was blocking the tumor's ability to put out the growth factor and recruit the new blood vessels it needed to thrive. The tumor had been so voracious it had made Tonya weak and anemic—"eating up all her blood," in her mother's words—requiring her to have almost monthly blood transfusions. But interferon ended that problem.

Finally, two years after she had first felt a pain on Halloween night, Tonya could think about the future. She had begun college at the University of Vermont, planning to become an elementary school teacher. She was working part-time in her sister's day care center. She talked of going on to earn a master's and even a Ph.D. "I thank God every single day that my doctors were there listening to Dr. Folkman that day," Tonya said. Folkman reflected on the irony of all that publicity that had made some of his colleagues wince. Had it not been for all the hubbub in spring 1998, Alan Homans probably wouldn't have attended Folkman's lecture in Burlington. He wouldn't have heard about interferon, and Tonya probably would have died.

Seven months after that lecture, Tonya was very much alive, witnessing the arrival of a new life, the birth of her niece. "I saw her come into this world!" she says. "I was right there when she was born. I just have this bond with her, because this was the child I was never supposed to see. She was born on January 31, 1999. Her name is Maggie. She is my goddaughter."

Chapter Seventeen

———

IN SEPTEMBER 1998, A NOTICE was posted on the World Wide Web claiming that Judah Folkman would soon be forced to retract the papers reporting angiostatin's and endostatin's spectacular results in mice. Folkman suspected the writer had sold short on EntreMed stock and was trying to drive the price down. The anonymous author was wrong—Folkman had no need to retract his laboratory's papers—but the note was not totally off the mark. It was true that Folkman was running into problems, in the sense that no other labs had yet published any reports confirming his results.

Soon after he began shipping endostatin to researchers around the country, Folkman heard that the drug had become inactive by the time it got to some of the laboratories, including Doug Hanahan's in San Francisco and the lab at the NCI. The recipients reported that the drugs were having little or no effect on cancer-bearing animals. Folkman was alarmed, needless to say. Any such report carries with it the suggestion that somehow the original research was wrong, or worse, that the results had been embellished. "You can tell when they're angry," Folkman says. "They call collect."

Folkman and his colleagues soon noticed that the problem seemed to be only with batches that were shipped to distant places. The endostatin being tested in local labs was fine. So the problem, in all likelihood, was in the shipping. Like many drugs or biomedical compounds, the endostatin was being frozen in small plastic vials, packed in dry ice, and sent out via Federal Express. Folkman and O'Reilly began doing experiments to figure out what might be going wrong. First, they found that the problem was not caused by freezing. When they froze a vial of endostatin, then thawed it, the drug worked normally. So how could transportation hurt it? Hoping to find clues, they packed a sample in dry ice, stowed it in the trunk of a car, and drove around Boston with it. Sure enough, when they brought it back into the lab and thawed it, the endostatin didn't work. But why?

As they tried to figure out what was going on, Folkman and his colleagues found themselves facing a public relations crisis. On November 12, 1998, a couple of months after the anonymous Internet note, *The Wall Street Journal* published a long front-page article headlined: NOVEL CANCER APPROACH FROM NOTED SCIENTIST HITS STUMBLING BLOCK. The subhead added: "So Far, Others Can't Match Folkman's Feat: Ending a Tumor's Blood Supply." A third of the way down the page was a sketch of Folkman, looking very worried. In the story, reporter Ralph T. King Jr. wrote that after all the anticipation and hype, there had yet to be any reports of replication. More ominously, the scientists at the National Cancer Institute were openly frustrated that they couldn't make the drugs work. King did point out that Bristol-Myers Squibb's researchers had succeeded in making small batches of angiostatin "that reliably slow tumor growth in mice," though they were having trouble making useful amounts of the drug.

Folkman was terribly pained by the article, and so was his wife. For decades, Paula Folkman had shared the ups and downs of her husband's career, reveling in the triumphs but also sharing the resentments that boiled below the surface. Folkman once remarked how Paula had kept his psyche intact in low moments, always reminding him of all the lives he'd saved in the operating room and of all the young surgeons he'd trained. But rarely had he felt as angry as he did on the day he read Ralph King's article in *The Wall Street Journal*. He answered it quickly, in a news release put out by Children's Hospital. Not only had his results with mice been confirmed in laboratories in Boston, Chicago, and San Francisco—though not yet published—but he was now able to announce that a Harvard colleague, Bjorn Olson, had also inhibited rat brain tumors with endostatin. And Dr. Vikas Sukhatme, across the street at the recently merged Beth Israel Deaconess Medical Center, had since used antiangiogenic therapy to suppress the growth of kidney tumors in mice. "Unfortunately, Mr. Ralph King, a reporter for *The Wall Street Journal,* chose to focus only on the challenges of translating the successes in our laboratory to other laboratories," Folkman was quoted saying in the news release. "We spent a significant amount of time with him trying to help him better understand that hurdles such as these are typical in any new research effort."

Indeed, replication of scientific results sometimes takes years, often for the most trivial reasons. Folkman related an early experience with angiostatin and mice. An outside researcher called and complained that the angiostatin was toxic—it was killing the mice. Did you do an autopsy? Folkman asked. No; there was no pathologist available. So Folkman invited the researcher to his lab and watched his technique. The researcher injected five mice with angiostatin, but even before he'd finished injecting the last mouse, two of them had already died. Folkman opened them up, and saw that they were full of blood—there was a clear tear in the spleen. The treatment was indeed lethal: The animals had been stabbed to death.

"When you first inject an animal, that first day is fine," Folkman said later. "But the second day they know you're coming. They have learned. They recognize your shadow and they turn around and bite." The injections were given with a very fine needle, a number 30, which can quickly slip right through the skin and into the spleen if the mouse jumps or jerks, causing a hemorrhage. He demonstrated the proper way to give the injection: Hold the mouse gently by the nape of the neck so it can't turn around and bite. He counted four people in his lab who gave excellent mouse shots—but there were four others he wouldn't allow near the mice. "They're so scared, they kill the animals all the time," he said. "They break their necks."

In the wake of the *Wall Street Journal* story, support for Folkman came from a researcher who had been able to confirm his results. Dr. Gerald Soff, at Northwestern University Medical School in Chicago, wrote to the newspaper to say he had made his own angiostatin and had been able to confirm its effectiveness against some metastatic and primary tumors in mice. Soff wrote that his results "serve as completely independent confirmation" of Folkman's work.

Folkman's spirits were also lifted significantly after a ten-day visit to his lab by a team of National Cancer Institute researchers. They had accepted his invitation to send a contingent to Boston to get hands-on help in replicating his results. Folkman's people trained the federal scientists in the use of antiangiogenic agents, and they were able to confirm his results with another group of mice. They still hadn't confirmed the work in their own laboratories, but Richard Klausner and the agency's leadership decided that was no longer necessary. They were satisfied that the new drugs did, in fact, eradicate tumors in mice, and that toxicity tests in larger animals—moving toward human trials—should start as soon as possible.

Meanwhile, Folkman's lab continued trying to figure out what was happening to the drugs in transit. The first real clue came serendipitously, in a report in *Nature Biotechnology* about this very problem. Researchers had found that packing drugs and compounds in frozen vials in dry ice—frozen carbon dioxide—essentially bathed the vials of drugs in carbon dioxide gas. It had the unexpected ability to seep right through the walls of the plastic vials. The result of contact with the carbon dioxide was a dramatic change in the pH (the acidity) of the drugs, which apparently rendered them inactive. One obvious answer seemed to be to ship the drug in glass containers, rather than in plastic—with a lot of extra packaging.

EVEN AS FOLKMAN WAS STRUGGLING with such issues, Michael O'Reilly continued searching for more antiangiogenesis agents. He found one within the same complex biological fluids that had yielded angiostatin and endostatin. This inhibitor seemed even more potent than the two proteins discovered earlier. He and Folkman named the agent angiodormin, and it turned out to be a molecule full of surprises.

One day, O'Reilly's wife, Val, who was then a resident in orthopedic surgery at Massachusetts General, was chatting with a researcher at the hospital, Lawrence Weisbach, who had been working on chemicals derived from cartilage. Aware of the Folkman lab's history with cartilage, she thought her husband should meet Weisbach. The two researchers did get together, and it led to an important connection for O'Reilly and the Folkman lab: A colleague of Weisbach's, Harvard physician Mark Goldberg, was vice president for medical affairs at Genzyme Corporation, a biotech company based nearby in Framingham. After an introduction, Goldberg invited O'Reilly out.

Over lunch, Goldberg told O'Reilly and some other members of the Folkman laboratory about the company's exciting new work, especially in genetic engineering. In fact, Genzyme's lead compound—antithrombin-3, or AT-3, which was already in clinical trials as a blood clot buster—was being made in genetically altered nanny goats. Clotting is facilitated in part by a protein called thrombin; antithrombin-3's role is to act as a braking system that can quickly turn off thrombin's action and avoid too much clotting—the kind that can be dangerous if it interferes with blood flow. Antithrombin-3 was being tested by doctors in Europe to combat recurring blood clots in people's legs, and Genzyme expected to soon be able to sell it in the United States.

As Goldberg discussed AT-3 and described its molecular structure, O'Reilly was making a connection in his mind. "As we were walking out," Goldberg recalls, "I was talking with Michael, just the two of us, when he said, 'You know, I might have something we should talk about.' At first he wouldn't tell me. But he did say that something related to antithrombin-3 may be antiangiogenic. But the experiments were very early on, and he would get back to me. Well, you know, this is a guy who works day and night, so he e-mailed me on a Sunday to say that antithrombin-3 is antiangiogenic." Just as O'Reilly had silently suspected during their meeting, angiodormin and antithrombin-3 were the same weight, the same size, and had the same structure. They were essentially the same molecule.

Goldberg invited Folkman and O'Reilly back out to Framingham, and there O'Reilly revealed that he had found a slightly altered version of antithrombin-3, and it was an extraordinarily powerful inhibitor of blood vessel growth. The Folkman lab's molecular analysis showed that only a very small change in AT-3's structure was enough to convert it, irreversibly, into the angiogenesis inhibitor they were calling angiodormin. By changing one small molecular loop, tucking it inside the molecule rather than leaving it dangling outside, antithrombin-3 was turned into angiodormin. In scientific terms, the discovery meant that nature had found an efficient way to use one molecule to do two vital jobs. In commercial terms, because Genzyme was already making antithrombin-3 in large amounts, and was pushing it through clinical trials, the company could produce and get angiodormin into the pipeline as well. "Their data sounded extremely interesting to me, and it looked very strong," Goldberg later said. "Our people were immediately impressed, and we started telling them what we knew about AT-3, the chemistry. The fit was just beautiful."

So was the timing. By the time angiodormin was discovered, O'Reilly's research was being supported by NCI money, which freed Folkman to steer the commercial rights to someone other than EntreMed, which already was knee-deep in angiostatin and endostatin work and wouldn't be able to develop angiodormin nearly as quickly as Genzyme through its transgenic nanny goats. Genzyme had been hoping for a six-million-dollar annual market for AT-3 in the United States and Europe. O'Reilly's discovery had the potential to open up a six-hundred-million-dollar annual market for angiodormin. Genzyme was excited, to put it mildly.

Thus the deal was struck, with Harvard holding the patent and Genzyme getting the license. In the meantime, Folkman, O'Reilly, and their collaborators submitted their paper on angiodormin to *Nature*, in England. It quickly ran into trouble. To begin with, one anonymous reviewer didn't like the name angiodormin, arguing instead that it should be called "antiangiogenic antithrombin-3," or aaAT-3. The editors of *Nature* agreed, and also asked for a huge number of changes, as well as more research, more tests, and more analysis. After several months of back-and-forth haggling, Folkman and O'Reilly pulled their paper, reconfigured it, and mailed it off to *Science*, where it would be published in September 1999.

GENZYME'S GOAT-RAISING FARM is set among the rolling hills in Charlton, Massachusetts, about fifty miles west of Boston. At the front door, visitors are required to dip the soles of their shoes into a bath of pink antiseptic fluid. "These are the best-cared-for goats in the world," remarks the director of operations, Christopher Hendry, leading a tour one day through the barns, milking sheds, embryo transfer facilities, and laboratories. They are also probably the most expensive and valuable goats in the world.

The goats, the property of Genzyme's subsidiary, Genzyme Transgenics, are pioneers in the new form of biotechnology called "gene-pharming." Each animal is injected with a new gene—the gene for AT-3—that is specifically designed to be active only in mammary tissue, so that the protein is made along with the goats' milk and can be produced in large amounts and retrieved very easily. In fact, Genzyme's production system can extract two grams of aaAT-3 from every liter of goat's milk, and a good goat can make eight hundred liters of milk a year. The best Bristol-Myers Squibb achieved with angiostatin, through fermentation, was only thirty milligrams per liter—and it was tough to make a liter.

Inadvertently, Genzyme was very well prepared to jump into the antiangiogenesis business. As Folkman's lab discovered, changing the clot-buster protein AT-3 into the antiangiogenesis agent aaAT-3 was easy. Simply cooking it gently and adding a chemical called citrate changed the protein's molecular shape slightly, converting a clot buster into a very strong nontoxic angiogenesis inhibitor and antitumor agent. With its goats, Genzyme had a herd of living factories on the hoof: The goat-based production process had already been approved by the Food and Drug Administration, and Genzyme had amassed almost a decade of experience with antithrombin-3. It wouldn't take long, it seemed, for Genzyme to get aaAT-3 into the clinic for tests against cancer. Indeed, within a few months, Genzyme was able to give Folkman and O'Reilly about four ounces of aaAT-3, whereas it had taken three years for Bristol-Myers Squibb to squeeze out a similar amount of angiostatin. Genzyme was moving fast, and the excitement within the company rose as executives realized how much profit they stood to make without having to invest large amounts of money in research and development.

Their good fortune was practically an accident, the result of a series of chance events. O'Reilly's isolation of what was now being called aaAT-3 (or triple-AT-3) was such a surprise that he and his colleagues at first suspected it had to be an error. There seemed to be so much potent activity for so little fluid that they felt some contaminant must have slipped into the liquids they were extracting from the cancer cell culture system. It took another postdoctoral fellow in the laboratory, Dr. Steven Pirie-Shepherd, to figure out that the vital ingredient, antithrombin-3, was not a tumor product at all, but an agent that came into the system as a natural part of the culture medium, fetal calf serum. A processing agent, an enzyme called elastase, was responsible for transforming antithrombin-3 into aaAT-3, the potent inhibitor. The discovery opened the door to a whole new family of bloodborne molecules they hadn't explored before called serpins.

It was known that serpins, which help with blood clotting, comprise five of the forty known proteins that are part of the emergency blood-clotting system. The team began a series of laboratory experiments to see if the other known serpins also had antiangiogenesis activity. The first one they looked at—anti-alpha-2-antiplasmin—turned out to be a powerful angiogenesis inhibitor. The whole family of serpins would soon be on the noteboard in Folkman's conference room among those burning questions for postdoctoral fellows to tackle. There would be no shortage of work, especially because Genzyme's scientists were still struggling to scale up production of reliable aaAT-3.

For Folkman, the most remarkable part of the emerging story was seeing how nature had found ways to use specific biomolecules for multiple purposes, all within the wound-healing process. Antithrombin-3 is constantly present in the bloodstream, ready to help clear out blood clots after a wound starts to heal. Meanwhile, its residue, aaAT-3, stays a little longer to keep blood vessel growth from going too far. As an emergency system, the blood-clotting mechanism is vital, but it's equally vital to shut it off in time, before serious damage—stroke, for example—arises from lack of blood to vital organs. Ironically, triple-AT-3's antiangiogenesis activity could not have been noticed in the AT-3 clot-busting trials. Under the rigid rules of the research protocol, all cancer patients were excluded.

GIVEN THE LEVEL of enthusiasm and achievement in the laboratory, it wasn't easy for Folkman to get back on track in the office, answering queries from patients all over the world, advising doctors who asked about antiangio-genesis, and arranging travel to give talks and collect awards. One thing he still had to deal with was the all-too-familiar public relations problems that the *Wall Street Journal* article had caused on his home turf. Many people within the Harvard and Boston medical community had looked askance at the explosion of publicity detonated by the *New York Times* story in May, and the *Journal* article six months later gave them cause to say, "See?" The story's im-plication was that something was messy in Folkman's laboratory, or at least that Folkman wasn't telling the full story. The *Journal*'s article left such a neg-ative impression that Folkman began hearing disturbing rumblings from within Children's Hospital, and the nearby Dana-Farber Cancer Institute. It was said that doctors were worried about "the Folkman problem." The phrase made him furious. "People were asking, 'What should we do about the Folk-man problem?' as though we had started it," Folkman says. He saw himself as a victim of bad journalism—and carping colleagues.

The simmering fuss reached a boil on a major committee at Dana-Farber that had recently been appointed by David Nathan to coordinate the insti-tute's ten-year grant from the National Institutes of Health. By now, thirty-six different labs within the Harvard system were at work on angiogenesis research, and Folkman was their representative on the committee. The group had been meeting every other week when the *Wall Street Journal* article came out. "Somebody on the committee, who had not read our papers, but just the newspaper, said maybe we shouldn't have [angiogenesis research] on the grant, and what are we going to do about the Folkman problem?" Folkman says.

Tired of the backbiting and the bellyaching, Folkman stood up at a meet-ing in mid-December and read a statement. "About four weeks ago," he said, "there was a very misleading and erroneous article in *The Wall Street Journal*, which was devastating to me and made my wife ill. The article focused on one of the most recently published angiogenesis inhibitors, endostatin, and why some labs find it so hard to reproduce its powerful antitumor effect. In fact, we routinely make recombinant endostatin every week, and four different re-search groups in the lab use it as a potent angiogenesis inhibitor and anti-tumor agent. Other labs in addition to ours make their own protein, and also find it very reproducible. The first confirmatory papers from other labs will be in the January issue of *Cancer Research*, with others to follow. But it is not trivial to learn how to produce and use this protein, and we are in the midst of teaching a group at the National Cancer Institute how to make endostatin and how to use it in tumor-bearing animals. I have every confidence that in a couple of months they will be up to speed. However, many colleagues at Harvard have informed me that certain individuals connected with Dana-Farber and the Medical School . . . have been less than supportive, and have been openly critical of me and my work . . . behind my back! Therefore, I do not wish to collaborate further on this grant application. I have my own work to do. I am confident that there are enough good people working on angiogenesis at Harvard to do the work for this section of the grant. I will be available at any time as a consultant if you need it. But, I do not want support from the grant."

And then Folkman walked out. He had been able to withstand scientific criticism for three decades because he had never allowed himself to take it too seriously. But now it did strike a nerve. To face the murmurings, the rolled eyes, and the sideways glances from colleagues at this stage of his career—when his work was known worldwide and awards were coming in steadily—was more than he was willing to ignore.

But doubts were still in the air, and two months later, in February 1999, Bristol-Myers Squibb, which had sublicensed some of the rights to angiostatin from EntreMed four years before, dropped a bombshell, announcing it was abandoning development of angiostatin and ending its agreement with EntreMed. It was a huge disappointment for Folkman, O'Reilly, and other members of the research team in Boston, not to mention John Holaday and his colleagues at EntreMed. The value of EntreMed's stock dropped almost in half, with about 3.3 million shares changing hands the day of the announcement, about ten times more sales than usual. Bristol-Myers shares fell only twenty-five cents. (EntreMed's stock rebounded back to twenty-five dollars a share when the NCI announced that its own researchers, working in Folkman's laboratory in Boston, had succeeded in duplicating his original work, shrinking tumors in mice by using endostatin.)

Though the decision by Bristol-Myers was a major setback, there were some in Folkman's laboratory who thought it might not be a bad thing. They had long felt a lack of enthusiasm on the part of the big drug company, and it was holding back progress. The five-year agreement with EntreMed that had started with such promise had deteriorated into an untenable scientific partnership, with two groups of scientists going in different directions. To develop a reliable production system for angiostatin, EntreMed had first tried using genetically altered yeast cells, then switched to Chinese hamster ovary cells, and finally came back to yeast. Bristol-Myers, meanwhile, had started out and stayed with genetically engineered bacteria. "We went around and around about that, each pursuing our own ideas," a member of Folkman's lab later said. "Bristol-Myers didn't want to play like the rest of us did."

One of the things Bristol-Myers demanded as part of the angiostatin contract was that EntreMed immediately destroy its angiostatin-making cultures, even though Kim Lee Sim and her staff had already spent several years engineering the yeast cells so the cultures made the protein efficiently. "That was very hard," she recalls. "On the day we had to do it, we held a funeral for our cultures. As we dumped everything into a biohazards bag" to be destroyed, "we poured in a little champagne—it was very good champagne—and closed it up. That was very sad." It turned out to be doubly sad, because Bristol-Myers soon threw in the towel, making the scientists at EntreMed vow to never again destroy valuable cultures. They also breathed a big sigh of relief that their company had not signed away the rights to Folkman's second antiangiogenic agent, endostatin.

The big drug company had gotten its bacterial system going in 1998 and was putting some resources into it, but everything changed when Leon Rosenberg left the company for Princeton University, taking his enthusiasm for angiostatin with him. Rosenberg's replacement, Peter Ringrose, was "a consummate drug development guy," in the words of a member of Folkman's team, "and he wouldn't allow the stuff that Rosenberg would"—meaning that Bristol-Myers would now pursue drugs offering more immediate promise. The company had decided that angiostatin was still too far from the clinic, not as close to market as some of the other products the company was pursuing. "At this time, angiostatin protein in its present form does not meet our criteria for molecules that advance to clinical trials," Robert Kramer, head of the cancer drug discovery program at Bristol-Myers, told the public. "We have chosen to direct our resources to other programs in our broad oncology pipeline."

Kramer did note that the firm had other potential antiangiogenesis agents in the research pipeline, which the company intended to keep on pursuing. The company also made it clear it was keeping one foot in the door. Its announcement said it "will have the option to re-assume development and marketing rights for angiostatin protein once clinical proof of principle has been demonstrated." In other words, let someone else—maybe the government— pick up the research tab, and get angiostatin close to clinical trials, and then we'll reassess whether to wade in again.

It wasn't clear that EntreMed would welcome Bristol-Myers's return, if it came, because in the meantime EntreMed's scientists had refined their yeast-cell system to produce enough pure angiostatin for research, and was awarded an IND—an investigational new drug permit—by the Food and Drug Administration early in 2000. Winning the permit meant clinical trials could be set up, but there was no sign Bristol-Myers would soon find angiostatin alluring enough to have another go. Still, as the firm's public relations representative, Tracy Furey, stated: "If it has to do with cancer, we're involved." That, of course, remained to be seen. Bristol-Myers had closed down its only facility that was making the drug, and in February 1999 informed EntreMed that it was returning the licensing rights without having filed for an IND permit with the Food and Drug Administration. Some thought it was a case of NIH syndrome—"Not Invented Here"—and that the few people within the company who were enthusiastic about angiostatin were finally outrun by those who cared very little. "We were competing with the naysayers" within Bristol-Myers, Holaday says. In the end, after Rosenberg's departure, the company's leadership couldn't visualize angiostatin as a commercially viable drug.

For EntreMed, it was a loss of tremendous financial support, but the company managed to survive the transition and began to accelerate its own work, trying to make angiostatin in large amounts. The company's small group of scientists concentrated on a species of yeast cells called *Pichia pastoris*. They began by inserting the gene that makes angiostatin into each yeast cell, then growing the cells in huge vats while the cells—acting as if the new gene were one of their own—obeyed its instructions and produced the pure drug, angiostatin. After months of work fine-tuning the yeast-based production system, it began to work reliably enough that the clinical trials for angiostatin came within grasp.

By this point, EntreMed was even farther ahead in the drive to scale up production of Folkman's second antiangiogenesis agent, endostatin, and bring it to clinical trials. EntreMed had not gotten entangled with Bristol-Myers on endostatin—the drug company hadn't offered Holaday enough money—but instead hired an independent company, Covance Laboratories, to make it in bulk. Covance was able to make enough for the National Cancer Institute to do something essential before human trials could begin: run toxicity tests in animals other than mice. The NCI arranged to use monkeys, but at first the toxicity testing was slow. The doses being given were tiny, increasing only in small steps. Impatient, and certain that endostatin would show no signs of toxicity, Folkman urged the NCI to go right to the top and give the monkeys doses one hundred times higher than would be used in humans. As

Folkman predicted, the massive doses didn't show even a hint of toxicity. It was an important step toward clinical trials.

There was, however, more trouble from *The Wall Street Journal*. On September 13, 1999, Ralph T. King Jr. fired another salvo at Folkman's team, declaring that "the National Cancer Institute has failed to reproduce the highly publicized effects of [endostatin] after months of attempts in its labs," and that despite this, the institute had decided to begin human trials. It was in fact true that NCI scientists had not replicated Folkman's results in their labs in Bethesda. But it was also true—as the institute said in a quick and direct response to the *Journal* story—that after its technicians went to Folkman's lab and were able to confirm the work there, NCI was satisfied that the drug was ready to be tested in humans. "Given the reports of antitumor activity of human endostatin in mice and its documented lack of toxicity," the institute said, "NCI believes that the only way to begin to rigorously evaluate this unique compound in people with cancer is to move it into clinical trials."

And so the time drew close when Folkman, along with the rest of the world, would know whether the great goal would be achieved. Covance came through with enough for the National Cancer Institute to schedule the first human toxicity trials to begin in fall 1999. Folkman saw the first one-kilogram bottle of endostatin and marveled. It was worth seven million dollars. How many lives might be saved with the contents of that bottle? No one could know. But it would be too late for many of those who had desperately called or even appeared in Boston in the days and weeks after Gina Kolata's story heralded a potential cure for cancer. Mike McAlary, the New York *Daily News* columnist who had written, "Maybe we don't have to die," would never know if the news was true or not. He died eight months later, on Christmas morning, 1998.

Chapter Eighteen

———

AS THE DREAM of conquering cancer—or at least controlling it—seemed to grow tantalizingly close, something else was emerging from Judah Folkman's years of work, something much less evident than antiangiogenesis but equally profound and important. Cardiovascular specialists were exploring ways to exploit the opposite effect—angiogenesis, the stimulation of blood vessel growth—as an emergency repair for hearts and legs. Eye specialists, too, were coaxing clues from angiogenesis research to learn why diabetics so often go blind and to seek ways to prevent it. Judah Folkman's long years of research into all the aspects of blood vessel growth had suddenly spawned an explosion of ideas, even the start of another biomedical revolution.

By the mid-1990s, a handful of heart doctors had begun experimenting with the idea that the growth-stimulating factors discovered a decade earlier—FGF and VEGF—might help restore blood circulation to failing hearts and endangered limbs. The few cardiovascular specialists who first dared try it ran head-on into disbelief and dismay, even outright hostility, from many of their colleagues.

Even those bold enough to make the attempt had serious misgivings. When Doctor Jeffrey Isner first injected genes that make a growth factor into a patient's leg in an effort to restore circulation, he wondered whether he was going too far, too fast.

Ever since graduating from the Tufts University School of Medicine and serving his residency in cardiology at the Georgetown University Medical Center in Washington, Isner had been consumed by a fierce drive to achieve something important in medicine. He was a cardiovascular surgeon with the drive and tenacity to take on the seemingly insurmountable problems of his field. One of these was the dismal predicament of patients whose arterial blockages were so extensive that normal catheterization and bypass operations were impossible. Patients with failing legs were severely disabled, and heart patients' lives were in danger.

In the mid-1990s, as a lead surgeon at St. Elizabeth's Medical Center in Brighton, a Boston neighborhood, Isner began to wonder if there was an answer in the developing field of angiogenesis. Over the past decade, Folkman and his colleagues at Children's Hospital, and others in the growing field, had gradually uncovered hormonelike factors that specifically cause blood vessels to grow. Folkman, of course, was putting all his resources into finding angiogenesis *inhibitors,* looking at every way possible to make blood vessels *stop* growing and thus block cancer. But Isner had his eye on the opposing factors, the angiogenesis stimulators. Could they somehow be exploited to induce new blood vessels to grow exactly where he wanted them, in just the right places to restore failing circulation? It was an entirely new approach, so Isner and his research colleagues needed a quick course in the budding science of angiogenesis. Being in Boston, Isner decided to seek advice from the master, right across town at Children's Hospital. Although he had never met Folkman face-to-face, he was well aware that his contribution to medicine was already immense, and he respected Folkman's dogged determination to pursue his ideas by going from one logical step to the next.

The patients Isner's team was immediately interested in were those suffering from serious circulatory failures in a leg, of the kind often associated with diabetes. They often had severe pain, ulcers, and impaired ability to walk. And they sometimes got hooked on narcotic medications to help cope with the pain. In fact, studies had shown that patients with failing leg circulation often were in such severe pain that their quality of life was comparable to that of cancer patients in the terminal phases of their illness. It was an intractable problem, and hardly an uncommon one. Isner set out to see whether the newly discovered blood vessel growth factors such as VEGF and b-FGF might be used to cause new blood vessels, a collateral circulation system, to grow.

A sketchy answer began to emerge one day in 1996 when a sales representative from the biotechnology firm Genentech was making a call at St. Elizabeth's. The salesman was in town to push a new clot buster, but Isner was more interested in Genentech's new version of FGF, which the company was just then beginning to make available for experimentation outside its own labs.

The salesman asked what he wanted it for, and Isner told him his idea. The suggestion reached Genentech researchers in South San Francisco, and they found the idea interesting enough to give Isner a small amount of the scarce growth factor so he could run a few animal experiments.

A Japanese postdoctoral fellow working with Isner, Satoshi Takeshita, agreed to take on the project, and soon after the FGF arrived from California, Takeshita injected small doses of the growth factor into the femoral arteries of a dozen rabbits. Then he closed the arteries to starve the downstream tissue of oxygen, setting up conditions for new blood vessel growth—the tissues demanded it. Satoshi waited three days to sacrifice the first rabbit, and when he saw the results he came running to Isner, all out of breath. "You've got to see this angiogram!" he said. Isner put the angiogram—showing the positions, sizes, and numbers of blood vessels in the rabbit after the treatment—up on his X-ray view box. "Sure enough," Isner recalled later, "this animal was just loaded with collateral blood vessels."

Next Isner and his colleagues tried the other stimulator, VEGF, and also gave placebo injections to control animals. When they compared the angiograms, they saw that VEGF, like FGF, induced the growth of new blood vessels in the animals. But did that mean that simply injecting the growth factors could save somebody's leg? Isner thought it might, and was soon hell-bent on getting Genentech to set up a clinical trial to try to find out. They had positive animal experiments, and plenty of desperate patients looking for anything that might help them avoid amputation. But Genentech demurred, unwilling to get into a project that had so little data to go on, and no amount of cajoling or wheedling could change the company's mind.

The corporate roadblock was frustrating for Isner, but in the end it turned out to be a blessing, because it forced him into new thinking. Coincidentally, the St. Elizabeth's team had been exploring the possibilities for pioneering new therapies that might someday emerge from the burgeoning new field of gene transfer, or gene therapy. Dr. Betsy Nabel, at the University of Michigan, had recently shown that it was possible to insert some extra genes and get them to function inside endothelial cells, the vital cells that line the inside of arteries and begin growing to form new capillaries. This hinted that endothelial cells might be responsive to gene therapy. Isner considered Nabel's work "a seminal observation," though in retrospect it shouldn't have been a big surprise. Many kinds of cells were being altered by giving them new genes for making all manner of proteins, such as human insulin, human growth factor, and blood-clotting factor.

The idea of somehow inserting genes into endothelial cells led Isner's team to start thinking that maybe they could begin to exploit all this new genetic technology and this emerging science in a way that would allow them to actually rebuild parts of failing circulatory systems in their patients. They might even be able to do it through genetic engineering, with genes alone, rather than having to go to Genentech and beg for the scarce growth factor proteins. A California company, Vical, Inc., had reported that genes didn't even need to be forced into special cells or into viruses to activate them. Genes, "naked" because they were not being carried into cells by a virus or any other vehicle, could simply be injected into muscle tissue. A few muscle cells would soak up some of the genes and somehow turn them on, making them active. This reaction was a major surprise—"outrageous science," as one expert remarked—and it provided a direct and simple avenue for Isner's team to explore. They suspected the muscle cells that were living there anyway and were being starved for oxygen might be the best candidates for making VEGF, the protein that would stimulate new blood vessel growth. They could use the "naked" DNA—copies of the gene that makes VEGF—to produce the growth factor itself. It was a bold gamble; this strange naked-DNA technology invented by Vical was essentially untried for this purpose. But if it worked, it might cause the cells to make VEGF for several weeks and perhaps awaken dormant capillaries and get them growing. There was an obvious— and ironic—source for the DNA representing VEGF: Genentech, which had refused all requests for the proteins themselves. Napoleone Ferrara, the Genentech scientist who had just beaten Folkman to the discovery of VEGF (née TAF), was happy to share the gene.

Satoshi Takeshita began testing the idea with animals. Instead of injecting the protein VEGF into the rabbits, he simply injected the naked DNA that makes VEGF into the animals' muscles. And it worked beautifully. By using the genes, they got new blood vessel growth every bit as good as they got with the pure protein. Success with the gene injections meant that they didn't have to grovel for Genentech's blessing anymore. They would go directly to the government for approval of human trials.

That was no small thing in itself. Human trials of gene therapy were a brand-new research field in which experiments had been tried on only a few patients, none of whom needed new blood vessels, so they were subject to more than the usual governmental oversight. Seeking permission was a formidable task, not to be undertaken by a neophyte. Lacking direct experience in such matters, Isner decided to consult someone for help. He called Dr.

James Wilson, a leading gene therapy experimenter who had just moved to the University of Pennsylvania, and told him his idea. After a phone conversation, Isner and his colleagues dispatched to Wilson a package explaining the results in rabbits, discussing the therapy proposal with all the details. Wilson sent back a blunt opinion that Isner's idea would never work because they were using the "naked DNA" technique. But Isner, like Folkman, refused to to be discouraged.

Jim Wilson wasn't the only expert whose doubts about naked DNA made it difficult for Isner to go ahead with his treatment in patients. The disapproval, in fact, was sometimes brutal. That naked DNA had begun to revolutionize vaccine technology—offering a new way to make vaccines, as well as a safe, cheap, and effective way to use them—failed to alter the opposition to Isner's seemingly radical, unproven idea. He was using an untried technique in an untested new field of medicine, hoping to treat what were considered hopeless cases of cardiovascular disease. But, of course, there were good reasons to be cautious—as Wilson himself would realize only too well a few years later. Early in 2000, Wilson's work at Penn, tailoring viruses to be carriers of genes to correct inherited deficiency disorders, would be shut down by the federal government after an eighteen-year-old, Jesse Gelsinger, died of a massive immune reaction in a gene therapy trial. As part of the fallout, Isner's work was also interrupted while the government agencies sorted out how gene experiments should proceed.

Isner was running a very limited and closely monitored study involving only a few patients for whom there seemed to be no alternative other than losing a leg to amputation. But the assurances failed to make his critics any less uncomfortable. One day in 1997, Isner stood before an audience of experts at the annual clinical meeting of the American Heart Association and was roundly scolded for even suggesting such an experimental treatment. Having detailed his findings and his rationale, Isner found himself under assault by colleagues who lined up to heap abuse upon him. Heart specialists, among the best in the world, queued up behind aisle microphones to fiercely denounce the questionable notion that genetic engineering and a simple injection could induce blood vessels to grow and replace clogged arteries. Worse, to begin treating real patients so early, without benefit of more animal trials and rigorous, large-scale, double-blind trials, was seen by many as reprehensible. Here was Isner going directly into patients hoping for efficacy, rather than first running months-long trials testing for toxicity and side effects. He also seemed to be reporting results too early: Were new blood vessels really there? If so, would they last? And what about the placebo effect? Was this all imaginary?

But the opposition didn't stop Isner. He was convinced he and his colleagues were on to a potentially revolutionary treatment that might alleviate some of the most vexing and intractable problems in cardiovascular medicine. They were gambling they could save hearts, legs, and even lives if they succeeded in getting enough new blood vessels to grow where they were needed. His persistence helped win grudging permission from the Food and Drug Administration to try his treatment on a few patients.

ISNER GOT HIS FIRST patient in the modern way. A schoolteacher from the Bronx, Nancy Perez, had called his office in Boston after spotting a brief television report from the AHA meeting. Isner's idea sounded interesting and plausible, and Perez was absolutely desperate: She was about to lose a leg to amputation because of failing circulation. She asked her own doctor in New York if he'd heard of Isner's work. He had, indeed; her doctor had been one of the most vociferous of the physicians who'd stood up to condemn Isner at the AHA meeting. Isner remembered him. "This is the most unethical thing I've ever heard," the doctor had said. "It will never work. I can't believe you guys would waste your time."

So the doctor was aghast when his patient asked what he thought about Isner's work. Forget it, he told Nancy Perez bluntly. But she didn't forget it; it was her leg, not the doctor's, and she was ready to try anything to save it. She contacted Isner's office in Boston and said she wanted to be one of the first patients to test Isner's idea. Isner and other cardiovascular specialists constantly saw patients like Perez. For them, standard treatments, including multiple artery bypass operations, had usually failed because once blood circulation in the legs has stopped, it is very difficult to get it reestablished, even with sophisticated operations. It was not uncommon for such patients to go through several surgical procedures and still have no choice but amputation.

When she arrived in Boston, Nancy Perez was in terrible shape—in a wheelchair, almost completely immobile, and hooked on narcotic painkillers. A zombie, Isner thought when he saw her. He began the procedure, giving a few simple injections of the special gene directly into Perez's leg muscles, near where the artery was blocked. The procedure was quick and relatively painless, and a few days later Perez would be on her way home to New York.

But as Isner finished the procedure, he was plagued with doubts. After he treated her and he walked out of the room, he felt as if he were wearing dirty underwear. He thought to himself, What have you degenerated into? This is the closest thing to voodoo medicine. Injecting this stuff and expecting to see something happening is really pathetic. I mean, what's the chance this is going to work?

When Perez came back to Boston two weeks later, she announced: "There is something happening." Isner, seeing no obvious signs of change, asked her what she meant. "I don't know," Perez replied. "But something is happening in my leg. I feel something going on."

Isner's first thought was the obvious: Maybe it was the placebo effect, just wishful thinking. It was a common and powerful phenomenon in desperate patients; just being admitted to a clinical study could make some people feel better, even without treatment. But when Perez came back a week later for another checkup, his doubts evaporated. Tests showed that the blood pressure in her leg had started to increase, and that alone was amazing. Improved blood pressure in a stricken limb was rarely if ever seen in such patients, and it indicated that something important was indeed happening in tissue that had been dangerously starved of blood. Her pain was also subsiding, enough so she could be weaned off the painkilling drugs. And within a year, this young woman who had been all but resigned to being crippled for life, whose arteries were so clogged that she was a week away from being scheduled for an amputation, was out of her wheelchair and resuming normal activities, including running, all after only one series of shots.

It was hard to know exactly what was happening inside Perez's leg because the tiny capillaries presumably being triggered to grow by the shots couldn't be seen on X rays. Angiograms indicated that a host of new small vessels had grown past the area of blockage, but it seemed only an autopsy—preferably many years later—would show what had actually occurred. In the meantime, the improvement in symptoms was all the evidence that Isner and his colleagues needed to indicate that they had pulled off a medical miracle. Quietly, a door opened on to a new era in the treatment of cardiovascular disease. Much of the doubt of skeptics disappeared with Nancy Perez's wheelchair, and in the next three years, Isner and his team successfully treated more than one hundred people struggling with severe circulatory problems in their legs. Inevitably, Isner and other doctors began thinking seriously about whether angiogenesis therapy had an even more important use—in the heart.

Every year several hundred thousand Americans undergo coronary artery bypass surgery to route blood around clogged arteries, while thousands of others go through angioplasty to open those arteries. The costs are enormous—forty-five thousand dollars or more for each bypass procedure— and still other patients can't be helped at all. One such seemingly hopeless patient was Floyd Stokes. He had been the picture of the rugged west Texas peanut farmer, but at age fifty-eight he was almost completely disabled because of heart disease. His chest pains were so severe that he could hardly pull his boots on.

Stokes had undergone a coronary artery bypass operation fifteen years earlier, but his doctors at Harris Methodist Fort Worth Hospital had recently found that the blood vessels that should have been feeding his heart were clogged again. This time there wasn't anything further they could do; they determined that another surgery might be dangerous, harming his already weakened heart and maybe doing more harm than good. A second specialist confirmed the opinion. But then Stokes's wife, Jean, read an article in *Newsweek* about Isner's naked-DNA experiments on patients in Boston whose legs needed new blood vessels. Tagged onto the end of the article was word that Isner was seeking permission from the FDA to give these shots to heart patients. "That's what I need," Stokes told his wife after reading the article.

But when they contacted Isner's staff in Boston, the answer was blunt and crushing: no. The experiments hadn't yet progressed to heart patients. "I understand that," Stokes told Isner's assistant. "But when you do get approval I want to be on your list. I want that procedure, because I've been turned down everywhere to get another bypass, or anything to do me any good. I'm a farmer and a rancher, and I can't do my work." A big, barrel-chested man, Stokes had come to the point where he'd had to hire extra farmhands to work his peanut fields, while he supervised. "All I can do is sit in my pickup at the end of the rows," he said mournfully.

It took many months for Isner to get permission from the Food and Drug Administration to try the therapy on a few heart patients, and almost as soon as it came through, Floyd Stokes was on his way to Massachusetts. On the operating table, Isner gave him twenty small injections of naked DNA, shooting multiple copies of the gene that makes VEGF into the big Texan's oxygen-starved heart muscle. After a few days in the hospital for observation, the peanut farmer and his wife flew back to their ranch in Texas, waiting, hoping, praying, for good results.

They didn't have to wait long. In about three weeks Stokes felt better.

Then, one Sunday morning, he woke up and told his wife, "I feel fantastic!" He couldn't believe it would work that quickly. He called Isner and his staff and told them how good he felt, asking, "Can this be it? Can it be working this quick?" Well, yes, they said, they had people say they felt better after two or three weeks. "Man, this is something else!" Stokes shouted. He resumed active work on his farm, and six months after treatment he was vigorously striding around, looking hearty, bubbling with enthusiasm. "I don't have any pain, and I can work as hard as I want," he told a visitor. "I walk anywhere I want to."

Albert Laurent was a retired construction foreman who lived in a four-family building in Lawrence, Massachusetts, in an apartment whose living room was decorated with his own homemade oak woodcraft treasures and photographs of his twelve children. Laurent was seventy-two, short and friendly. But he was a man who'd been so disabled with heart disease that he could barely creep up the stairs to the apartment where he lived with his wife of fifty years, Eileen. His angina (chest pains) hurt so badly that Laurent could only struggle up two steps, take a couple of nitroglycerin pills, sit and rest a few minutes, and then take another two steps, pop more pills, and rest again. Laurent had already gone through a coronary artery bypass operation, which eventually failed, plus several catheterization procedures that had temporarily reopened the clogged arteries feeding his heart. The vessels had then reclosed, and Laurent was only being kept alive on nitro pills and other potent medications. He was a man of habits and had long made a point of attending Mass every day, but now that was impossible. Just making it through the day was an ordeal. "I was sure I was going to die at any moment," he says.

Laurent's physician, Dr. Robert Shulman, was alert to new possibilities, and in 1998 he asked Laurent if he was willing to try something that was completely new and virtually untested. "I said yes, because there was nothing else," he recalls. "I didn't have much to lose." So his name was given to Isner's team at St. Elizabeth's Hospital, and Laurent was soon enrolled as one of their first heart patients. The results were swift and amazing.

Within weeks of getting the naked-DNA injections directly into the heart muscle, he was experiencing far less angina pain and feeling stronger. He had told Isner the one thing he really hoped was that he would just get well enough to resume work in his home woodshop. One day a few weeks after therapy began, Laurent got up, went to his shop, and didn't come back out again. Worried, his wife went to check on him, imagining that she might find his body. But she found him beavering away on his wooden trinkets. A week later Laurent felt even better, so much so that he made his way down to the church. His bothersome angina pain was gone, though his condition was still not perfect. "I can tell when I overdo it," he says. "If I work too hard and don't rest, I feel a burning sensation in my chest. But it goes away if I sit down and take a rest." The nitro pills, though kept handy, seemed to be a thing of the past.

Jeffrey Isner wasn't the only one pursuing angiogenesis. A few other doctors soon followed with their own variations. Rather than take the naked-DNA approach, Dr. Ronald Crystal and Dr. Todd Rosengart, at the Cornell University Medical Center in New York City, genetically engineered the adenovirus, a cause of the common cold, so that it contained the gene for VEGF but no longer could cause disease when it infected the patients' cells. The redesigned virus was injected into the heart muscle, whose cells then made VEGF, released it locally, and stimulated new blood vessel growth. Meanwhile, Dr. Michael Simons, a Russian émigré who headed the angiogenesis research center at Beth Israel Deaconess Medical Center in Boston, was using the other growth factor, FGF, and a slightly different approach. Simons and his colleagues used tiny, leaky plastic pellets to deliver the FGF to heart muscle cells of patients with blocked coronary arteries. (He had practiced first on pigs, but one broke loose in the operating room and began running around the hospital's cardiac ward. There was pandemonium.)

All the teams reported early and sustained signs of success. Within two years of starting the angiogenesis gene therapy in 1997, Isner would report that 90 percent of the seventy-two heart patients he treated with VEGF infusions of naked DNA felt either reduction or complete elimination of heart disease symptoms. Fully half no longer had any angina pains at all for at least a year. But the treatments could not save everyone, especially older patients. One, an elderly woman who also had severe kidney and respiratory problems, died four months after being treated. Another, who had been suffering through four to six angina episodes daily, died only twenty hours after the VEGF injection procedure. Still, it was a mortality rate of less than 3 percent. According to Isner, patients of the same ages with the same problems, if left untreated because nothing else worked or they were waiting for a transplant, would be expected to have a 16 percent mortality rate, meaning eleven patients, rather than two, would probably have died. And many of those who were treated with angiogenesis weren't just *not dying*. Like Floyd Stokes and

Albert Laurent, they were thriving. Even a woman awaiting a heart transplant, treated with VEGF gene injections instead, recovered and remained free of symptoms.

The results were so impressive that the American Heart Association—sponsor of the meeting at which Isner was so harshly scolded for suggesting angiogenesis therapy—named the so-called natural bypass procedure one of the top-ten research advances in heart disease for 1998. To emphasize the point, that year's clinical meeting in Dallas was attended by Floyd Stokes, who had gotten his DNA injections only half a year before and was eager to show how well they had worked. To its adherents, there seemed every possibility that if the successes in both the lab and the clinic continued, angiogenesis treatment might become the first choice instead of the last. And if it could significantly reduce the need for dangerous and expensive coronary artery bypass operations, it would be one of the great advances not only of the decade but of the century.

And yet many cardiovascular specialists and other experts remained unconvinced. Chief among them was Harold Dvorak, the Harvard pathologist who was one of the éminences grises of blood vessel research. "I don't believe that work at all, and nobody else does either," Dvorak declared, obviously overstating the case. "You certainly can initiate new blood vessels with this material, but they are the kind of vessels that tumors and wounds initiate. They aren't worth much." Dvorak was a pioneer in the field, having suggested many years before that a substance which turned out to be VEGF had to exist. But now he argued that the formation of new blood vessels is a complex process, requiring many different growth factors, and that correct growth probably required that they be present in a particular order and in the correct amounts. "So it's naive to think that a single one is going to be able to do it. VEGF forms vessels, but they are not normal. I think the concept of growing new vessels is a very good one. But I don't think we're going to get very far with a single growth factor. Jeff has published a lot of papers on this, and I wish he were right. It would be very nice if he were right. I just don't think he is."

How did Dvorak explain patients like Floyd Stokes and Albert Laurent? "I think there is a huge placebo effect that has to be taken into consideration in these things. Especially in something as variable as heart disease and artery disease that can vary for many reasons." Indeed, for Isner and his colleagues, proving effectiveness was difficult because only tiny capillaries are induced to grow by VEGF, and they can't be seen in X rays or other imaging techniques. But the animal experiments had clearly shown that massive growth of new blood vessels could be induced, and this same growth seemed to be occurring in patients.

Michael Simons, Dvorak's colleague at Beth Israel who was trying to spur blood vessel growth by injecting FGF, thought that Dvorak might not have fully explored and considered the latest work in the field, perhaps dismissing it too casually. Dvorak's eminence in the field—he was a world expert, after all—had led others to share his skepticism. But it was also true that it was a young field, and revolutions in medicine seldom happen overnight. Isner found that despite his successes, very few of his patients were referred by other doctors; most came to him on their own after hearing about his work in news reports.

Maybe having a new set of abnormal blood vessels was simply better than nothing. Simons conducted a double-blind, randomized, controlled study in twenty-four heart patients, and he found a direct correlation between exposure to FGF and improved heart function. Patients who got the highest doses during bypass operations (when the chest was open anyway and the heart was easy to get at) showed the most improvement in their symptoms of heart disease. They were no longer short of breath and had less fatigue. Patients who got low doses, or no doses, did not show as much improvement. But also reporting some improvement were three of the seven placebo patients—perhaps lending credence to Dvorak's position.

In another study, sixty-six heart patients were given doses of FGF in their hearts via catheter, rather than during bypass operations, and about 80 percent showed a reduction in their symptoms and an increased capability for exercise—though among the 20 percent who saw no benefit were some who actually got worse. Of course, these were the first experiments in a brand-new field—the expertise was still to come—but it was already clear to Simons that more selective and potent growth-stimulating agents would become available even in the first few years of the twenty-first century. He compared the work being done in a few patients' hearts to blasting a little bird out of the sky with a bazooka; you can do it, but it's overkill. Simons believed, in fact, that medical scientists would soon be able to stimulate new blood vessels to grow specifically where they wanted and to make them develop properly to serve the heart without problems. "It's all coming," Simons predicted. "The science is good."

———

WHEN A BEAUTIFUL IDEA is released into the world, it can evolve in ways that surprise even its inventor. Judah Folkman never expected that his years of work on angiogenesis—much of which was financed by the National Cancer Institute—would pay off first and most dramatically in the battle against cardiovascular disease, rather than cancer. The cardiologists were sprinting past the cancer researchers, he reflected one day, feeling a great deal of pride mixed with a tinge of ruefulness. But mostly pride: He knew that if angiogenesis therapy could help even a fraction of the hundreds of thousands of people with coronary artery disease, or some of the 200,000 or so patients whose legs were amputated each year, the benefits would be mind-boggling.

Isner and the other angiogenesis practitioners were not unaware of Folkman's scientific altruism. They knew him as a rare kind of researcher—never territorial or overly protective of this field he had invented; happy to help other scientists push ahead, even if they were competitors. "I don't think I've ever met anybody in academic medicine who is more of a gentleman in that regard. Nobody," Isner says. "He's exceptionally generous in terms of sharing ideas, reviewing papers." Soon after Isner sent his first research paper on angiogenesis to the *Journal of Clinical Investigation*, he got a call from someone at the National Institutes of Health, saying that Folkman had just been in Bethesda, and he was telling people about Isner's results and urging that the work be supported. Folkman had obviously been one of the reviewers of Isner's paper. Later, Folkman gave a talk at Isner's research institution, St. Elizabeth's Medical Center, and he mentioned he had just been on a lecture tour and everybody was asking about Isner's work on angiogenesis for hearts and legs. "Plenty of other people in that position, had they reviewed that paper, would have rejected it and then set their own laboratories to work on that subject," Isner says. "Or they would maybe have stalled the paper, or done anything they could to have stomped out any potential competition. But he did just the opposite. He promoted it."

As a veteran Boston-area clinician and researcher, Isner had a vivid memory of Folkman's long battles to create and advance the field of angiogenesis. "The idea, the first vague notion about blood vessels being required for tumors to grow, and that there must be mediators for that in the body, was totally wacko," Isner reflects. "He was really hamstrung by the lack of what are now contemporary techniques, which would have made it so much easier to identify all these growth factors. So they continued to look at him as being a little bit crazy." Isner could appreciate the position, of course. Though they had little personal contact aside from long discussions at scientific meetings, he regarded Folkman as a mentor in spirit. There was at least one important difference in their perspectives, however. In 1999, Isner joined the biomedical gold rush, founding a company called Vascular Genetics in Durham, North Carolina. Among his critics there was some annoyance that he sometimes neglected to mention his pecuniary interests when speaking of the wonders of gene therapy for cardiovascular diseases.

EVEN IN FOLKMAN'S laboratory, there were some who were interested in using the principles of angiogenesis to combat conditions other than cancer. While Isner, Simons, and others were avidly pursuing ways to save patients by growing new blood vessels for hearts and legs, in one small part of Folkman's lab ophthalmologist Anthony Adamis was quietly working on a way to block angiogenesis to save people's eyes. By the late 1990s, abnormal angiogenesis was finally being seen as a key player in conditions as varied as blindness, arthritis, psoriasis, and other ailments involving inflammation. Folkman had opened new avenues, and many researchers were eagerly exploring them, including some who had once been critics.

Like many of the researchers who took up residence on the tenth floor of the Enders Building, Anthony Adamis came to Folkman's team almost by happenstance. A decade earlier, in 1989, the newly trained ophthalmologist wandered a few blocks from his office for a lunchtime lecture at the Schepens Eye Research Institute. The talk was one in a series of research seminars, and Adamis, then finishing up his clinical training and thinking about how he wanted to apply it, liked to amble in with a brown bag lunch, find a seat, listen, and learn. If the speaker was less than stimulating, he'd manage to catch a few winks. Adamis didn't know anything about Folkman and wasn't expecting much. He got his lunch and was ready to fall asleep. But then he sensed there might be something different about this lecture. He saw the entire auditorium begin to fill up and heard a low buzz that suddenly hushed as Folkman stepped up to the microphone. Then Adamis heard Folkman talk about angiogenesis, about the idea that a factor induced capillaries to grow on demand. It fit exactly with what Adamis was seeing in patients with diabetic retinopathy—an excess growth of tiny capillaries, a problem that struck as many as twenty-four thousand diabetics a year. It was the most common form of blindness in people still in their working years. Adamis got no sleep that day. He took copious notes, writing small because he was running out of paper and he wanted to get every word down. A decade later, he still had the notes.

For Adamis, a young doctor hoping to do important eye research, Folkman's discussion was a bolt of lightning. Everything clicked for him. With his clinical background as an ophthalmologist he knew that the major causes of blindness in the developed world are diseases where blood vessels grow in an uncontrolled fashion. He realized then what he was going to do with the rest of his life: He was going to study this. His dream was to have some sort of impact on blindness.

But first he had to meet Folkman. He tried to squeeze up to the podium after the lecture, but the crush of the crowd was too much for any one-on-ones. He left the lecture hall resolving to contact Folkman and find a way to win a berth in his laboratory. A colleague at the Massachusetts Eye and Ear Infirmary was able to arrange an introduction, and one Saturday morning Adamis went across town and sat with Folkman for almost two hours, batting ideas back and forth with him. Folkman told Adamis all about angiogenesis, and Adamis told him he wanted to find a treatment for diabetic retinopathy, a form of blindness that was especially severe in people with type 1, or insulin-dependent, diabetes. In Folkman, Adamis found a man who was comfortable thinking decades ahead, who made quick connections that others missed, and who was extraordinarily generous with his time, his ideas, and his enthusiasm. He also found that Folkman had long been interested in the physiology of the eye, in part because it was within the eye, in the light-sensing organ called the retina, that tiny blood vessels could most easily be seen and studied. In fact, by then Folkman had worked with so many rabbit and mouse eyes that he could almost be counted as an expert. "It was just a marriage that was so appropriate," Adamis says, looking back. "The eye and blood vessels. Vascularization and angiogenesis. The main reason people go blind."

But winning a research spot in Folkman's laboratory wasn't easy. By the end of the 1980s there was fierce competition to be on his team. Lab space was so tight, the place was already so chock-full of researchers and technicians, that Folkman was making jokes about researchers falling over from carbon dioxide poisoning. But at the conclusion of their Saturday morning meeting, Folkman told Adamis he'd like to show him around the lab. Adamis later recalled that when an applicant took that step, when Folkman said he wanted to show the person around the laboratory, that meant they were in. Adamis told Folkman he wanted to learn all there was to know about angiogenesis—and Folkman said there was only one way. Adamis needed to eat, sleep, drink, and dream angiogenesis. That's how he would learn, by marinading himself in angiogenesis. So Adamis did. All he needed now was enough money to support his work. He wrote his first grant proposal and sent it to a special program at NIH that supported physicians trying to gain experience in biomedical research. He got it on his first try: a five-year grant that would pay for his salary and supplies.

Diabetic retinopathy had been known and studied for a long time when Adamis began exploring whether antiangiogenesis in some form could be used to counter its effects. For decades its symptoms were known to generally arise about ten years after the initial diagnosis of diabetes, when for some reason the tiny blood vessels in the retina (the filmlike layer that sits at the back of the eye, similar to the way photographic film is loaded into the back of a camera) become especially weak and leaky. As the damage gradually begins killing off the retinal cells, the number of cells available to sense the light that comes into the eye declines, an irreversible process eventually leading to blindness.

The process was well known simply because the fine network of blood vessels that feed the retina is easily visible to ophthalmologists. They can actually see the damage occurring and map its progress. They can see signs of increased permeability of the capillaries in the retina: tiny bulges, breakages, and excess fluids leaking from fragile blood vessels. For many years, the standard treatment was to carefully monitor diabetic patients for signs of damage, and then try to cut off the flow of blood to areas where the capillaries were most leaky. In the last quarter of the twentieth century, precise pulses of laser light were used like an optical scalpel to "photocoagulate" vessels feeding the damaged areas. By blocking blood flow to small areas, sparing much larger parts of the retina, doctors were able to slow the process and preserve sight for many thousands of people. But it was ultimately an inadequate treatment. With each laser procedure, the patient would lose a little more of the retina and a little more sight. Laser treatments could slow down the damage, but they could not completely stop it.

Some scientists, especially Harold Dvorak, had postulated an elegant theory over the years. They thought that diabetes somehow damaged the cardiovascular system, causing the cells in the retina to run short of oxygen. Under stress, these retinal cells released a chemical signal that stimulated blood vessel cells to begin sprouting new branches in order to get more oxy-gen. But these new blood vessels were weak and permeable, Dvorak theo-rized, because only capillaries grew in—without supporting cells such as pericytes—when VEGF was the sole growth factor present. These incom-plete blood vessels were the same kind tumors drew, explaining why some tumors seem to be such bloody messes. In eyes, meanwhile, this condition caused damage to the retina, reducing its ability to sense light. Thus, the theory went, in an effort to save itself, the retina called in blood vessels that ended up doing more harm than good. The eye's emergency response to oxy-gen starvation was actually disastrous—it eventually erased vision.

Dvorak's idea was logical but hard to prove. In fact, it went unconfirmed for more than two decades, not in the least because the chemical signal he sus-pected of triggering the faulty blood vessels—a molecule he dubbed VPF, for vascular permeability factor—was one of those mystery growth factors that were for a long time arguably only theoretical. But then, in 1989, Dvorak announced he had isolated and purified VPF. It turned out to be the same molecule that Napoleone Ferrara, at Genentech, found and identified as a stimulator of angiogenesis. With that, Dvorak and others made VEGF, as the molecule became most widely known, the primary suspect behind destruction of the retina. Adamis, arriving very soon after this important moment, began trying to confirm whether VEGF was in fact the key to blindness in diabetics.

Adamis began cooperating with Dr. Pat D'Amore, in Folkman's lab, and Dr. Jan Miller, a colleague at the Massachusetts Eye and Ear Infirmary who was using monkeys to study diabetic retinopathy. She could mimic what hap-pened in diabetic patients by using a finely tuned beam of laser light to dam-age a small zone of blood vessels in the monkey's retina and block blood flow to part of the organ. As the cells in that zone became ischemic—that is, lack-ing adequate oxygen—they began producing the chemical "help" signal to stimulate the growth of replacement blood vessels. And the new vessels that arrived in response were indeed the kind of fragile, leaky vessels seen in dia-betic retinopathy. But was it really VEGF that caused diabetic retinopathy?

To test the idea, Adamis and Miller grew retinal cells in laboratory dishes, stressing them with low oxygen to see how they responded. Sure enough, they pumped out VEGF. Now they needed to know whether the VEGF was actu-ally the agent calling in new capillaries. To find out, Miller and Adamis injected the animals' eyes with so-called monoclonal antibodies, highly spe-cific molecules that could seek out and inactivate VEGF molecules. So if

VEGF was actually the villain in diabetic retinopathy, then the injection of antibodies into the eye would stop the growth of new blood vessels. And that was exactly what they saw. The antibodies blocked the action of VEGF and prevented the damage that would have been done to the retina. To check their results, Adamis and Miller injected VEGF itself and found the growth factor on its own could cause all the symptoms characteristic of diabetic retinopathy.

At about the same time, just across Brookline Avenue from the Children's Hospital complex, Dr. Lloyd Paul Aiello, a research ophthalmologist at the Joslin Diabetes Center, was finding identical evidence using rats. Aiello came from a whole family of eye doctors. His father and grandfather were ophthalmologists, and so was his wife and his wife's father. Aiello's father and grandfather, in fact, had developed the treatment called photocoagulation therapy, in which intense, narrow beams of laser light were used to burn blood vessels, closing off the capillaries that were leaking blood and slowing the process of diabetic retinopathy. When he was younger, Aiello thought he'd break the mold and go into something other than eyes. But then he found himself doing an ophthalmology residency at Johns Hopkins. A few years later he, too, was working on diabetic retinopathy.

The idea that lack of oxygen is what starts the deterioration process in the retina had been around since the 1960s, when it was observed that damage to the tiny blood vessels that bring in oxygen precedes the loss of vision. So Aiello began looking for a molecule that could account for the damage. He grew retinal tissues in a laboratory dish, then put the dish into a special incubator in which the amount of oxygen could be controlled. When he reduced the oxygen concentration in the tissue to match conditions in the eye when it is diseased, he found that VEGF levels went up. "They say, 'Help! I need oxygen!' and they start spinning out the VEGF," Aiello explains.

His next step was to take samples of vitreous fluid to see if the eyes of patients with active diabetic retinopathy contained excess VEGF. They did, while those who had no active disease, or who didn't have diabetes, had very low levels of the growth factor. He also found strong hints that the major cause of blindness in the elderly, macular degeneration, also involves excess production of VEGF, but in a slightly different part of the eye. The result in macular degeneration cases is progressive loss of peripheral vision.

All this was good to know, but it didn't explain what caused or stimulated the production of VEGF in the eye. It didn't explain why cells in the retina become starved for oxygen, setting off this whole cascade of disastrous events.

That was the fundamental question, and an important part of the answer soon began to surface. Careful studies of the process in the retina began to show that oxygen starvation began when the capillaries feeding the retina got clogged. What clogged them turned out to be white blood cells getting stuck inside the tiny blood-carrying channels. Then, using fluorescent dyes and pictures taken through a microscope, Adamis and Aiello showed that some white blood cells (leukocytes) in diabetics seemed to be stickier than normal and couldn't pass easily through the tiniest blood vessels. The errant leukocytes seemed to be coated with so-called adhesion molecules on their surfaces, as if they were covered with Velcro. "They actually stick, and stay stuck," Adamis explains. Once the clogging begins, the oxygen-starved retinal cells become stressed and begin to call for help, trying to reestablish the supply of blood they need to function and stay alive. VEGF is then made and released, and the damage begins.

The next step was to search for whatever was making the leukocytes stickier than they should be. The main candidate was a molecule dubbed ICAM-1, for intercellular adhesion molecule-1, a substance that seemed to be overly abundant on the white blood cells in diabetics. In rats, this overexpression of the ICAM-1 molecule was detectable within days of the animals being made diabetic. And Adamis, Aiello, and their colleagues found a way to abolish the effect by using specific monoclonal antibodies to stop ICAM-1's activity. It was the first suggestion that there might be a simple and benign way to avoid diabetic retinopathy, a major step forward in eye research.

Meanwhile, Adamis, Aiello, and others were trying to devise ways to deliver effective drugs to the eye, and only to the eye. They knew that discovering the targets of treatment was only part of the goal—just as important was figuring out a benign way to deliver the treatment. They focused on using plastic patches—akin to nicotine patches—that could be inserted under the lower eyelid and gradually release compounds locally. "You could put in a year's worth of drug, and then just put in the patch," Adamis says. "So I envision in the future that if you are diagnosed with diabetes, and you have no complications yet, you go to the ophthalmologist, put the patch on, and you never get the disease."

Remarkably, within just ten years, by struggling to dissect and understand why abnormal blood vessel growth occurs in the eye, Adamis and his research colleagues had all but unraveled one of the most difficult riddles in vision research. Better still, their research was showing that the blinding disorder could probably be prevented in ways that were both inexpensive and easy. In

1999, Adamis, Aiello, and seven colleagues published a landmark paper in the *Proceedings of the National Academy of Sciences* that seemed to explain exactly how and why diabetics became blind, and what could be done about it. Adamis, it seemed, was on the verge of accomplishing exactly what he'd set out to do that day back in 1989, when he'd taken his lunch over to Schepens Eye Research Institute and heard Judah Folkman talk about angiogenesis.

Chapter Nineteen

———

HIGH EXPECTATIONS ARE HARD to live up to, especially if they're someone else's. Judah Folkman found himself in that position as his two big antiangiogenesis drugs, endostatin and angiostatin, finally headed toward clinical trials near the end of 1999. Folkman was expected to cure cancer—it said so in *The New York Times*. Now all he needed was for the drugs to work in people as unequivocally as they had in mice. But it was not so simple, of course, and the results would not be known quickly. The first phase of the trials, as in tests of all drugs overseen by the Food and Drug Administration, was designed to test for safety, not efficacy. So those receiving the first test doses would be patients with the most advanced cancers, patients for whom everything else had failed, and they would receive very small doses to start. Moreover, the experience with mice, as well as with patients like Jennifer LaChance and Tonya Kalesnik, who had been treated with interferon, indicated that antiangiogenesis drugs have a slow, cumulative effect, taking up to a year to eliminate tumors. It stretched the limits of reasonable expectation to think that critically ill patients in the first trials would take a few injections of low-dosage, slow-acting drugs and waltz out of their hospital wards, cancer-free.

Obviously, such waltzing wasn't likely. A study that had recently been done at the Johns Hopkins Medical Institutions, in Baltimore, showed starkly that very little about a drug's potential is discernible from the results of Phase I trials. Because the patients admitted to such trials are desperately ill, and because the doses of drugs given are so small, half of the patients fail—they drop out—within 1.8 months, even if the drug being tested ultimately turns out to be effective. In contrast, in trials of drugs that turn out to be flops—never making it to the market—half of the patients drop out by 1.6 months. Statistically that's almost dead even, and the take-home lesson is that Phase I toxicity trials generally don't say much about a candidate drug's ultimate success. Thus by any measure, the expectations for Folkman's antiangiogenic agents were far beyond reason.

Endostatin, the second of the antiangiogenic agents discovered by Michael O'Reilly less than half a decade earlier, was the first to be put to the test, in trials involving fifteen patients at each of three sites: the Dana-Farber Cancer Institute in Boston, the M. D. Anderson Cancer Center in Houston, and the University of Wisconsin Medical Center in Madison. The clinical researchers would start with very small doses—only fifteen milligrams per kilogram of body weight daily, measures so insignificant that they were unlikely to have any effect—and then gradually escalate them to see if there came a point when the drugs became toxic and should be stopped. The idea was to see if, and how much, endostatin could be given safely. If the drug passed that test, proving itself nontoxic, then the dosages would be increased to levels where they could begin to be tested for efficacy—to see if they actually worked against tumors. Even then, it could be another year before the results were in. Because antiangiogenesis works by shutting down the growth and migration of blood vessel cells, it's a far slower process than poisoning or blasting tumor cells with radiation or chemotherapy. The tests in mice had made it clear that the antiangiogenic drugs had to be continued for a very long time, and that stopping too early would allow the blood vessels to regrow, reigniting tumor growth. Slow and steady was the rule. So the first patients selected for the trials had to wonder how lucky they were: The protocols of the studies made it unlikely any of the first patients would be saved by the new drugs.

Still patients lined up, brave and desperate people who knew their chances were worse if they didn't try at all. The first endostatin trials were scheduled for October 1999 at Dana-Farber, and as news of that first opportunity got around, thousands of patients called, wrote, and e-mailed, frantically hoping to qualify for one of the fifteen slots in the small toxicity test. The same rush happened a few months later in Wisconsin, and again in Texas, when the two other Phase I endostatin trials were opened under the auspices of the National Cancer Institute. Most of the applicants were disappointed. Some patients arrived with complications beyond cancer, such as high blood pressure or diabetes, or even the wrong kind of cancer. People with brain tumors, for example, were excluded because the doctors could not know whether endostatin might weaken the blood vessels feeding a brain tumor so much that hemorrhaging in the brain might occur.

Unlike most clinical trials, in which all the treatment centers do exactly the same things, the doctors running the three endostatin trials were allowed to set some of their own rules, select the kinds of tumors they would treat, and decide how to enroll their patients. This was because antiangiogenesis was so new and untested that no one really knew how to use endostatin. "Since no one knows," explained Dr. Mark Kieran, director of pediatric neuro-oncology at Dana-Farber, "having one person write the protocol would be very arbitrary." In Boston, patients were selected almost on a first-come, first-served basis, while in Houston and Madison they were chosen from among patients who were already under care at the hospitals. There were only two things patients in all three trials had to have in common: Their malignancies had to have defied all previous treatments, and the patients couldn't be so near death that they might succumb in just a week or two, before they could be evaluated for signs of drug toxicity. Such an immediate death would be seen as a waste of the precious drug, while raising serious questions about why the patient died. Was it the cancer or the drug?

Folkman was delighted that clinical trials had finally begun for the antiangiogenesis drugs, and he was optimistic about their long-term promise. But he also knew exactly what to worry about. Most central was the simple possibility that the human body might metabolize the drug differently than the mouse body, rendering it impotent. That's what he'd had in mind when he'd quipped to *Times* reporter Gina Kolata that if you were a mouse with cancer, he could take good care of you. The clinical trials, meanwhile, were out of his control. He was just an intensely interested observer. So he worried about how they were being run and how they were being perceived. Someone might give the wrong doses and derail the trials. Or people wouldn't truly understand the process, especially with a new kind of drug like endostatin, which needed time and patience. Some of these drugs—whether those developed by his lab or by others—might fail, he thought, perhaps leading some people to doubt his entire premise. "It's the same as the *Challenger* space shuttle," he told people. "*Challenger* crashed because of a frozen O-ring. But that does not overturn Newton's principles. Some drug failures are the result of bad O-rings."

The clinical researchers worked hard to learn all they could from the first patients. In all three centers, the patients were tested almost incessantly with MRI scans, blood tests, positron-emission topography (PET) scans, and a battery of other diagnostic measures meant to watch for signs of damage to their vital organs. It seemed to evoke the experience of astronauts setting out on a dangerous test flight. For some of the patients who found their way up Binney Street in Boston to get their daily endostatin infusions, the hardest part was the loneliness. Some patients had come from as far across the country as Alaska, leaving family and friends—all their support—behind. And when they realized that the low doses were unlikely to cure them, some gradually began to lose hope and concluded that the isolation wasn't worth it. A man from Alaska gave up and went home to be with his eight children, and face the dire consequences of his cancer. Another patient missed her young children so much that she, too, went home.

In Houston, each patient was fully evaluated every four weeks: Each got a PET scan, an oxygen isotope scan, and an MRI for blood flow, along with tumor biopsies and other tests. Then a committee of physicians got together every week to assess how the patients were doing and whether progress was being made. But they did not share their results with anyone outside the clinical setting. While the identities of the patients were carefully guarded in all three research centers, a few names and other details did begin to leak out. In Boston, one woman, who was from the Midwest, had come east for the trial and moved in with relatives to the south of Boston, in Plymouth, Massachusetts. The drive up the traffic-choked Southeast Expressway was such an ordeal that her doctors in Boston contacted the Massachusetts State Police, getting her a special pass to display in her car window so she could use the less-congested high-occupancy-vehicle lane on the highway. There was even an offer to send a limousine down to Plymouth to ensure she could make the trip seven days a week through the winter of 1999–2000. She declined use of the limousine, and kept driving back and forth for several months. But by that point, it was clear that her tumor was growing, not responding to the very low doses of endostatin, and she had to leave the trial. The rules of the trial protocol required that any patient whose tumor expanded by more than 50 percent, despite endostatin, had to drop out. The rule was designed to allow these patients to seek other treatment. In the early going, when the doses were smallest, the dropout rate was high.

Meanwhile, the drug was showing zero toxicity in all the Phase I trials. The doctors caring for these patients were amazed that they saw none of the typical episodes of vomiting, diarrhea, nausea, and loss of hair normally experienced by patients in cancer drug trials. In fact the oncologists, who usually spent much of their time trying to get their patients through the dreadful side effects of chemotherapy, had very little to do. Their patients felt fine, even wanting to put their clothes on and go home. Some went on shopping trips, and a few even began talking about taking vacations abroad. But some impatient cancer researchers outside the trials took the seeming lack of toxicity as a bad sign, an indication that the drug wasn't working. "Toxicity is equal to efficacy in most oncologists' minds," Roy Herbst, the oncologoist who was leading the endostatin trial in Houston, said in the early going. "That's cancer. That's the way our drugs work." But this drug was different. It wasn't chemotherapy. It wasn't poison.

Meanwhile, though nothing was revealed officially, a few patients who were bumped from the trials emerged to say that endostatin had not worked for them. Chuck Killian, a forty-two-year-old insurance agent from Mundelein, Illinois, was a colon cancer patient whose earlier chemotherapy treatments had failed. By spring 1999, before the endostatin trials, he was certain he would be dead by Christmas. But when he learned that one of the endostatin trials would be conducted in Madison, Wisconsin, he quickly applied, and he became one of the first patients enrolled.

Killian began receiving his daily injections of endostatin early in 2000—sometimes showing up in a T-shirt with a color picture of Judah Folkman printed on the front, prepared by his wife, Lori, an advertising executive—and over the next few months he started to feel better. But in fact his tumor was still growing. The very small doses of endostatin had given him no side effects, but neither could they contain Killian's already advanced cancer. The Wisconsin research protocols dictated that patients could not continue in the trial once their tumors expanded by 50 percent, and Killian reached that point in early May 2000. He was crushed when he realized he was out.

Because the first few patients weren't instantly cured—although that would have come as a complete surprise to anyone connected with the studies if it had happened—endostatin suffered an early and continuing public relations problem. Word began going around in the press that the treatments weren't working. *The Boston Globe*'s Richard Saltus reported, for example, that James Pluda, at the National Cancer Institute, saw no signs of progress among patients in the three trials. In the context of the study, of course, Pluda's statement was not surprising. He was not at all pessimistic about the eventual prospects for success. But partly because the trials were so shrouded in secrecy, a hint of failure seemed to be emerging. It didn't help that Pluda's comment came just as Chuck Killian was publicly saying that his tumor had grown and he'd been forced to leave the Wisconsin trial. Investors in particular seemed to assume the worst. In the absence of encouraging news, EntreMed's stock plummeted. The publicity was also causing some patients to lose hope. A few wondered if they should drop out.

What wasn't being reported, except sub rosa among researchers and hospital staff, was that there were already small signs of efficacy. Little by little, as the doses of endostatin were increased during the winter, reports began to leak out of the three medical centers that a few patients were doing better. In addition to the complete lack of toxicity, the doctors were saying quietly to each other that in some patients the tumors seemed to have stopped growing. The nurses knew it, too, and the word had it in Boston that one man's tumors—both his primary tumor and its metastases—had begun to shrink. Even at tiny doses of endostatin—in relative terms only one seventh the doses that had been effective in mice—his metastases were down 50 percent. Word from the clinic was that he was feeling so good, despite being an end-stage cancer patient, that he would come in for his daily injection and then head off to work.

And he was not alone in showing progress. Another patient in the Boston trial, described only as a sixty-year-old woman from Chicago fighting metastatic breast cancer, was also showing signs of tumor shrinkage. Tests indicated that the interior of her tumor was deteriorating, as if it were liquefying and dying. She, too, was feeling far better than when she arrived in Boston months earlier. But in July 2000 she shocked the doctors by deciding to go home to Chicago, needing to take care of pressing personal business. Daily doses of endostatin were needed, but her doctors found no way to arrange for her injections while she was out of town. So there was real fear that an interruption in endostatin treatments would free her tumor to regrow explosively. But eleven days later, when she reported in again for treatments at Dana-Farber, the relieved doctors found that her cancer had not regrown. While visiting home, she had stopped in her office to see fellow workers, who were amazed at how good she looked and by her energy level and high spirits. She obviously felt good, as did several other patients in the trial, who reported much-improved quality of life.

Strangely enough, these quiet signs of success had apparently not leaked widely enough to reach the National Cancer Institute in Maryland. When the NCI's director, Dr. Richard Klausner, visited Harvard Medical School in late June 2000 to discuss the agency's research plans, he was asked why he hadn't mentioned angiogenesis research. Klausner's reply, according to members of Folkman's team, was that antiangiogenesis "is a pseudotreatment," and that angiogenesis was going to be harder to figure out than carcinogenesis. It was another example of the doubts and barriers that Folkman and his work had been colliding with through three decades. In any case, the results were beginning to speak for themselves.

Such hints of success were not officially announced, however, for fear of setting off a massive rush of patients seeking a drug that was unproven, and in any event unavailable. In April 2000, doctors and the Food and Drug Administration decided it was better to wait and be sure, allowing time for the drug-manufacturing process to be scaled up before breaking any news. There wouldn't be much solid evidence until the trial ended, and even bigger, more convincing trials could begin.

It was at that point, in mid–March 2000, that the FDA asked the doctors at Dana-Farber to stop increasing the doses until the two other centers could catch up. The agency wanted everyone to keep treating at 240 milligrams per kilogram of body weight per day for a while, to let the patient numbers build up, while the debate continued over whether to escalate higher, to 300, 400, or 500 milligrams per day. An intense argument also erupted over whether—and what—to report. Half of the experimenters wanted to present the data on toxicity at the upcoming American Society of Clinical Oncology meeting in mid-May, in New Orleans. Others in the research group argued that even the data showing early signs of efficacy in a few patients should be included. It was evidence, albeit preliminary, that small, regular doses of endostatin were associated with improvements, especially in patients with the slowest-growing types of tumors. This seemed to support Folkman's prediction that less-aggressive cancers would be most sensitive to the drug.

As this was occurring, trials began at Thomas Jefferson University in Philadelphia for angiostatin, the other antiangiogenesis drug developed in Folkman's lab. The early results offered a surprise that had nothing to do with cancer—a surprise to everyone but Folkman. One of the first patients enrolled in the trial saw her decades-long struggle with the skin disorder called psoriasis suddenly resolve. Psoriasis is caused by abnormal blood vessel growth in the skin, and it was one of the ailments that Folkman had suggested might yield to antiangiogenesis treatment. Although the results were serendipitous—and seen in only one patient—the discovery set off immediate interest in testing angiostatin as a potential treatment for the very bothersome skin condition. And it offered unexpected but welcome evidence that antiangiogenesis treatment was offering value in medical settings.

FOLKMAN'S TRIUMPHS WITH MICE and the expectations for the drugs that had been developed in his lab had gotten most of the antiangiogenesis-related publicity. But about a dozen small biotechnology companies, and a few big ones, were avidly but quietly exploring their own versions of antiangiogenesis drugs, some of which had already been in clinical trials for years. In some instances, the ideas spawned by Folkman were even leading clinical researchers to use existing anticancer drugs and treatments in new ways or in new combinations that turned out to be antiangiogenic.

The list of companies trying to develop antiangiogenic drugs was extraordinary, considering how unsuccessful Folkman had been in drawing support just a few years earlier. Genentech, Sugen, Agouron, British Biotech, Aeterna, Cytran, Calgene, Medimmune, TAP Holdings, ImClone Systems, EntreMed—all were in the hunt, targeting cancers of every variety by testing their own new antiangiogenesis agents in combination with standard, already approved chemotherapy agents. (In one instance, a legal battle developed between Folkman, Children's Hospital, and EntreMed on one side and Chicago's Abbott Industries on the other over the patent ownership for a molecule called kringle 5, part of plasminogen, the parent compound, from which angiostatin was extracted. Children's had licensed the patent to kringle 5 to EntreMed, but Abbott claimed that the molecule had actually been discovered by one of its scientists. After three years of fruitless negotiation, the company filed a ten-million-dollar federal lawsuit against the hospital in spring 2000. Folkman and Children's strongly disagreed and countersued Abbott. It is an ironic symbol of just how interested the giants of the pharmaceutical industry had finally become in Folkman and his angiogenesis ideas.)

One of the most interesting developments involved a small drug research company in Sweden, OXiGENE, Inc., which had bought the rights to a new antiangiogenic drug called combrestatin. The drug had been developed by chemist G. Robert Pettit, the director of the cancer research institute at Arizona State University. Pettit had scoured the world looking for agents that might be useful against cancer, and one of those he came up with was, like the chemotherapy drug Taxol, a natural product extracted from the bark of a tree—in this case a species of willow that grows in South Africa. Unlike endostatin, which was thought to block the formation of new blood vessels, combrestatin seemed to have an ability to erase the existing blood vessels already supporting a tumor. Pettit, a widely respected researcher, was participating in the National Cancer Institute's new biological evaluation system in the early 1980s, joining the search for natural agents in plants and other organisms and seeing whether they had any anticancer activities when tested in culture dishes with brain cancer cells. Pettit and four colleagues found that the root bark of the South African tree *Combretum caffrum*—used "as a Zulu charm for harming an enemy," he wrote in the *Canadian Journal of Chemistry*—did have some effect.

Originally, combrestatin was viewed as a potential adjuvant therapy, something to use in combination with other drugs or with radiation treatments. In 1998, Arizona State University licensed the drug exclusively to OXiGENE, which a few months later signed a letter of intent with Bristol-Myers Squibb to develop and market it. For Folkman, there was a bit of irony in the deal. Bristol-Myers was giving OXiGENE seventy million dollars for combrestatin, shortly after dropping its interest in Folkman's angiostatin. Pettit's drug may have seemed a surer bet, since combrestatin had already been synthesized chemically in the laboratory and was much closer to being a commercial product. And indeed, combrestatin did get into clinical trials a year ahead of Folkman's endostatin, and by the time the endostatin trials were finally up and running, results from combrestatin were beginning to surface. In some cases the patients' tumors seemed to have stopped growing, and in one case the results were truly exciting.

Clayton Twigg was a fifty-six-year-old retired telephone engineer from Westlake, Ohio, who went to his doctor with what he thought was laryngitis in September 1997. He had also been having some terrific headaches, but his doctor didn't detect anything serious and thought the problems would quickly pass. Reassured, Twigg and his three grown sons embarked on a ten-day fishing adventure in Canada, and when he came home, his doctor suggested a thorough massage. Maybe that would help him relax. The massage would feel great, anyway. The masseuse vigorously kneaded Twigg's back and arms, and worked on the muscles in his neck, twisting, pulling, squeezing, getting taut muscles loosened up. But during the massage, the alert masseuse noticed a small lump on Twigg's neck and advised him to have it checked.

Twigg's doctor didn't like the look of the lump and sent him to an ear, nose, and throat specialist. By then, his laryngitis was much worse; his voice was nearly gone. Looking down Twigg's throat, the specialist spotted a tumor that had already paralyzed one vocal cord. It was growing on his thyroid gland, pushing against his windpipe and making it hard to breathe. Exploratory surgery revealed that the growth had spread like a spider's legs, growing down into his chest. It was a relatively rare type of cancer called an anaplastic thyroid tumor—a very stubborn and aggressive cancer that doesn't

respond well to treatment and usually kills a patient within six months of diagnosis. When Twigg asked about his chances, his oncologist, Dr. James Cunningham, was blunt. The prognosis, Cunningham said, was poor. There were
drugs and procedures that could keep him comfortable, but that was about all.
Still, Twigg wasn't interested in giving up without a fight. He agreed to have
aggressive chemotherapy and radiation late in 1997, but still the treatments
failed. The tumor did shrink slightly, but then it began expanding again,
crowding ever harder against his windpipe. He could also feel it restricting his
neck movements; during evening walks with his wife, Rose, Twigg could feel
a tightness, as if his head were being held down by a rubber band, whenever
he tried to look up and to the side. "I didn't want to be strangled by this
thing," Twigg said later. "I didn't want to go that way."

Twigg was fighting for his life, and his wife, sons, and friends were fighting alongside him. Like others suddenly overtaken by an infamous disease
they knew little about, they gathered as much information about cancer as
they could. Twigg began taking regular doses of vitamins, eating garlic, and
doing everything else he could think of that seemed even halfway logical. In
his research, he kept coming across mention of Judah Folkman and antiangiogenesis. The idea looked interesting, but the bad news from Boston was that
Folkman's drugs were at least two years away from clinical trials, and it was
unlikely Twigg could hang on that long. Cunningham suggested that another
round of chemotherapy, this time with doxorubicin, might be worth a try, and
other doctors whom Twigg consulted in Cleveland concurred. But none of
the doctors was very optimistic. "I was told that in six months, I'd be gone,"
Twigg recalls. "It was the first time anyone had given me a time frame."

Twigg agreed to start getting large doses of doxorubicin, visiting the clinic
regularly to sit for a few hours while the drug was infused through a port that
had been installed in his chest. He took courage wherever he could find it. On
his refrigerator was a cartoon poster of a heron struggling to swallow a large
frog, only to have the frog reach down to squeeze the bird's neck shut, keeping it from swallowing. The caption: "Never give up!" Twigg, as determined
as the frog, kept searching for something new, scanning the National Cancer
Institute's website listing cancer trials. He found a trial starting in Ken-
tucky—but the subjects could not be taking any other drugs. Then he got
lucky. Cunningham made a habit of attending weekly tumor board meetings
at the University Hospitals Health System in Cleveland on Fridays and had
discussed Twigg's case a number of times. During one session he heard that a
new trial, involving an antiangiogenic drug, was about to get under way. The

study was being headed by oncologist Scot Remick, and when Cunningham proposed Twigg as a subject, Remick agreed—if for no other reason than that Twigg was seriously ill but still healthy enough to live through the trial. The drug he would test was combrestatin. The trial was expected to begin in the fall of 1998.

As they began to learn the ins and outs of drug trials, Twigg and the other patients who were accepted into the study quickly realized there was a paradox: The first patients to be admitted to the trial were not necessarily the luckiest. If you were desperately ill but near the front of the line, getting the lowest dosages in the toxicity phase of the trial, the drug might have little or no effect. But if you were near the end, you might not live long enough to get the highest, presumably most effective doses. Twigg figured his odds were better with the higher doses and hoped he'd be placed near the end of the Phase I study. This was not an uncommon hope among the patients in the trial. When another patient, fifty-five-year-old Dorothy Datta, learned that she would be the second to receive combrestatin, she worried it would do her no good. "It would really suck," she remarked to Twigg, "if here I am, number two, and they get to patient number seven before they find the correct dose, and then I can't get it." Her worry was prophetic. Later, after Datta had finished her part of the trial, she tried to get back in but was refused. Twigg and others contacted members of the Ohio congressional delegation in her behalf, but to no avail. "We recently went to her memorial service," Twigg said later.

Twigg was scheduled to be number eight, a member of the third group of threes in Phase I, but because of a delay in getting the drug, he did not begin treatments until February 1999—well over a year after he was accepted into the study and more than *two* years after he had been diagnosed and begun the aggressive chemotherapy and radiation treatments. Finally, in the dead of winter 1999, the call came. Twigg went up to Cleveland and found himself being infused with the experimental drug in a room bathed in yellow light. The FDA, concerned there would be a light-sensitivity reaction in patients getting combrestatin, had required that all natural light be blocked out. So Twigg took the medicine sitting in a room that glowed an eerie yellow.

Almost immediately, Twigg felt a common side effect: an intense itch in the groin area and on his buttocks. He was also tired and had some fever and chills, but he managed to get through that first night without serious harm. In the morning Twigg was examined carefully by his doctors, and by noon was on his way home, where Rose had homemade soup warm and ready. He continued to feel tired for the next few days but wasn't terribly ill. Soon he was up and out of bed, resuming his daily walks with Rose, and going back to the hospital every three weeks for another combrestatin treatment, each time feeling the same suite of relatively mild side effects. (Other patients reported more severe side effects, including pains in the chest and diarrhea.)

About two weeks after the first treatment, the Twiggs were out for one of their walks when Clayton remarked that the feeling of a rubber band pulling on his neck seemed less severe. He didn't know if the tumor was actually shrinking, but he did believe something good was happening. A few weeks later, when he was in Cleveland for his third treatment, Remick ordered an MRI scan to see if there was any change in the tumor to match what Twigg was reporting. The new pictures confirmed the good news: The tumor was a third smaller. Remick was ecstatic—"He was jumping around, all smiles," Twigg recalls—which was nothing compared to Twigg's reaction. After the next infusion of combrestatin, another MRI exam showed the tumor had shrunk even more, down by two-thirds. "You could see it was disappearing from my neck," Twigg says. Remick was elated. Such dramatic progress was not expected in a Phase I clinical trial, where clinical researchers were usually happy if the drugs proved safe. After the sixth infusion, Remick was anxious to take a close look and told Twigg he wanted to perform exploratory surgery to examine the tumor, or its remains, directly. Remick went in on August 2, 1999, and found nothing—no tumor at all. When Twigg got out of the hospital, he went home and prayed some more. He thanked God, and he prayed the tumor wouldn't come back. Then he went fishing with his sons.

Just to be safe and to satisfy the protocols, Twigg was given two more infusions of combrestatin, bringing the total to eight over about seven months. A year later, in the middle of 2000, he was still cancer-free. Would the tumor recur? No one could say. But to Remick, the success was amazing. "Clayton Twigg," he observes, "is our poster boy." Still, he and his colleagues realized Twigg was just one patient; the results had exciting implications for him but not necessarily for everyone else. Indeed, they later rewrote some of the protocols because they were seeing signs of heart damage in some of the combrestatin patients.

Folkman had more than a passing interest in the early, unofficial reports on combrestatin. This was because the drug was in molecular terms very similar to yet another fledgling drug that had come out of his own lab. The drug was called 2-methoxyestradiol (2ME2), and although no one could predict whether it would work as well and as quickly as combrestatin, 2ME2 did have one major advantage: It could be taken orally. Moreover, since it was a product of the human body—rather than an extract from tree bark, as combrestatin was—it might not cause the same uncomfortable side effects.

The potential value of 2ME2 was thoroughly overshadowed by the other antiangiogenesis drugs that had come from Folkman's laboratory with great fanfare. But even as the hubbub about the discovery of angiostatin and endostatin swirled around the Folkman lab and Children's Hospital, work had been proceeding very quietly on 2ME2, a little-known metabolite, or by-product, of estrogen that was now turning out to be a potential treatment not only for cancer but for other unrelated diseases as well. The idea first emerged from Folkman's suspicion that estrogens, in one form or another, should have antiangiogenic effects, a logical presumption because a woman's body changes so dramatically in concert with her menstrual periods, and especially during pregnancy. Tissues in the uterus grow, and then regress, all choreographed by an expanding and contracting blood supply, over and over again, without doing harm. It made sense that angiogenesis could be in control of such changes, at least partially.

Folkman had begun asking that question as early as 1983, and some of his coworkers had run a few experiments hinting that he might be right, publishing more than once on the topic. Still, the research really didn't get very far until ophthalmologist Robert D'Amato joined Folkman's team in 1992. D'Amato, another young scientist who got hooked on Folkman's ideas during a lecture, came in on a shoestring, ready to find money on his own if only he would be allowed to work at Children's. He was backed by excellent training in biology, medicine, and neuroscience, and he sought out especially difficult work. As it turned out, D'Amato also had a critical connection: It was his long relationship with John Holaday that led to EntreMed's key role in funding and developing antiangiogenesis drugs.

As an ophthalmologist, D'Amato was eager to study the fundamental biology of age-related macular degeneration, the leading cause of blindness in the elderly. He wanted to work with Folkman, because they agreed that macular degeneration looked very much like a problem of excess blood vessel growth—of unruly angiogenesis. Folkman told D'Amato he hoped to find oral angiogenesis inhibitors to fight the condition because getting a shot in the eye every day was not a very appealing treatment. Intrigued, D'Amato agreed to give it a try. But where to begin? He decided to try to imagine what was going on inside his own body, trying to visualize how various known drugs might affect him, starting at his head and progressing down to his feet. Nothing seemed to relate to angiogenesis, or antiangiogenesis, until he started thinking of reproductive problems—especially when he considered not his own body, but that of a woman. What about birth defects? When he compiled a list of drugs, vitamins, or agents that seemed to be linked to birth defects, one name stood out: thalidomide. When he thought about it, D'Amato became terrifically excited about the idea that thalidomide might be antiangiogenic. He began running experiments to see if he could support his thesis and see if thalidomide could redeem itself. If so, maybe it could be used as an antiangiogenesis drug.

At first, in tissue culture experiments, the drug didn't seem to do much. But then D'Amato realized that tissue culture was too unnatural; it was the drug's metabolites, the chemicals that were left over as thalidomide was being processed in the body, that were the likely birth defect culprits. This meant thalidomide had to go through the gut and be processed in the body before it began causing its notorious birth defects. Before long, he found in chemical testing that twelve different metabolites were produced as thalidomide was gradually broken down in the body, some of which were active in angiogenesis assays, such as chicken eggs and mouse eyes, and some of which were not. Triumph came when D'Amato was able to show that giving oral doses of thalidomide to rabbits could actually block the growth of new blood vessels in the eye.

D'Amato and Folkman published the findings in the *Proceedings of the National Academy of Sciences* in 1994, and the idea immediately raised all the old fears about thalidomide and birth defects. D'Amato's research colleagues told him that he was foolish even to be interested in the drug, a sentiment that was widely shared by pharmaceutical firms. But D'Amato and Folkman finally managed to interest one biotech executive in developing thalidomide far enough to bring it to clinical trials for macular degeneration. The savior was, once again, D'Amato's longtime friend, John Holaday at EntreMed. Thus began thalidomide's journey toward clinical trials for macular degeneration. Of course, it was emphasized over and over again that *no* women of childbearing age should ever use the drug. But by 2000, after the first patients were given their doses of thalidomide, there were clear signs that the drug and the principle of antiangiogenesis might have real impact on one of the world's major vision problems.

D'Amato's discovery about thalidomide, and his determination to explore the notorious drug, soon led to a bold step by another doctor in Boston. Taking note of thalidomide's antiangiogenic properties, Dr. Mark Kieran, the director of pediatric neuro-oncology at Dana-Farber, began carefully using thalidomide to treat incurable brain stem tumors in a few children. These were tumors that usually killed about half their victims within six months of diagnosis. But in mid-2000 Kieran found that by combining precise radiation treatments with doses of thalidomide, he was able to keep seven of his ten young patients alive and well nine months after diagnosis, with no recurrences of their tumors. At the University of Arkansas, meanwhile, Dr. Bart Barlogie was using thalidomide, combined with stem-cell transplants, on patients with multiple myeloma. Forty-five percent of his 169 patients were still alive two years later, and 10 percent of them had not experienced significant relapse of their tumors. Barlogie believed that without thalidomide most of his patients would have died within six months. Hoping to learn whether thalidomide alone might work, and whether it could help newly diagnosed patients, rather than end-stage cases, Barlogie began setting up a new, larger trial that would involve five hundred patients. How much of a future thalidomide had as an anticancer drug was uncertain. But the early results were indeed remarkable.

Just as remarkable, meanwhile, was that thalidomide wasn't the most promising drug to emerge from D'Amato's work. Folkman's interest in estrogen as a possible source of angiogenesis inhibitors had led to research by D'Amato identifying 2ME2 as the last metabolite made from estrogen as it is broken down. He also determined that 2ME2 is almost absent from a woman's urine until the last trimester of pregnancy, when the 2ME2 level bounces a thousand times higher; it gets especially high in the last week of pregnancy. Folkman speculated that its specific job is to slow down—or turn off—blood vessel growth in the placenta just prior to birth. Without 2ME2 to keep blood vessel growth under control, he wondered, might the highly vascularized placenta erupt into a massive tumorlike growth such as a hemangioma, perhaps spurred by the flood of growth hormones coursing through the baby's blood system? D'Amato's experiments soon showed that 2ME2 was an exquisitely specific inhibitor of angiogenesis. Collaborating with Ernest Hamel, a noted expert on steroids at the National Cancer Institute, he discovered that 2ME2 only stops the growth of two kinds of cells: endothelial cells and, surprisingly, breast cancer cells. It seemed that 2ME2 was inactive against every other type of cell in the body.

Given such exciting results, John Holaday jumped at the chance to license the drug, and after much experimentation and scaling up for production by EntreMed, 2ME2 entered clinical trials in Indianapolis against breast cancer in April 2000. The word leaking out of the trials was that the results with 2ME2 were immediate and impressive. In their very first patient, a woman with metastasized breast cancer whose lymph nodes were expanding massively in areas around her upper chest and neck, the tumors soon began shrinking visibly. At EntreMed, John Holaday was ecstatic. He hoped 2ME2 might be his grand-slam homer.

Even more ecstatic was the Montreal radiologist Dr. Heidi Patriquin, who had kept herself alive with regular doses of thalidomide, plus chemotherapy and other treatments, since her advanced case of cancer had been diagnosed five years before. Nothing seemed to be working anymore, and Patriquin had hoped to find a way into one of the three endostatin trials, and had failed. She had lined up again for the angiostatin trial in Philadelphia, but without success. Then, finally, in late spring 2000, the door opened and she was admitted into the Indiana University breast cancer trial of 2ME2, in Indianapolis. She hurried to Indiana for tests and analysis, collected her medicine, and then returned to Montreal to swallow her own daily doses of 2ME2. There was, of course, no guarantee the treatment would work. But at least it was another chance, and only time would tell.

SPURRED BY ALL the excitement, research continued apace in Folkman's laboratory. Even as endostatin, angiostatin, and the various other drugs began clinical trials, even as Folkman seemed to spend half his time accepting awards and giving talks around the world, he continued to lead his regular Friday morning lab meetings whenever he could. The intensity of the discussions never waned. Folkman and the members of his team were still looking ahead, still spinning off ideas, still dreaming.

One idea that struck home had first arisen a few years earlier, when Folkman had been asked by biologist Robert Kerbel, at the University of Toronto, why cancer drugs such as Taxol and vinblastine didn't seem to be antiangiogenic. Logic would suggest that such poisonous drugs would harm blood vessel cells along with cancer cells. Folkman posed this question to his troops: "Why doesn't chemotherapy treat the endothelium? After all, that's the first cell it sees. The drugs have to cross through blood vessels to get to the tumor cells. So, in theory, anticancer drugs should be antiangiogenic, or at least have some antiangiogenic component."

That was one of the important questions Folkman asked a young pediatrician, Dr. Tim Browder, when he came to work in the lab in the mid-1990s. As a thoroughly experienced hematology-oncology specialist—a "heme-onc," in the vernacular—Browder took the question as a challenge. It took him only a few days to come up with an answer—one so loaded with potential, and so certain to be controversial, that it took several more years of work and research before he and Folkman felt comfortable going public with it. What Browder suggested was that some of the standard drugs being used in chemotherapy were in fact antiangiogenic. It's just that they had always been used incorrectly. Browder was boldly pointing out that many of the drugs employed in the preceding half century could have been given in a different way, and they might have saved more lives if their antiangiogenic properties had been known.

The problem, Browder suggested, was modern medicine's absolute reliance on the phenomenon called MTD—a drug's maximum tolerated dose. In other words, all the poison you can stand. Ever since the 1940s, it had been carved in stone that the way to use chemotherapy was to hit tumors as hard as possible, as early as possible. If the patient was lucky, most of the tumor cells would be killed before the patient was killed. One hitch was that these drugs were aimed at cells that were dividing—tumor cells—and that meant that the poisons would also target and damage all other cells that were dividing, such as those in the intestinal lining, the bone marrow, and the hair follicles. That's why cancer patients' hair falls out, why intestinal damage causes severe diarrhea, and why bone marrow is sometimes damaged enough to cause anemia and reduced immunity. In fact, one of the reasons for doing bone marrow transplants in cancer patients is to rescue them after their original bone marrow has been wiped out by the potent treatments. Consequently, oncologists must spend much of their time coping with the deleterious side effects of chemotherapy.

Under standard protocols, chemotherapy was stopped to allow the vulnerable tissues to gradually recover. After this "resting" period, treatment would then resume. The chemotherapy would again drive the patient almost to death before another rest period. For some patients this approach worked; the cancer was defeated. But for many others, it was a disaster: They would become horribly sick as their tumors were bombed, and then the tumors would regrow during the rest period. Worse, eventually the tumors would become drug resistant and untreatable. Browder's theory was that this entire treatment procedure was simply masking what was really going on. He felt that some of the standard chemotherapeutic drugs were in fact antiangiogenic, or partially antiangiogenic, but had never been recognized as such because little thought had been given to what actually happened during the resting period. Perhaps the blood vessels feeding a tumor were also ravaged in chemotherapy, but that the resting period that had to be given to allow the patient to survive also provided time for the injured blood vessels to rebuild themselves, bring in fresh blood, and allow the tumor to resume wildfire growth. What if, rather than giving chemotherapy in the traditional way—in large, short busts—it was given as an antiangiogenic drug, in low, steady doses, over a long period?

Browder brought this idea back to Folkman after one of their regular Friday morning lab meetings, and Folkman got so excited that he started hopping around. "You don't see that too often, him hopping around," Browder remarked later. The idea certainly smacked of heresy, but that did little to deter Folkman. When he later called Robert Kerbel in Toronto and described Browder's idea, Kerbel, too, thought it was terrific. "I put down the phone," Kerbel recalls, "and I said to myself, 'Dammit, why didn't I think of that?'"

The theory of maximum tolerated dose had been the basis for chemotherapy ever since the days when Sidney Farber was fighting to push the treatment into the mainstream. To open up a whole new paradigm, to suggest using standard chemotherapy in low, long-term doses aimed at the blood vessels instead of the tumor, Browder knew he'd need to present powerful evidence. He and Folkman thought a big piece of that evidence would come if they could show that the new, antiangiogenic approach would circumvent the vexing problem of drug resistance, which was the major reason chemotherapy so often failed. Kerbel had earlier suggested that antiangiogenesis might overcome drug resistance. He believed that because endothelial cells, unlike tumor cells, were stable and normal, not mutating, they were far less likely to develop drug resistance. Browder agreed, and with Folkman set out to try to prove it in mice. They decided they had to create mice in which the tumors were absolutely drug resistant—so drug resistant their cancer could withstand doses of drugs that would certainly kill the host animals. It took months of work, transplanting increasingly resistant tumors from mouse to mouse, but once he had created enough mice burdened with tumors that could not be stopped by chemotherapy, Browder tried giving the animals small doses of Taxol or vinblastine. By experimentation, he found that rather than daily or constant infusions, the optimum dose schedule seemed to be one small dose every six days. And as he and Folkman hoped, they could see that the repeated small doses gradually made the aggressive, highly drug-resistant tumors stop growing as their life-support systems dried up. In contrast, when Browder used the conventional hit-and-rest approach on another group of mice, the tumors couldn't be stopped. It confirmed that the antiangiogenic method was, in Browder's words, "gangbusters better." It didn't eliminate the resistant tumor, but it kept it flat for thirty-six days, which is a long time in the life of a mouse.

Browder's findings meshed nicely with those of biologist Kerbel, who thought that antiangiogenesis therapy might offer the first way to get around drug resistance, the big killer. The reduced-dose chemo approach was not ready for the public, but even as Browder was beginning to give seminars and lectures on his ideas, strong, human, and wholly ironic evidence was right down the hall.

Michael Retsky was a physicist and electron microscopist who lived south of Boston in Trumbull, Connecticut, and liked to drive to Boston's outskirts and then bicycle the rest of the way to work at Children's Hospital. His research focus was breast cancer, specifically how breast cancer cells grow and how the blood vessels may be involved in supporting such growth. But he was also vitally and personally interested in cancer—his own. Retsky had taken to heart the idea that Tim Browder was pursuing so avidly, that frequent low doses of chemotherapy might be an effective approach to cancer control. In fact, he had believed in the principle for a decade.

Retsky was diagnosed with Stage III colorectal cancer in 1995, when he was working in his own research business. He was no neophyte on the subject. He had been studying tumor growth since 1983 when, in Colorado Springs, Colorado, he had joined a discussion group whose members were trying to understand cancer and the properties of tumor growth. While combing through the older literature on cancer back then, he had encountered a fundamental piece of work called the Gompertzian theory, which held that tumor growth is a steady, continuous process. But newer data in the literature, as well as his own research, strongly suggested that tumor growth is not a steady process. Tumors grow in spurts—resting, growing, resting, and then growing some more, depending on conditions. In the context of cancer treatment, it meant that modern chemotherapy was based on an unsupported assumption. Because it seemed so fundamentally important, Retsky and several colleagues published an article on their findings in *Cancer Research* in 1984. The paper caused a major stir among cancer specialists because it challenged the entire foundation of chemotherapy. Finally, in 1992, Retsky was invited to a meeting in Switzerland to present a paper to eight hundred top breast cancer doctors. Essentially, he was there to defend his very disturbing conclusions. "They were going to have me for lunch," he recalls. Before his talk, Retsky dug even deeper into the literature and came up with a startling discovery. He found that the evidence for the idea that tumors grow steadily rested on a set of papers published in the 1950s and 1960s by Anna Laird, at the Argonne National Laboratory near Chicago. Laird's papers had been so convincing at the time that cancer researchers had relied on her findings completely; there were more than five hundred references citing the Laird papers in the cancer literature. But it seemed to Retsky that few people had bothered to actually read the Laird reports in detail. "Her conclusion was based on only eighteen rodents and one rabbit," Retsky said. "And on that basis she'd concluded that the Gompertzian equation was a general biological phenomenon, a general rule. Thousands and thousands of people have been treated on that basis— just nineteen animals and very scattered data. That is a very shaky foundation."

Retsky's report in Switzerland was surprisingly well received, and it was convincing enough to be published in the journal *Cancer Investigation* in 1993. Two years later, his own cancer diagnosis yanked his findings out of the realm of the abstract. Suddenly the Gompertzian equation and Laird's few animals came into very stark focus. He had to think very carefully about how he wanted to treat his own cancer. There was no shortage of advice; Retsky knew hundreds of cancer doctors the world over. But the expert he consulted first was an old friend from his Colorado Springs days, Dr. Jack Speer. Speer had used an unusual schedule of chemotherapy to treat several patients, and he had seen some success. With almost continuous infusions of low doses, a few patients, including some with metastasized tumors, lived longer. Speer also advised Retsky to discuss his case with two other specialists—Dr. Bill Hrushesky, at the Veterans Hospital in Albany, New York, and Jacob Lokich, in Boston—both of whom had been experimenting with the drug 5-FU (fluorouracil). Instead of giving 5-FU in massive doses, followed by weeks of rest, both doctors had been trying it in a different dose regimen, giving it almost constantly in smaller doses. Retsky decided to go with a regimen that required him to wear a small pump that constantly infused the drug.

Retsky was aware of Folkman and his work, had seen some of his lab's many papers, and made it a point to be in the audience when Folkman made a presentation at the annual meeting of the American Society of Clinical Oncology in 1996. Afterward he approached Folkman and asked if he could come to Boston for a visit. He wanted to discuss Folkman's data on tumor dormancy and to see if there might be some opportunity for collaboration. Retsky didn't mention that he himself had cancer and that as they spoke he was receiving chemotherapy in a constant trickle from his drug pump. He tended to keep his disease to himself, because he didn't want people feeling sorry for him. Eventually, though, the subject had to come up, and Retsky assured Folkman that he could be both a patient and a scientist.

Retsky soon set up his own treatment protocol. He found the twenty-four-hour-a-day pump uncomfortable, and he hooked himself up only at night before bedtime and removed it in the morning. He was convinced that what he was getting was antiangiogenesis treatment. The going was slow, but after two and a half years, Retsky's colon tumor shrank and disappeared. Like most cancer patients, he worried it would return, but he knew that if it did, he could simply go back to the drug pump. Nearly three years after taking the pump off for the last time, however, the cancer had not recurred. Retsky saw himself as evidence to support Folkman and Browder's idea that some established drugs might be working through antiangiogenesis. "I am the anecdotal story that it works," Retsky says. For his part, Folkman felt that even though one patient hardly represented a clinical trial, Retsky's experience was enough to offer doctors a new avenue that they could try when all else had failed. And "when all else fails" was key, as far as Folkman was concerned. "It can be used only on patients who are drug resistant, for whom nothing else is left," Folkman says. "And we warn everybody that we don't know what the best dose for you is."

AS ALL OF THIS was occurring, Folkman's star was constantly on the rise. He was gathering in prestigious awards worldwide, almost one a week in 1999 and 2000. It was clear that he had finally not only broken through the barrier to scientific respectability but to real stardom. At the huge American Society of Clinical Oncology meeting in New Orleans in May 2000, Folkman lectured twice in a six-hundred-seat hall, both times to standing-room-only crowds of cancer doctors. It could not be said that Folkman failed to enjoy the attention and accolades. Finally it seemed that his peers were judging him to be persistent, not obstinate. This was a distinction he had long sought. Now it seemed clear that great strides had been made largely because one man worked, pushed, and badgered one idea for so many years. Step by painful step, at first alone and then with colleagues he had engaged in the struggle, Folkman had faced the objections and surmounted all the barriers that inflexible critics and doubters threw in his path. This experience had bred an enduring confidence and had even given him a sense of peace. He didn't yet know how the big question would turn out—how smoothly the idea of antiangiogenesis would move from the bench top to the bedside—but still, he was as close as he had ever been to real satisfaction.

One reason Folkman was able to persist so long, and remain on the staff at Children's Hospital and on the Harvard Medical School faculty, despite so much controversy and criticism, was his consummate skill as a physician, teacher, and pediatric surgeon. Critics had always sniped at his ideas and his style as a researcher, but there was never any question about Folkman's skill as a physician and teacher. Year after year Folkman won medical students' votes as one of the best teachers on the Harvard Medical School faculty. He was regularly tapped to lecture first-year medical students on what it means to be a doctor, occasions on which he emphasized over and over again the importance of being alert and alive to the patients' feelings. He repeatedly argued that a physician's bond with his or her patients should be so close that it transcends a strictly professional relationship. When you walk into the hospital room when your patient's family is visiting, he lectured the medical students, the patient should immediately say to his relatives, "I want you to meet *my* doctor." If they don't, something's wrong.

"You are their doctor," Folkman tells the students. "There's a certain point at which they begin to trust you, and you won't abandon them. You won't go on vacation and disappear. Or they can't reach you. They're scared to begin with, and if they get that sense, then they're *very* scared." Folkman would never have his patients feel disconnected from their doctor. He always made sure they had his home telephone number. "Here is my telephone number; here is my beeper number," he would say. "I never want to hear that you couldn't get hold of me." He found that patients almost never abused his extraordinary solicitousness. "They don't have to test it," he said. "They only abuse it when they can't get hold of you." When young residents in training objected to that idea, groaning about never having any time of their own or about being awakened late at night, Folkman's answer was blunt: "You chose medicine. It's a service career. Long hours are part of the job. If you want a different kind of life, think about becoming a banker."

Another fundamental lesson Folkman always tried to impart to medical students was never to destroy hope. There are moments when hope is all that remains for a patient to cling to. Although many doctors worry about raising false hopes, Folkman found that patients don't really punish their doctors for that. There are desperate moments when even false hope is better than no hope. He recalled the case of a young medical student who was himself burdened with a brain tumor. The young man said he didn't like it when people used the term "false hope." "They have no right to do that," he told Folkman. "They don't have this tumor."

Everyone has an obituary date, Folkman would tell his students, and then he would ask: "Suppose we knew your date?" He would pull out a list of the students and feign reading. "Jones, you're in the year 2000, March 31, at three P.M.," and on down the list. After a few names, sensing the students had had enough, he would look up and say, "You don't want to hear any more? So what are you going to do in the meantime if you know the date? You've destroyed hope. So now if a patient asks you, 'How long do I have to live, Doctor?,' are you going to tell him two weeks, two months, or two years? You put a time on it, and it just destroys hope." He urged his students never to utter the words "I can't do anything more for you." They could always do something. They could make the patient feel more comfortable. Or go to the window of his or her hospital room and point outside. "Do you see that building over there? That's the research building. We're working on it."

Even when Folkman was in hot pursuit of the secrets of angiogenesis, he had time for people. Traveling often, he would carry a list of some two hundred cancer patients who had called seeking his advice. They weren't necessarily *his* patients, but he made a commitment to call at least ten of them every night, wherever he was, to discuss their concerns and offer what advice he could. As a doctor, he felt he could do no less.

A

Abbott Laboratories, 235, 276, 335
academia, commercialization of, 138–52,
  170, 181
Adamis, Anthony, 321–27
adenovirus, 317
adrenaline, 130
agribusiness, 213
Aiello, Dr. Lloyd Paul, 325–27
Algire, Dr. Glen, 79–80, 82, 93, 94
Alpha Omega Alpha, 37
Alpha-v, Beta-3, 290
Alza, 177, 178
American Association for Cancer
  Research, 242, 281
American Cancer Society, 23, 105,
  109–17, 160, 212, 286
  history of, 109–10, 159
  press seminars, 109–11, 115–24, 181
American College of Surgeons, 17, 33
American Heart Association, 212, 312,
  318
American Society of Clinical Oncology,
  334, 347, 348
Amgen, 150
amino acids, 97, 199, 206
  sequencing, 206–8, 210, 253, 255
amputation, avoided with angiogenic
  treatment, 308–13, 320, 321
anaplastic thyroid tumor, 336–38
anatomy, 28, 29, 30, 84, 158
Anderson, Dr. W. French, 112–13, 114
Anderson (M. D.) Cancer Center,
  Houston, 186, 233, 235–36
  endostatin clinical trials, 329–32
Andrews, Bess, 284

aneurysmal bone cyst, 269
angioblastoma, 274, 276, 279
angiodormin, 299–301
angiogenesis, 4, 80
  accepted by research community, 198,
    236–37, 260, 281, 289–90
  angiostatin and, 256–57, 280, 281, 283,
    296–99, 303–7, 328–29, 336
  cartilage research, 167–69, 173–76,
    192, 201–5
  cell migration, 195–97
  chicken assay, 104–5, 124, 135, 175,
    199, 216, 248
  diffusing factor, 101–4
  endangered limbs and, 308–13, 320,
    321
  endostatin and, 3–5, 264–67, 280, 281,
    283, 296–99, 303–7, 328–48
  endothelial cell growth, 81–90,
    125–33, 188–98, 199–217, 223,
    232–67, 296–319, 343–48
  eye disease and, 321–27
  gene therapy, 310–21
  heart disease and, 308–9, 312, 314–19,
    320, 321
  hemangiomas and, 221–37, 245
  inhibitors, 99–100, 120, 173–76, 194,
    201–3, 215–17, 233–36, 239–67,
    268–80, 290–99, 303–7, 309, 328–48
  inhibitor-stimulator balance, 242–67
  interferon and, 221–34, 236, 237, 245,
    268–76, 279, 281, 290–95, 328
  invention of, 80–81, 90
  in vitro research, 124–33, 136, 166–67,
    188–97, 201–5, 215–17, 252–53

angiogenesis *(cont'd)*:
  leaky plastics research, 176–79
  Monsanto-Harvard research funding
    deal, 136, 138–52, 163–64, 166, 170,
    180–83, 188, 207, 213, 214
  natural inhibitor theory, 245–46
  onset of, 240–41
  perfusion experiments, 86–90, 116
  plasmin role, 255–57, 261
  postsurgical eruption of metastases
    and, 238–41, 244–48
  press on, 283–87, 294, 296–97, 303,
    307, 332, 335
  rabbit eye experiments, 93–96, 101–2,
    135, 169, 174, 177, 199, 248
  research, 80–90, 93–105, 116–36,
    163–79, 181–98, 199–217, 223,
    232–67, 268–80, 283–84, 288–90,
    296–307, 308–27, 328–48
  stimulators, 99–100, 120, 122, 202–9,
    213, 241–67, 271–74, 279–80,
    308–19
  TAF, 96–99, 116, 118–36, 164–69,
    173–79, 181–88, 194–97, 199–205,
    208–11, 215–17, 253, 263
  Takedo funding, 214–17, 276
  terminology, 80–81, 210
  TNP-470, 216–17, 235–36, 239–40,
    243, 249, 279–80
  tumor suppression of metastases and,
    239–67
  VEGF, 209–11, 234, 240–44, 249,
    289–90, 308–27
  see also antiangiogenesis; blood
    vessels; growth factors; inhibitors;
    stimulators
angiogenin, 206–8, 213
angiostatin, 256–67, 271, 280, 281, 283,
  296–99, 303–7, 328–29, 336
  clinical trials, 306, 328–29, 334, 343
  invention of, 256–57
  press on, 283–87, 303, 307
animal research, 25, 79
  angiostatin and endostatin, 257–67,
    280, 281, 296–98, 306
  blood substitute, 50, 54, 81, 82
  chicken assay, 104–5, 124, 135, 175,
    199, 216, 248
  diabetic retinopathy, 324–26
  dog experiments, 25–30, 31–37
  Folkman's early tumor cell
    experiments, 51–57, 78–90, 93–105
  fumigillin experiments, 216–17
  legislation, 25–26
  rabbit eye experiments, 93–94, 95–96,
    101–2, 135, 169, 174, 177, 199, 248
  rabbit thyroid experiments, 52–54, 74,
    81, 82, 116
  reduced-dose chemotherapy, 345–48
  TNP-470, 217, 235, 239
  tumor-feeding blood vessel
    experiments, 79–90, 93–104,
    116–24, 217, 235, 239, 241, 251,
    310–11
  tumor suppression of metastases,
    251–67
  see also research; *specific researchers
    and experiments*
Annals of Surgery, 86
antiangiogenesis, 99–100, 197, 221–37,
  249
  AT-3, 299–302
  angiostatin, 256–67, 280, 281, 283,
    296–99, 303–7, 328–29, 336
  cancer treatment, 3–5, 256–74,
    283–89, 303–7, 328–48
  combrestatin, 335–59
  Denis case, 274–80
  drug shipping problems, 296–99
  early treatments, 268–82
  endostatin, 3–5, 264–67, 280, 281,
    283, 296–99, 303–7, 328–48
  EntreMed funding, 250–51, 259,
    262–63, 266, 286–87, 304–6,
    332–35, 340–43
  hemangioma cases, 221–37, 245
  industry interests in, 249–51, 259,
    262–63, 266, 276–77, 286–90,
    299–306, 332–36, 340–43
  interferon, 268–76, 279–81, 290–95,
    328
  Kalesnik case, 290–95
  LaChance case, 271–73, 274, 281, 284
  marimastat, 276–79
  marketing concerns, 251, 286–87,
    299–306, 332–36, 340–43
  natural agents, 245–46
  pediatric, 268–80

press on, 283–87, 294, 296–97, 303, 307, 332, 335
reduced-dose chemotherapy, 343–48
research, 3–5, 221–37, 247–67, 268–80, 283–84, 288–90, 296–307, 328–48
search for agents, 247–67
thalidomide, 342–43
TNP-470, 216–17, 235–36, 239–40, 243, 249, 279–80
2ME2, 339–43
see also inhibitors
antibiotics, 20, 110, 216, 268
antibodies, 170, 239
monoclonal, 289–90, 324–26
anticancer drugs, 157, 163, 236, 239, 335, 343
anticogenes, 156, 162–63
aorta endothelial cell experiments, 126, 190, 193
Arizona State University, 336
arteriovenous malformation, 275–79
Associated Press, 116, 121, 285
aspergillis, 216
Atkinson, Stephen, 88, 147, 214, 217, 227
AT-3 (antithrombin-3), 299–301
Auerbach, Dr. Robert, 104, 223

B
Baltimore, David, 151, 162
Barger, Dr. Clifford, 29, 34
Barlogie, Dr. Bart, 342
Bausch & Lomb, 177
Becker, Dr. Fred, 46–57, 62, 69, 82, 119
Beckman, Arnold, 147
Beckwith, Jonathan, 138
BeneFin, 176
Beth Israel Deaconess Medical Center, Boston, 297, 317
Beth Israel Hospital, Boston, 34, 71, 98, 117, 156, 210, 223
b-FGF, 233, 240, 241, 309
Biochemical and Biophysical Research Communications, 209
biochemistry, 82–83, 134–36, 138–39, 163, 199–200
researchers vs. doctors in, 87–88
Biochemistry, 207

Biogen, 150, 151, 152
biology, 82–83, 138
blood vessel, 51–57, 78–90, 93–105, 116–36, 163–79, 181–98, 199–211, 215–17, 223, 232–67, 268–82, 388–90, 296–99, 303–7, 308–27, 328–48
biomedicine:
academia vs. industry in, 138–52, 170
pharmaceutical industry and, 212–13, 248–49
biotechnology, 149–52, 299
industry interests in angiogenesis, 249–51, 259, 262–63, 266, 276–77, 286–90, 299–306, 309–11, 332–36, 340–43
research, 138–49, 149–52, 170, 213, 262
revolution, 149–52, 170, 209, 213
bladder cancer, 234, 267
blindness, 288, 321
angiogenic treatment for diabetic retinopathy, 321–27
Blood, 236
blood clotting, 261, 310
AT-3, 299–302
blood pressure, 81, 314
blood pump, 24–27, 33–34, 37, 47–48
Gross, 24–27, 34, 37
Lindbergh-Carrel, 50
blood substitutes, Folkman's research on, 49–54
Blood Vessel Club, 131
blood vessels, 5, 56, 64, 84, 134
growth of, and relationship to tumors, 51–57, 69, 78–90, 93–105, 116–36, 163–79, 181–98, 199–211, 215–17, 223, 232–67, 268–82, 288–90, 296–99, 303–7, 308–27, 328–48
see also angiogenesis; antiangiogenesis; capillaries
Blumberg, Baruch, 162
Blumgart, Dr. Herman, 19
Boehm, Thomas, 265, 281
Bok, Derek, 140–41, 143, 146, 150–51
bone:
disappearing bone disease, 274–79
growth, 278
tumor, 268–74

bone marrow, 190
  leukemia and, 234–36
Boston, 4, 19, 20, 41, 45, 57, 58, 60, 64,
  73, 112, 149, 150, 152, 208, 228
  medical community, 20–24, 98,
  122–23, 145, 169–70, 172, 303
  see also specific hospitals
Boston City Hospital, 23, 46, 70, 72, 168
  Folkman as instructor at, 70–72
  Folkman's lab at, 77–88, 89, 116
Boston Globe, The, 26, 119, 121, 144,
  148, 332
Boston Herald American, 144
Boston Lying-In Hospital, 65, 127, 155
Boston University, 126
Bouck, Noel, 241–44, 247
  Cell paper, 243, 247
brain, 255
  cancer, 168, 267, 329
breast cancer, 5, 38, 159, 168, 267, 333,
  342–43
  reduced-dose chemotherapy
  approach, 346–48
Brem, Steven, 168, 169, 174, 239–40
Briggs, Tommy, 221–26, 229, 234, 236,
  237, 271, 280, 293
Brigham Hospital, Boston, 23, 40, 71,
  134, 206, 234
Bristol-Myers Squibb, 262–63
  angiogenesis interests, 263, 297, 301,
  304–6, 336
British Biotech, 276–77, 335
British Journal of Cancer, 86
Brody, Jane, 119–21
Brouty-Boye, Danielle, 197
Browder, Dr. Tim, 343–46, 348
Burch, B. H., 19
Burkitt's lymphoma, 162
Burrows, Dr. Patricia, 228, 229, 275–78
Butterfield, Kit, 175, 189

C
calcitonin, 270
Calgene, 335
CAM (chicken chorioallantoic
  membrane) assay, 104–5, 124, 135,
  175, 199, 216, 248
Canada, 228, 232, 233, 250, 343, 345
Canadian Journal of Chemistry, 336

cancer, 3, 23, 51, 110, 156–57
  angiogenesis stimulator-inhibitor
  balance, 242–67
  angiostatin treatment, 256–67, 280,
  281, 283, 296–99, 303–7, 328–29,
  336
  antiangiogenic treatment, 3–5,
  256–74, 283–89, 303–7, 328–48
  bladder, 234, 267
  bone, 268–73
  brain, 168, 267, 329
  breast, 5, 38, 159, 168, 267, 333,
  342–43, 346–48
  causes of, 156–60, 197
  cell division, 51–57, 114, 159, 167
  cervical, 110, 279
  chemotherapy, 112–15, 331, 343–48
  colon, 267, 284, 332, 346
  dormancy, 239–67
  endostatin treatment, 3–5, 264–67, 280,
  281, 283, 296–99, 303–7, 328–48
  eye, 103
  Folkman's early tumor cell research,
  51–57, 69, 78–90, 93–105
  genetics and, 150, 156–63, 206, 241,
  251, 281
  giant-cell sarcoma, 290–95
  growth factors, 86, 87, 89–90, 96–102,
  118–36, 163–79, 181–97, 199–211,
  215–17, 229, 232–67, 271–74,
  289–90, 296–307, 328–48
  history of treatment, 112–14, 156–63
  interferon treatment, 197, 223, 224,
  290–95, 328
  liver, 52, 162
  lung, 110, 158–59, 160, 251–52,
  257–59, 264, 279
  Monsanto-Harvard research funding
  deal, 136, 138–52, 163–64, 166, 170,
  180–83, 188, 207, 213, 214
  ovarian, 89
  pediatric, 75–76, 112–15, 156, 160,
  268–73
  postsurgical eruption of metastases,
  238–41, 244–48
  primary tumor, 264–65
  prostate, 267
  reduced-dose chemo approach,
  343–48

research, 51–57, 78–90, 96–105,
    118–36, 156–79, 181–97, 199–211,
    212, 215–17, 232–67, 281–82,
    288–95, 303–7, 328–48
skin, 52–54
terminology, 157
testicular, 160
TNP-470 treatment, 235–36, 239–40,
    243, 249, 279–80
tumor relationship to blood vessels,
    51–57, 69, 78–90, 93–105, 116–36,
    163–79, 181–98, 199–211, 215–17,
    232–67, 268–74, 288–90, 296–99,
    303–7, 328–48
tumor suppression of metastases,
    239–67
"two-years" comment controversy,
    282, 283–87, 290, 307
viral transmission, 160–63, 197
War on, 163
Cancer Investigation, 347
Cancer Research, 303, 346
capillaries, 84
    endothelial cells, 188–97, 209
    growth of, 87, 95–96, 99, 101, 104,
        167, 169, 188–97, 209, 234–35, 314,
        322
    hemangioma cases, 221–37
Carlotti, Dr. Al, 268
Carrel, Dr. Alexis, 50
cartilage research, 167–69, 173–76, 192,
    201–5
CEA, 117
Cell, 243
    Bouck paper, 243, 247
    O'Reilly paper, 259–60, 261, 263–64,
        280
Cell Biology, 86
cells, 158
    discovery of, 158
    division of, 51–57, 114, 158, 159, 167,
        193–94, 201–3
    migration, 195–97, 223
    recoiling, 215–16
cervical cancer, 110, 279
Cetus, 150
Champion, Hale, 180
chemotherapy, 4, 5, 52, 53, 87, 110,
    112–15, 130, 156, 160, 163, 224,

236, 265, 267, 270, 274, 276, 280,
    329, 337, 338
early use of, 112–14
maximum tolerated dose, 344–45
reduced-dose approach, 343–48
side effects, 331, 344–45
Chen, Lan Bo, 190
Chicago Tribune, 119, 121
children:
    antiangiogenic treatment, 268–80
    bone disease, 268–79
    cancer, 75–76, 112–15, 156, 160,
        268–73
    cystic fibrosis, 64–66, 75
    heart defects, 24–27, 30–32
    hemangioma cases, 221–29
    surgery, 24–27, 30–37, 71–76
Children's Hospital, Boston, 23, 24, 32,
    54, 64, 71, 73, 88, 105, 111, 115,
    223, 236, 303
    Enders Research Building, 94–98,
        105, 133, 143, 172, 175, 184, 205,
        321
    Folkman as chief-of-surgery, 71–72,
        76–77, 88, 95, 122, 133, 164,
        183–87, 198, 213
    Folkman labs, 88–90, 93–98, 105, 116,
        133, 143, 165–66, 172, 181, 196,
        200, 217, 238, 246, 254, 321–23, 343
    giant-cell tumor cases, 290–95
    Gross research lab, 23–27, 30–37, 64
    hemangioma cases, 226–37, 275
    "two-years" comment controversy,
        283–87
Children's Hospital of Philadelphia,
    73–76, 228
chondrosarcomas, 168, 201, 204–5
Churchill, Dr. Edward, 39, 42, 62–63, 67
circulatory system, 5, 80
    blood vessel/tumor relationship,
        51–57, 59, 78–90, 93–105, 116–36,
        163–79, 181–98, 199–211, 215–17,
        223, 232–67, 268–82, 288–90,
        296–99, 303–7, 308–27
    construction of, 81
    failing, angiogenic treatment for,
        308–14, 320, 321
Circulis, Janis, 192
cleanliness, basic ideas of, 154–55

clinical trials, 213, 231, 328
  angiostatin, 306, 328–29, 334, 343
  AT-3, 299, 300
  combrestatin, 336–39
  endostatin, 3–5, 306–7, 328–34, 336,
    343
  Phase I, 328–29, 338–39
  TNP-470, 235–36, 279–80
  2ME2, 342–43
Cobb, Carl, 119, 121, 148, 182–83
Cohen, Stanley, 200
Cold Spring Harbor Laboratory, Long
  Island, 200, 241, 282, 287
Collaborative Genetics, 150
collagenase, 276
Collateral Therapeutics, 276
colon cancer, 267, 284, 332, 346
combrestatin, 335–39
congenital heart defects, 24–27, 30–37
Corkery, Joe, 85, 89, 91
Cornell University, 149, 171, 180
Cornell University Medical Center, New
  York, 317
Cotran, Ramzi, 91, 125–26, 128, 131,
  187, 191
Covance Laboratories, 306, 307
cow aorta endothelial cell experiments,
  126, 190, 193
Crick, Francis, 282
Crystal, Dr. Ronald, 317
C-type viruses, 161–62
Culliton, Barbara, 181–82
Cunningham, Dr. James, 337–38
Curie, Marie, 9, 160
cystic fibrosis, 64–65, 75
cytokines, 131

D
D'Amato, Dr. Robert, 5, 249–50, 340–42
D'Amore, Dr. Pat, 324
Dana-Farber Cancer Institute, Boston,
  4, 112, 189, 190, 191, 231, 234, 246,
  267, 286, 291, 293, 303, 304, 342
  endostatin clinical trials, 329–34
Datta, Dorothy, 338
Davis, Alan, 109, 112, 115–18
Denis, Bianca, 274–80
DePriest, Oscar, 43
Dextor, Aaron, 21

diabetes, 130, 150, 309
  angiogenic treatment for diabetic
    retinopathy, 321–27
Diamond, Dr. Louis, 114–15
DMSO, 111
DNA, 83, 159–60, 161–63, 202, 210, 281,
  282
  naked, 311–19
Doll, Richard, 158–59
doxorubicin, 337
Dunn, Dr. Thelma, 52
duodenal ulcer, 60–61
DuPont, 140, 212
Dvorak, Dr. Harold, 210–11, 223,
  318–19, 323–24

E
Ebert, Robert, 140–41, 144, 146
EGF (epidermal growth factor), 131,
  200
Einstein, Albert, 11
elastase, 302
electron microscope, 84, 128, 144
endangered limbs, angiogenic treatment
  for, 308–14, 320, 321
Enders, Dr. John F., 94–95, 105
endostatin, 3, 264–67, 271, 280, 281,
  283, 296–99, 303–7, 328–48
  clinical trials, 3–5, 306–7, 328–34, 336,
    343
  discovery of, 264–65, 280
  press on, 283–87, 303, 307
  shipping problems, 296–99
  toxicity, 4, 329–34
endothelial cells, 81, 84, 85–86, 99, 125
  gene therapy, 310–19
  growth research, 81–90, 125–33,
    188–98, 199–217, 223, 232–67,
    268–80, 288–90, 296–319, 343–48
  hemangiomas, 221–29
  inhibitors, 201–3, 215–17, 233–36,
    239–67, 268–80, 290–99, 303–7,
    309, 328–48
  inhibitor-stimulator balance, 242–67
  migration of, 195–97, 223
  stimulators, 99–100, 120, 122, 202–9,
    213, 241–67, 271–74, 279–80,
    308–19
England, 158–59, 276–77, 289, 300

EntreMed, 250, 300, 335
  antiangiogenesis research and funding,
    250–51, 259, 262–63, 266, 286–87,
    304–6, 332–33, 335, 340–43
  share price fluctuations, 286–87, 296,
    332–33
enzymes, 134, 138, 150, 164, 170, 195,
  199, 206, 255, 276
Epstein-Barr virus, 162
estrogen, 131, 340, 342
Europe, 202, 233, 285, 299; *see also*
  specific countries
Ewing, Dr. James, 113
Experimental Cell Research, 86
eyes, 93–94, 177, 288, 321–27
  angiogenic treatment for diabetic
    retinopathy, 321–27
  cancer, 103
  macular degeneration, 340, 341
  rabbit eye experiments, 93–94, 95–96,
    101–2, 135, 169, 174, 177, 199,
    248
  research, 321–27, 340–41
Ezekowitz, Alan, 226, 228, 232

F
Farber, Dr. Sidney, 109, 111, 112–15,
  121, 124, 160, 345
  use of chemotherapy, 114–15
Fawcett, Donald, 84
Fedder, Joe, 166–67
Ferrara, Dr. Napoleone, 209–11, 289,
  311, 324
Feynman, Richard, 173
FGF (fibroblast growth factor), 130, 190,
  205, 207, 208, 213, 232–34, 240,
  244, 249, 271–74, 276, 279, 293,
  308–10, 317, 319
  gene therapy, 317, 319
fibrin, 210–11
fibroblasts, 125, 127–31, 190, 205
Fidler, Dr. Isaiah, 96, 233–34
Fine, Dr. Howard, 267, 280
Fine, Dr. Jacob, 71
Fleming, Alexander, 216
Flory, Paul, 178, 179, 180
folic acid, 160
Folkman, Benjamin (grandfather), 7–8,
  13, 36

Folkman, Bessie (mother), 7, 8, 9, 15, 17,
  18
Folkman, David (brother), 7, 10, 13–15,
  18, 20, 41
Folkman, Jerome (father), 6–16, 18, 20,
  67
Folkman, Joy (sister), 7, 10, 13, 15, 41
Folkman, Judah, 3–6
  altruism of, 105, 121, 147, 165, 195,
    196, 238, 320
  at American Cancer Society Press
    Seminars, 115–24, 181
  angiogenesis theory and research,
    80–105, 116, 118–36, 163–79,
    181–98, 199–205, 208–11, 215–17,
    223, 232–67, 271–72, 280–84,
    288–89, 296–99, 303–7, 309,
    320–23, 328–48
  awards, 37, 72, 262–63, 348
  birth of, 9
  blood substitute research, 49–54
  Boston City Hospital lab of, 77–88, 89,
    116
  Briggs case, 223–26
  cartilage research, 167–69, 173–76,
    192, 201–5
  celebrity of, 121, 124, 237, 260,
    281–82, 348
  chicken assay, 104–5, 124, 135, 175,
    199, 216, 248
  childhood of, 6, 7–15, 67
  as Children's Hospital head of surgery,
    71–72, 76–77, 88, 95, 122, 133, 164,
    183–87, 198, 213
  Children's Hospital labs of, 88–90,
    93–98, 105, 116, 133, 143, 165–66,
    172, 181, 196, 200, 217, 238, 246,
    254, 321–23, 343
  compassion for patients, 66–68, 76,
    294, 349–50
  critics on, 87–89, 98, 102–5, 117,
    122–24, 184–92, 229–32, 260–61,
    296–98, 303–4, 332, 348
  Denis case, 276–79
  Director's Lecture (1997), 281–82, 287
  early tumor cell research, 51–57, 69,
    78–90, 93–105
  education of, 9–14, 15–19, 20–44
  endostatin clinical trials, 3–5, 329–34

Folkman, Judah (cont'd):
  EntreMed funding, 250–51, 259,
    262–63, 266, 286–87, 304–6, 340–43
  as a father, 64–66, 75, 133, 186
  first academic paper, 19, 22
  fraud allegations against, 231–32
  Gross research lab work, 23–37, 64
  at Harvard Medical School, 19, 20–30,
    37, 70
  Harvard professorship, 70–72, 186–87,
    213, 349
  heartbeat project, 33–37
  hemangioma cases, 223–37, 271
  Kalesnik case, 290–95
  Karnovsky Lecture (1996), 280–81
  LaChance case, 271–73, 274
  leaky plastics research, 55–56, 142,
    173, 176–79
  marriage of, 41–43, 64, 133, 186, 303
  Massachusetts General residency,
    37–44, 58–70, 78
  Monsanto-Harvard funding deal, 136,
    138–52, 163–64, 166, 170, 180–83,
    188, 207, 213, 214
  naval duty, 44, 45–57, 68, 142
  NCI funding, 80–81, 133–35, 320
  pacemaker invention, 35–37
  pediatric surgery training, 72–76
  perfusion experiments, 85–90, 116
  personality, 67, 76, 165–66, 192
  press on, 115–16, 118–24, 145, 148,
    176, 181, 281–87, 297–99, 303,
    307
  published work, 19, 22, 102, 123, 175,
    183, 195, 207, 210, 341
  rabbit eye experiments, 93–94, 95–96,
    101–2, 135, 169, 174, 177, 199, 248
  rabbit thyroid experiments, 52–54, 74,
    81, 82, 116
  reduced-dose chemotherapy research,
    343–48
  Seminars in Medicine talk (1971),
    98–100
  stimulator-inhibitor balance theory,
    242–47
  as surgeon, 16–19, 28–44, 56–57,
    58–76, 133, 164, 183–87, 198
  TAF theory and research, 96–99, 116,
    118–36, 164–69, 173–79, 181–88,
    194–97, 199–205, 208–11, 215–17,
    253, 263
  Takeda funding, 214–15, 216–17
  2ME2 research, 339–43
  "two-years" comment controversy,
    282, 283–87, 290, 307
  -Vallee collaboration, 134–36, 139–43,
    163–66, 167, 180–83, 199, 206–8,
    263
Folkman, Kenneth (son), 65–66
Folkman, Laura (daughter), 64–65, 66,
    75, 133, 186
Folkman, Marjorie (daughter), 66, 186
Folkman, Paula Prial (wife), 41–43, 48,
    62, 64–65, 71, 75, 133, 186, 283,
    297, 303
Food and Drug Administration (FDA),
    224, 226, 277–79, 301, 306, 313,
    315, 328, 334, 338
Ford Foundation, 212
fractionation, 96
Frank, Dr. Howard, 19
Freiberg, Richard, 27–28, 29, 30, 42
fumigillin, 216–17
fungi, 215–17, 289
Furey, Tracy, 306

G
Galen, 157
Gaspodarowicz, Denis, 126, 129–30,
    189–91, 205, 209
Gelsinger, Jesse, 312
Genentech, 150, 152, 209, 276, 289, 335
  antiangiogenic drug development,
    289–90, 309–11
gene-pharming, 301
General Electric, 212
General Motors Prize, 262–63
genetics, 83, 97, 138, 150–52, 193, 202,
    206–7
  AT-3 and, 299–302
  angiogenesis gene therapy, 310–21
  angiostatin and, 262
  biotechnology revolution, 149–52, 209
  cancer and, 150, 156–63, 206, 241,
    251, 281
  cloning, 210, 262
  gene-splicing, 150, 241, 262
  manipulation of plants, 213

Genetics Institute, 150, 151
Genzyme Corporation, 299–301
  AT-3 research and production, 299–302
giant-cell sarcoma, 290–95
Gilbert, Walter, 151
Gilman, Alfred, 113
Gimbrone, Michael, Jr., 59, 83–90,
    94–96, 100–101, 125–29, 132, 169,
    176, 187, 188, 191
GM-CSF, 131
Gold, Dr. Phil, 117
Goldberg, Mark, 299–300
Gompertzian theory, 346–47
Goodman, Louis, 113
Greene, Harry, 93, 102
Gross, Dr. Robert, 23–38, 64, 65, 71–72,
    77, 88, 105, 179, 185, 192, 246
growth factors, 86, 89–90, 96–102, 163,
    181–97, 199–211, 215–17, 232–67,
    271–82, 289–90, 296–307, 308–27,
    328–48
  angiogenin, 206–8, 213
  EGF, 131, 200
  FGF, 130, 190, 205, 207, 208, 213,
    232–34, 240, 244, 249, 271–74, 276,
    279, 293, 308–10, 317, 319
  heparin and, 204–5
  inhibitor-stimulator balance, 242–67
  isolation and purification of, 133–36,
    139, 140, 166–69, 199–211, 253
  TAF, 96–99, 116, 118–36, 164–79,
    181–88, 194–97, 199–205, 208–11,
    215–17, 253, 263
  types of, 130–31
  VEGF, 209–11, 234, 240–44, 249,
    289–90, 308–27
growth hormones, 130–31, 209

H
hairy cell leukemia, 223
Hamel, Ernest, 342
Hanahan, Douglas, 241, 243–44, 296
Harris, Henry, 184
Harvard Medical School, 5, 17, 18, 19,
    20–30, 32, 37, 42, 46, 70, 72, 83, 84,
    85, 87–88, 91, 123, 134, 138, 150,
    184, 186, 284, 304
  commercialization of, 55, 138–52, 170,
    180–82, 213

Folkman's professorship at, 70–72,
    186–87, 213, 349
-Monsanto research funding deal, 136,
    138–52, 163–64, 166, 170, 180–83,
    188, 207, 213, 214
  "no-patents" policy, 141–43, 146–47,
    173
  oversight committee on Monsanto
    deal, 180–82
  research vs. doctors, 87–88, 123
heart block, 24, 26, 29, 34–37
heart disease, 261
  angiogenesis and, 308–9, 312, 314–19,
    320, 321
  in children, 24–27, 30–37
  dog research, 25–26, 28–30, 31–37
  gene therapy, 314–19
heart pacemakers, 33–37
Hellman, Dorothy, 30
hemangiomas, 221–37, 264, 271, 275,
    342
  Briggs case, 221–26, 229, 234, 236,
    237
  interferon treatment, 222–34, 236,
    237, 245
hemoglobin, 49–54
Hendry, Christopher, 301
heparin, 29, 34, 204–5
hepatitis B, 162
Herbst, Roy, 332
herpes, 162
Hertig, Dr. Arthur, 80
Hill, Austin Bradford, 158–59
Hippocrates, 157
Hodgkin's disease, 160
Hoffman-LaRoche, 224, 226, 248
Holaday, Dr. John, 249–50, 259, 262–63,
    304, 306, 341, 342
Homans, Dr. Alan, 290–95
Hooke, Robert, 158
hormones, 81, 83, 97, 129–31, 170, 199
Hospital for Sick Children, Toronto, 228
house calls, 75–76
Housman, David, 151
HPLC (high-performance liquid
    chromatography), 208
Hrushesky, Dr. Bill, 347
Huebner, Robert, 162
Huggins, Charles, 49

Hughes, Dennis, 294
hybridomas, 290
Hydron, 177
hypothalamus, 131

I
ICAM-1 (intercellular adhesion
    molecule-1), 326
Illig, Marjorie, 110
immune system, 93, 94, 211, 289–90
industry, 212–13
    vs. academia, in research, 138–52, 170,
        181
    biotechnology, 249–51, 259, 262–63,
        266, 276–77, 286–90, 299–306,
        309–11, 332–36, 340–43
    interests in antiangiogenesis, 249–51,
        259, 262–63, 266, 276–77, 286–90,
        299–306, 332–36, 340–43
    pharmaceutical, 212–13, 224, 226,
        227, 235, 248–50, 262–63, 301,
        304–6, 335
    research funding, 138–52, 163–64,
        180–83, 212–13, 248–51, 262–63,
        286–90, 332–36
    stock market and, 286–87, 296, 332–33
    see also specific companies
Ingber, Donald, 182, 214, 215–17,
    235–36, 239, 279
inhibitors, 99–100, 120, 167–69, 173–76,
    194, 201–3, 215–17, 233–36,
    239–67, 268–80, 290–99, 303–7,
    309, 328–48
    AT-3, 299–302
    angiostatin, 256–67, 280, 281, 283,
        296–9, 303–7, 328–29, 336
    endostatin, 3–5, 264–67, 280, 281,
        283, 296–99, 303–7, 328–48
    interferon, 222–34, 268–73, 290–95,
        328
    marimastat, 276–79
    plasmin and, 255–57, 261
    -stimulator balance, 242–67
    thrombospondin, 242–43, 244, 247,
        249
    TNP-470, 217, 235–36, 239–40, 243,
        249, 271, 276, 279–80
    tumor suppression of metastases,
        247–67

    see also antiangiogenesis; specific
        inhibitors
insulin, 22, 97, 130, 150, 170, 209, 241,
    310, 322
interferon alpha, 197, 223–26, 232,
    271
    antiangiogenic, 268–76, 279, 281,
        290–95, 328
    as cancer treatment, 197, 223, 224,
        290–95, 328
    as hemangioma treatment, 222–34,
        236, 237, 245
interleukins, 131
in vitro research, 124–33, 136, 166–67,
    188–97, 201–5, 215–17, 252–53
Isner, Dr. Jeffrey, 308–21
    gene therapy research, 310–19
Ixsys, Inc., 276, 290

J
Jaffe, Eric, 129, 131, 132
Japan, 202, 216, 233
    endothelial cell growth research,
        125–29, 216–17
    Takeda angiogenesis research, 214–15,
        216–17, 235
    TNP-470 research, 217, 235
Jenner, Edward, 21
Jimmy Fund, 112, 114, 115
Johns Hopkins Medical Institutions, 29,
    32, 68, 80, 204, 325, 328
Jones, Graham B., 113
Journal of Biological Chemistry, 130,
    132, 175
Journal of Clinical Investigation, 132,
    233, 320
Journal of Experimental Medicine, 93,
    102
Journal of Surgical Research, 55
Journal of the National Cancer Institute,
    79
Judaism, 8–11, 69, 72, 243

K
Kaban, Dr. Leonard, 268–73
Kalesnik, Tonya, 290–95, 328
Kaposi's sarcoma, 223, 224
Karnofsky, Morris, 191
Karnovsky Lecture (1996), 280–81

Kennedy, Donald, 150
Kerbel, Robert, 343, 345
Kieran, Dr. Mark, 330, 341–42
Killian, Chuck, 332
King, Ralph T., Jr., 297, 307
Klagsbrun, Michael, 166, 199–205, 232
    endothelial cell research, 201–5, 207
Klausner, Dr. Richard, 283, 286, 288,
    298, 333
Köhler, Georges J. F., 289–90
Kolata, Gina, 282, 330
    1998 antiangiogenesis article, 283–87,
    290, 307
Koop, Dr. C. Everett, 72–76, 88, 228
Kornberg, Arthur, 178
Kotulak, Ron, 119, 121
Kramer, Robert, 305
kringle 5, 335

L
LaChance, Jennifer, 268–73, 274, 280,
    281, 284, 290, 293, 294, 328
Ladd, Dr. William, 31–32, 72, 73
Laird, Anna, 347
Lane, I. William, 175–76
Langer, Robert, 170–79
    cartilage research, 173–76, 201
    leaky plastics research, 176–79
Lasker, Mary, 110
Laurent, Albert, 316–17, 318
leaky plastics, 55–56, 142, 173, 176–79
    Langer research, 176–79
    medicine-delivery system based on,
    178–79
Leighton, Joseph, 104
leukemia, 112, 156, 159, 224
    angiogenesis and, 234–36
    childhood, 112–13, 156, 160
    TNP-470 treatment, 236
Lewis lung carcinoma, 251–52, 257–59,
    264
Li Jin, 262
Lindbergh, Charles, 50
Lindskog, Gustav, 113
Lion, Kurt, 35
liver, 18–19, 204, 255
    cancer, 52, 162
Lokich, Jacob, 347
Long, Dr. David, 55–56, 142, 173, 177

lungs:
    cancer, 110, 158–59, 160, 251–52,
    257–59, 264, 279
    hemangioma, 221–26
    Lewis lung carcinoma, 251–52,
    257–59, 264
lymphatic system, 158

M
macular degeneration, 340, 341
Maniatis, Tom, 151
marimastat, 276–79
Mason, Richard, 111
Massachusetts Eye and Ear Infirmary,
    102
Massachusetts General Hospital, Boston,
    21, 23, 37–44, 58–70, 72, 78, 81, 90,
    123, 156, 268, 299
Massachusetts Institute of Technology,
    35–37, 123, 146, 149, 150, 151, 162,
    170, 189, 200
    Robert Langer and, 170–73, 178
Massachusetts Medical Society, 23–24,
    98
McAlary, Mike, 284, 307
McDermott, Dr. William, 70
McGrady, Pat, 109, 111, 115, 118, 119
McLaughlin, Loretta, 144–45
M. D. Anderson Cancer Center. See
    Anderson (M. D.) Cancer Center
Meadow, Henry, 140–43, 148, 150, 166,
    181
Medtronics, 37
Meister, Alton, 180
menstruation, 340
Merck, 248, 250
metastases, 244
    angiogenesis stimulator-inhibitor
    balance in, 242–67
    postsurgical eruption of, 238–41,
    244–48
    tumor suppression of, 239–67
microcinematography, 117
milk, growth-promoting agents in, 203
Miller, Dr. Jan, 324–25
Milstein, César, 289–90
molecular biology, 138, 149–50, 162–63,
    281
monoclonal antibodies, 289–90, 324–26

Monsanto, 137–38, 212, 250
  Agent Orange manufacture, 146
  -Harvard research funding deal, 136,
    138–52, 163–64, 166, 170, 180–83,
    188, 207, 213, 214
  oversight committee, 180–82
Moore, Dr. Francis, 71
Moss, Arthur, 41
MTD (maximum tolerated dose), 344–45
Mulliken, John, 226–29, 232, 271, 275,
    276
Murray, Dr. Joseph, 185

N
Nabel, Dr. Betsy, 310
naked-DNA experiments, 311–19
Nathan, Dr. David, 122, 184, 185, 187,
    229–32, 303
National Academy of Engineering, 170
National Academy of Sciences, 116, 135,
    170, 181
National Cancer Institute, 79, 80, 133,
    156, 248, 283, 286, 296, 300, 335
  angiogenesis research and funding,
    80–81, 133–35, 263–64, 283–89,
    297–98, 303–7, 320, 329, 333
National Institute of Medicine, 170
National Institutes of Health, 47, 68, 90,
    112, 126, 146, 162, 182, 183, 188,
    191, 198, 200, 212, 214, 230, 235,
    236, 288–89, 303, 320, 323
  1997 Director's Lecture, 281–82, 287
National Naval Medical Center, 45
Natural Science, 173
Nature, 86, 122, 196, 197, 232, 300
Nature Biotechnology, 298
Nature Medicine, 260
Naval Medical Research Institute, 46–57
nerve cells, growth of, 129, 130, 131, 190
New England Journal of Medicine, The,
    24, 98, 100, 117, 226, 228–30, 279
  Children's Hospital hemangioma
    report, 228–32
Newsweek, 286, 294, 315
Newton, Isaac, 9
New York Daily News, 284, 307
New York Hospital, 19
New York Times, The, 116, 119, 282
  on Folkman, 120–21, 283–87, 328

1998 Kolata antiangiogenesis article,
    283–87, 290, 303, 307
New York University Medical Center,
    274–75
NGF (nerve growth factor), 131
nitrogen mustard, 113–14
Nixon, Richard M., 141, 163
Nobel Prize, 56, 162, 178, 190, 200
Norplant, 147, 173
Northwestern University School of
    Medicine, Chicago, 242, 298
nuclear research, 160

O
Occusert, 177
Ohio State University, 14, 16–19, 22
oil, 137, 171
oligo, 210
Olson, Bjorn, 297
oncogenes, 156, 162–63
O'Reilly, Michael, 245–67, 281, 285, 304
  AT-3 discovery, 299–302
  angiostatin discovery, 257–67
  Cell paper, 259–60, 261, 263–64, 280
  endostatin discovery, 264–65, 280, 329
  tumor suppression of metastases,
    247–67
osteopathy, 74
ovarian cancer, 89
OXiGENE, Inc., 335–36

P
Palade, George, 182
pancreas, 241
Pasteur, Louis, 9, 154
patent ductus arteriosus, 31–32
patents, 55, 151, 173, 213
  Harvard's "no-patents" policy, 141–43,
    146–47
  kringle 5, 335
Patriquin, Dr. Heidi, 5, 343
pediatric surgery, 24–27, 30–37, 71–76
Peña, Dr. Alberto, 278–79
penicillin, 216
Perez, Nancy, 313–14
perfusion experiments, 85–90, 116
pericytes, 128–29, 193
pernicious anemia, 142
Pettit, G. Robert, 335–36

phagokinetic assay, 196
pharmaceutical industry, 212–13, 224,
    226, 227, 235, 248–49, 250, 262–63,
    335
  angiogenesis research funding, 263,
    297, 301, 304–6
  see also specific companies
Philadelphia, 73–76, 228, 334
Price-Shepherd, Dr. Steven, 302
pituitary gland, 129–30, 131, 209
placebo effect, 318–19
plasmin, 255–57, 261
plasminogen, 255–56, 257, 261–62, 335
platelets, 85–86
  growth-stimulating factor, 86, 89–90,
    96–102
plate tectonics, 154
Pluda, Dr. James, 283, 286, 332
polio, 22, 94–95
polymerase chain reaction, 262
postsurgical eruption of metastases,
    238–41, 244–48
Pott, Percival, 158
pregnancy, 340, 342
press:
  on antiangiogenesis, 283–87, 294,
    296–97, 303, 307, 332, 335
  on cancer research, 109–11, 115–24,
    144–45, 207
  disliked by scientists and doctors,
    115–16, 123
  on Folkman, 115–16, 118–24, 145, 148,
    176, 181, 281–87, 297–99, 303, 307
  on Monsanto-Harvard deal, 144–45
  "two-years" comment controversy,
    282, 283–87, 290, 307
  see also specific publications
Prial, Dr. David, 42
Proceedings of the National Academy of
    Sciences, 195, 327, 341
prostate cancer, 267
proteins, 97, 118, 161, 206, 209, 289
  growth factor, 86, 89–90, 96–102,
    118–21, 181–97, 199–211, 215–17,
    232–67, 271–82, 289–90, 296–307,
    308–29, 328–48
  plasmin, 255–57, 261
  in urine, 253–56, 262, 264
  see also specific proteins

Ptashne, Mark, 151
pulmonary hemangiomatosis, 221–26

R
rabbit eye experiments, 93–96, 101–2,
    135, 169, 174, 177, 199, 248
rabbit thyroid experiments, 52–54, 74,
    81, 82, 116
radiation, 5, 47–48, 52, 87, 157, 159, 160,
    163, 224, 236, 270, 274, 280,
    292–93, 329, 337, 338
rat aorta endothelial cell experiments,
    126–27
reduced-dose chemotherapy approach,
    343–48
Remensnyder, John, 40
Remick, Scot, 338, 339
research, 91–92, 211–12
  academia vs. industry in, 138–52, 170,
    181
  angiogenesis, 80–105, 116–36, 163–79,
    181–97, 199–217, 223, 232–67,
    268–80, 283–84, 288–90, 296–307,
    308–27, 328–48
  antiangiogenesis, 3–5, 221–37,
    247–67, 268–80, 283–84, 288–90,
    296–307, 328–48
  cancer, 51–57, 78–90, 96–105, 118–36,
    156–79, 181–97, 199–211, 212,
    215–17, 232–67, 281–82, 288–95,
    303–7, 328–48
  vs. doctors, 87–88, 123
  endangered limbs, 308–14
  Folkman's early tumor cell, 51–57, 69,
    78–90, 93–105
  funding, 116, 133–36, 137–52, 182–83,
    188, 211–15, 248–51, 262–64,
    303–7, 323
  gene, 310–21
  heart, 308–9, 312–19
  in vitro, 124–33, 136, 166–67, 188–97,
    201–5, 215–17, 252–53
  labs and styles, 91–92, 196, 211
  Monsanto-Harvard funding deal, 136,
    138–52, 163–64, 166, 170, 180–83,
    188, 207, 213, 214
  "pure" vs. applied, 169–70
  replication of scientific results, 297–98
  Takeda funding, 214–15, 216–17

research (cont'd):
    vision, 321–27, 340–41
    see also animal research; clinical trials;
        specific researchers, labs,
        procedures, and theories
restriction enzymes, 150, 209
Retina Foundation, Boston, 95
retinoblastomas, 103
Retsky, Michael, 346–48
reverse transcriptase, 162
Rhoads, Jonathan, 111
Richardson, Elliott, 141
Ringrose, Peter, 305
RNA, 83, 118, 161–62
Rockefeller Foundation, 212
Rockefeller University, New York, 198,
    263
Rodgers, Joanne, 118
Rosen, Dr. Fred, 88, 114–15, 122, 123,
    124, 134, 146, 167–69, 175
Rosenberg, Leon, 262–63, 305
Rosengart, Dr. Todd, 317
Rosenthal, David, 286
Rosenthal, Rosalind, 208–9, 210, 252
Rous, Peyton, 160–61
Rous sarcoma virus, 161
Ruckelshaus, William, 180

S
Sagan, Carl, 115–16
Sage, Helene, 252
St. Elizabeth's Medical Center, Brighton,
    Massachusetts, 309, 310, 316, 320
Salem Hospital, Massachusetts, 60–61
Salk, Jonas, 190, 271
Saltus, Richard, 332
Sanders, Dr. Jay, 66–67, 68–69
San Francisco, 126, 129, 150, 152, 189,
    190, 208, 209, 296
sarcoma, 270
Savage, Fred, 25
Schepens Eye Research Institute, 321,
    327
Science, 123, 175, 181, 197, 207, 210,
    223, 260, 301
    1977 angiogenesis article, 175, 183,
        186
    1980 interferon article, 197, 222
Seminars in Medicine, 98–100

Semmelweis, Ignaz Philips, 154, 155,
    156
serpins, 302
shark cartilage, 175–76
Shaw, Herb, 144–45
Shepro, David, 126
Sherwood, Dr. Louis, 98, 100
Shing, Yuen, 204–5, 207, 232, 252
Shulman, Dr. Robert, 316
Shwachman, Dr. Harry, 65
Simons, Dr. Michael, 317, 319
skin, 129, 131
    cancer, 52–54
    cell growth, 129, 131, 190
    psoriasis, 334
smallpox vaccine, 21
Soff, Dr. Gerald, 298
Sottrup-Jensen, Lars, 261
Soviet Union, 47, 54, 195
space program, 47, 68, 212
Speer, Dr. Jack, 347
Stanford University, 150, 180
Stanton, Frank, 180
Steiner, Rudolf, 80
steroids, 222, 276
stimulators, 99–100, 120, 122, 202–9,
    213, 241–67, 271–74, 279–80,
    308–19
    -inhibitor balance, 242–67
    see also specific stimulators
stock market, 286–87, 296, 332–33
Stokes, Floyd, 315–16, 317, 318
Sudduth, H. C., 49, 51, 52
Sugen, Inc., 276, 290, 335
Sugino, Yukio, 214
Sukhatme, Dr. Vikas, 297
surgery, 5, 17–19, 20, 28, 87, 238
    dog, 25–26, 28, 29–30, 31–37, 43
    eruption of metastases after, 238–41,
        244–48
    pediatric, 24–27, 30–37, 71, 72–76
Surgery (journal), 19, 22
SU6668, 290

T
TAF (tumor angiogenesis factor), 96–99,
    116, 118–36, 164–79, 181–88,
    194–97, 199–205, 208–11, 215–17,
    245, 253, 263

becomes VEGF, 210–11, 240, 311
cell migration to, 195–97
inhibitors, 99–100, 120, 167–69,
    173–76, 194, 201–3, 215–17,
    233–36
in vitro research, 124–33, 136, 166–67,
    188–97, 201–5, 215–17
isolation and purification of, 133–36,
    139, 140, 166–69, 199–211
leaky plastics research, 176–79
stimulators, 99–100, 120–22, 202–9,
    213
see also VEGF (vascular endothelial
    growth factor)
Takeda Chemical Industries, 214, 235,
    250
angiogenesis research and funding,
    214–15, 216–17, 235, 276
TNP-470 research, 217, 235
Takeshita, Satoshi, 310, 311
TAP Holdings, 235, 335
Taxol, 157, 236, 335, 343, 345
TCM (tumor-conditioned medium), 96
Technology Review, 170
Temin, Howard, 162
testicular cancer, 160
thalidomide, 5, 341–43
Thomas, Dr. Lewis, 46–47
3M, 36–37
Throdahl, Monte C., 137–43, 145, 146,
    148, 181
thrombospondin, 242–43, 244, 247, 249
thyroid, 50–51
    perfusion experiments, 85–90, 116
    rabbit experiments, 52–54, 74, 78, 81,
        82, 116
Time, 286
TNP-470, 217, 235–36, 239–40, 242,
    249, 271, 276, 279–80
    clinical trials, 235–36, 279–80
    postsurgical eruption of metastases
        and, 240
Todaro, George, 162
Tolsma, Sara, 243
Traphagen, D. W., 19
tritium, 201–2
Tufts University, 123, 246, 308
Twigg, Clayton, 336–39
2ME2 (2-methoxyestradiol), 339–43

U
ulcers, 60–61, 63
umbilical cords, endothelial cell growth
    extracted from, 127, 188, 193
United Press International, 121
U.S. Navy, 44, 45–57, 61, 68, 70, 142
University of Arkansas, 342
University of California, San Francisco,
    126, 129–30, 151–52, 183, 189, 209,
    241, 268
University of Massachusetts Medical
    Center, 246
University of Miami Medical Center, 68
University of Wisconsin, Madison,
    146–47, 162, 198, 200, 223
    Medical Center endostatin clinical
        trials, 329, 330, 332
Upjohn, 248, 250
uric acid, 102
urine:
    FGF levels, 271–74, 293
    proteins from, 253–56, 262, 264

V
Vacanti, Dr. Joseph, 187
vaccine technology, 312
Vallee, Dr. Bert L., 134–36, 139
    angiogenin research, 206–8
    -Folkman collaboration on TAF
        research, 135–36, 139–43, 163–66,
        167, 180–83, 199, 206–8, 263
Vanderschmidt, Fred, 35–37
Varmus, Harold, 183
Vascular Anomalies Program (VAP), 228
Vascular Genetics, 321
vascularization, 78
    cancer cells and, 78–90
vasculogenesis, 81
VEGF (vascular endothelial growth
    factor), 209–11, 234, 240–44, 249,
    274, 276, 289–90, 308–27
    diabetic retinopathy and, 321–27
    discovery of, 209–10
    gene therapy, 310–19
    TAF becomes, 210–11, 240, 311
    see also TAF (tumor angiogenesis
        factor)
ventricular septal defect, 24, 37
Vical, Inc., 311

vinblastine, 343, 345
viruses, 160–63, 233, 289
    cancer-causing, 160–63, 197
    C-type, 161–62
VPF (vascular permeability factor), 211, 324

W
Wall Street Journal, The, 297, 307
    articles on Folkman, 297–99, 303, 307
Warren, John Collins, 21
Washington University, St. Louis, 149
Waterhouse, Benjamin, 21
Watkins, Dr. Elton, 32–33, 34
Watson, James D., 157, 282
    "two-years" comment, 282, 283–87
"weeding and feeding," 193, 195
Wegener, Alfred Lothar, 153–54
Weinberg, Robert, 162
Weintrobe, Maxwell, 181
Weisbach, Lawrence, 299
Weisner, Jerome, 149
Welch, Dr. Claude, 61, 62

Wesley, Paul, 63, 91
Wheeler, Dr. Al, 246
White, Dr. Carl, 221–26
White, Dr. Paul Dudley, 25
Wigler, Michael, 162
Willock, Dr. Edgar, 64
Wilson, Dr. James, 312
Wolbach, William, 185–87
Women's Field Army, 110
World War II, 48, 109, 110, 137, 160

Y
Yale University, 68, 93, 113, 215

Z
Zauberman, Nahan, 95
Zetter, Bruce, 126, 129-30, 189–97, 208
    endothelial cell research, 190–97, 223
    interferon research, 197, 223
zinc, 134, 164
Zoll, Dr. Paul, 34–35
Zollinger, Dr. Robert, 16–23, 28, 59, 77

ABOUT THE AUTHOR

ROBERT COOKE, a native of Southern California, served four years in the coast guard before graduating from California State Polytechnic College and receiving a master's degree from UCLA a year later. Since then he has spent thirty-five years covering science and medicine for major newspapers, including *The Boston Globe, The Atlantic Journal and Constitution,* and *Newsday.* His fascination with science news began with the advent of the space age and matured with continuing exposure to the biological sciences. His interests are wide-ranging and include molecular biology, genetics, geology, astronomy, and archaeology and anthropology.

Cooke has been with *Newsday* for fifteen years. He is married to the former Sue Bailey Cato, whom he met just before he entered high school, and they have three grown children—Gregory, Karen, and Emily. He lives in Huntington, Long Island, New York.

ABOUT THE TYPE

This book was set in Ehrhardt, a typeface based on the original design of Nicholas Kis, a seventeenth-century Hungarian type designer. Ehrhardt was first released in 1937 by the Monotype Corporation of London.